PRINCIPLES OF QUANTITATIVE PERIMETRY

PRINCIPLES OF QUANTITATIVE PERIMETRY:
Testing and Interpreting The Visual Field

George W. Tate, Jr., M.D.
Assistant Professor
Department of Ophthalmology
Southwestern Medical School
University of Texas Health Science Center
Dallas, Texas

John R. Lynn, M.D.
Professor and Chairman
Department of Ophthalmology
Southwestern Medical School
University of Texas Health Science Center
Dallas, Texas

with an appendix by Ira H. Bernstein, Ph.D.

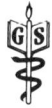

GRUNE & STRATTON
A Subsidiary of Harcourt Brace Jovanovich, Publishers
New York   San Francisco   London

Library of Congress Cataloging in Publication Data

Tate, George W.
  Principles of quantitative perimetry.

  Includes bibliographies and index.
     1. Perimetry.   2. Visual fields.   I. Lynn, John R.,
joint author.   II. Title.   [DNLM: 1. Perimetry.
2. Visual fields.   WW145 T216p]
RE79.P4T37   617.7'5   77-21065
ISBN 0-8089-1041-8

© **1977 by Grune & Stratton, Inc.**
All rights reserved. No part of this publication
may be reproduced or transmitted in any form or
by any means, electronic or mechanical, including
photocopy, recording, or any information storage
and retrieval system, without permission in
writing from the publisher.

Grune & Stratton, Inc.
111 Fifth Avenue
New York, New York 10003

Distributed in the United Kingdom by
Academic Press, Inc. (London) Ltd.
24/48 Oval Road, London NW 1

Library of Congress Catalog Number 77-21065
International Standard Book Number 0-8089-1041-8

Printed in the United States of America

To Our Teachers

Contents

1	The Concept of a Visual Field	1
2	Biophysics, Psychophysics, and the Visual Field	57
3	Available Visual Field Devices and Their Limitations	130
4	Indications for Perimetry and the Perimetrist	145
5	Testing the Visual Field with the Goldmann Perimeter: A Sequential Guide	152
6	Additional Techniques and Alternative Approaches to Goldmann Perimetry	179
7	Principles of Interpretation of the Visual Field	191
8	Visual Field Defects in Specific Diseases: Diagnosis of Specific Diseases by Visual Field Testing	230
9	The Principles and Practice of Automatic Perimetry	270
10	The Use of Perimetry: The Last Word	288
Appendix A	The Criterion Effect and Signal Detection Theory *Ira H. Bernstein, Ph.D.*	295
Appendix B	The Differential Diagnosis of Visual Field Defects	306
Appendix C	Toxic Agents that Affect the Visual Field	318
	Index	327

Acknowledgments

Writing a book, particularly your first, is an educational venture. Apart from the intellectual growth that you inevitably experience, you also develop an awareness of how dependent you can be upon your coworkers if text and illustrations of acceptable quality are to be produced. Those persons unable to perform are eventually recognized and shunned, while those who make the work proceed smoothly are treasured associates.

Of those who helped us prepare the text, no group worked harder than Mrs. Nancy Bain, Mrs. Jane E. Northcutt, and Mrs. Connie McAfee. These ladies worked tirelessly throughout the many text revisions, and without them the work would never have been completed.

Mr. Sigmund Andrews, Mrs. Leah Tubbs, Dr. Rosalind Frank, and Miss Ginger Nemir all contributed their artistic talents to produce illustrations for the book. Mr. Don Sticksel of House of Vision furnished several photographs of equipment. In addition, numerous authors around the world permitted illustrations that first appeared in their works to be reprinted here. We are grateful to all of these people for their generosity.

Special mention must also be made of Mr. Phillip Hearnsberger and his assistant, Miss Nancy Jenkins, who worked tirelessly to provide the photographic support necessary for the book. Every illustration in the book passed through their laboratory, and they greatly improved most of them.

We are also grateful to the staff at Grune and Stratton, Inc., for their help and patience. They aided us in the planning and suffered with us through several false starts, patiently translated the book from the original Texan into English, and helped us through the production.

Finally, we are very much aware of the debt we owe those who have taught us. To list all of the excellent teachers to whom this book is dedicated would be impossible, but thanking some who have especially touched our lives is appropriate.

Both authors have had the privilege to study with Dr. Paul Boeder, a fine gentleman to whom several generations of ophthalmologists owe their understanding of optics, and with Professor Dr. Elfriede Aulhorn, a gracious lady who is not only an able scientist and clinician but one who will be immortal for as long as perimetry is practical.

John Lynn is mindful of the many hours of excellent tutelage provided during his residency by Dr. Fred Blodi, Dr. P. J. Leinfelder, and Dr. Mansour Armaly; the latter also guided him through a fellowship and gave him his first exposure to perimetric research.

George Tate is grateful to many persons: to his father, for teaching him logic; to Dr. William D. Willis, who gave him the fundamentals of laboratory science and neurophysiology; and to his coauthor, who introduced him to ophthalmology. No one, however, has had so profound an effect on his career as Mrs. G. B. Wilson, an early instructor of mathematics who knew that if the teacher could teach the student to love the subject, the battle was won. Mrs. Wilson was so successful at this that she brought about a complete change in this student's likes and dislikes that still influence his career some twenty years later. Although she was among the first of a long procession of truly superb teachers, she remains the standard by which all others are judged.

Preface:
Why Test the Visual Field?

Visual fields are important because the pattern of deviation from their usual egg-shaped lines may localize the cause of the defect to a certain part of the eye or brain, help determine the activity and prognosis of the disease process causing the defect, and, in some cases, suggest the precise diagnosis.

Disease processes within the brain may be localized through perimetry, for visual nerve fibers are present throughout a large part of the brain, from front to back. A disease such as a tumor or a stroke often impinges on these nerve fibers and produces defects in the visual fields of both eyes. The patterns of these defects are characteristic because the fibers from the eye pass to the visual part of the brain through known tracts. That is, the fibers from the upper part of the eye remain in the upper visual pathway; half the visual fibers in each eye cross over to the opposite side of the brain; and the fibers from corresponding points in the two eyes gradually approach one another until they merge at the visual cortex in the back of the brain.

The activity of a disease process can be indicated by the distance between the isopter lines. If they are far apart, a three-dimensional representation of the flat visual field has a shallow slope in the area of the defect. Shallow slopes usually indicate an area of edema, pressure, or inflammation within the eye or visual pathway. On the other hand, a very steep slope (the isopters are close together) usually indicates a scar, an infarct, or some chronic disease process. The steepness of the slope in the visual field carries prognostic as well as diagnostic significance. The shallow slopes (acute inflammation, partial ischemia, etc.) have some hope of recovery if the cause of the defect is removed. The steep slopes (scar, infarct, etc.) indicate a poor chance of recovery.

All seven of the major causes of blindness in the United States (glaucoma, cataract, diabetes, other vascular diseases, uveitis, retinal detachment, and senile macular degeneration) have characteristic patterns of defects in the visual field and often show these defects early in the disease process. Visual fields are useful to the general practitioner in the management of endocrine disturbances, in the diagnosis of unexplained headaches, in the follow-up of vascular diseases, or in the diagnosis of blurry vision. At times it is even possible to obtain information from visual fields that might not have been available otherwise, such as the diagnosis of certain brain tumors (e.g., pituitary tumors).

One of the most important values of a visual field test is its ability to indicate the progression or regression of a disease process. This can serve as the basis for changes in treatment or reassurance that the current therapy is effective. For this reason, it is essential that visual fields be performed in such a manner that they can be reproduced reliably from one day to another, from one testing session to another, and, in this era of great mobility, from one geographic location to another. This poses the most stringent technical requirements of all of the possible uses of the visual field.

The purpose of this book is to aid the physician–perimetrist team in achieving the goals of high quality visual fields through the utilization of whatever means and techniques are most appropriate to particular patients. We have attempted not only to present the "plain vanilla" of clinical perimetry but also to give the reader insights into the underlying anatomy and physiology as well as into such experimental techniques as flicker, color, center-surround, and saturation perimetry. Automatic perimetry, a technique that we feel holds much promise, is discussed fully. Of course, many of these areas remain controversial, and even we differ on some points. We have tried, nonetheless, to achieve a reasonable balance among prevailing views and to achieve a consensus. Although we emphasize the Goldmann Perimeter and quantitative, reproducible fields, we hope those practitioners who use other equipment and have other needs will find the information we provide as useful.

George W. Tate, Jr., M.D.
John R. Lynn, M.D.

1
The Concept of a Visual Field

THE VISUAL FIELD: DEFINITIONS AND LIMITS

The visual field is all the space that one eye can see at any given instant. In current clinical testing of a visual field, the nonoccluded eye must remain stationary by looking steadily at a preselected target. The word perimetry, which is almost synonymous with visual field testing, means measurement of the periphery. The periphery of the visual field extends farther toward the temple than it does toward the nose. The nasal perimetric angle* where large tests may initially be seen ranges from 62° to 65°, and the maximum temporal perimetric angle normally ranges from 105° to 109° (Fig. 1-1). According to a recent report by Schmidt and coworkers, the portion of temporal retina that corresponds to the nasal field† *can* function between 65° and 80° if the eye is congenitally fixed in a position of extreme outward gaze so the nose is never seen.[13] As indicated in Figure 1-2, the normal limit of the nasal visual field is the retina, not the nose, despite the normal histological appearance of the extreme temporal retina.

COMPARISON OF THE CAMERA AND THE EYE: SIMILARITIES

Comparison of the human eye to a camera is appropriate in more ways than it is inappropriate (Fig. 1-3). The cornea and the lens of the relaxed emmetropic eye‡ are comparable to the camera lens when it is fully retracted; for both

---

*Perimetric angle is the angle at the center of the eye's pupil between a line that joins the object upon which gaze is fixated and another line that joins the object used to test the limit of the visual field.
†Since all light crosses in the pupil, nasal field corresponds to temporal retina, temporal field to nasal retina, superior field to inferior retina, and inferior field to superior retina.
‡Emmetropia is the normal state of an eye that has no refractive error, for it is not nearsighted (myopic), or farsighted (hyperopic), or astigmatic. Until they reach the age for bifocals (presbyopia), individuals with emmetropia do not wear glasses at all.

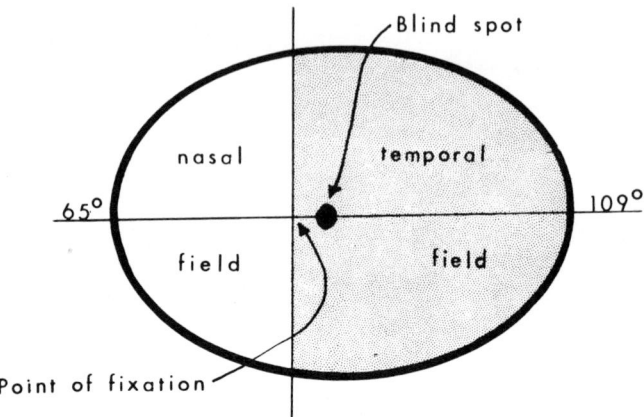

Figure 1-1 Limits of the normal visual field. A normal person's right eye can detect the presence of a large bright object at any location within the ovoid limiting line, except inside the blind spot near its center. Since the visual field of the left eye is a mirror image of the right and the eyes are aligned around the point of fixation, the blind spots do not overlap, and the normal person is not aware of them. (See the self-demonstration on page 10.)

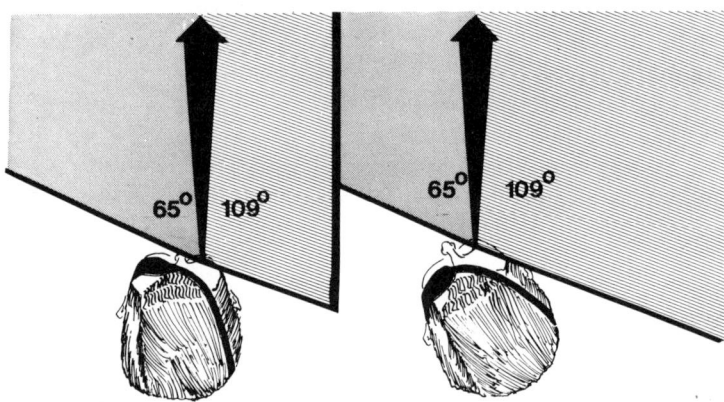

Figure 1-2 The retina, not the nose, limits the nasal field. Although the nose may be developmentally responsible for limiting the nasal visual field, that it plays no continuing role as a limit in visual adults can be proved by this self-demonstration. The reader should close the left eye; continue to look at an object straight ahead; find the limit of the nasal field by moving the left hand inward until it is barely seen; turn the head (but not the eye) to the left; *note the absence of significant change in the limit where the hand is seen; and, finally, compare the location of nose and left hand by looking at each.*

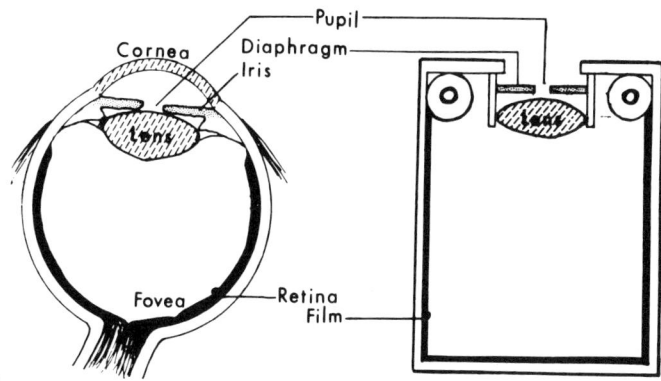

Figure 1-3 Comparison of eye and camera. The cornea and lens of the eye (shaded area) are equivalent to the lens of the camera (also shaded), for both lens systems bend light to make it focus on the retina and film, respectively. The iris and diaphragm both serve as variable-opening shields to let more or less light enter through the pupil. The retina and the film of the camera are similarly located at the back of each optical system. They are changed by light through photochemical processes to receive the picture. The retina and the camera film differ in very important ways, however, that are discussed in the text.

systems bring distant objects to focus. By moving slightly forward and by becoming thicker, the lens of the emmetropic eye remains equivalent to the camera lens when it shifts forward; for both movements bring nearby objects to focus. The iris diaphragm expands and contracts its opening—the pupil—to admit more or less light to the camera, just as the iris does for the eye. Even when their pupillary diameters are constant, the camera and the eye both receive more or less light, depending upon the perimetric angle of the source.

Thus, the test object may retain the same angular size† and the same intensity relative to the background, yet the pupil of constant diameter provides less area for admission of light as the test source moves from a central zone toward the periphery. Light from the test source passes through a circular pupil when the test object is located straight in front of the camera or eye, but the pupil is elliptical in shape when viewed from the periphery. Since the unchanged diameter of the pupil is the greatest dimension of the ellipse, the obviously smaller area of the ellipse allows less light to enter the eye or camera from the peripheral source, a fact that is recognized in photometry* (Fig.1-4) by the unit known as Troland.[8]

---

†The angular size or visual angle of an object within the visual field takes into account the plus or minus magnification effects of external corrective lenses and of changes in the distance between test object and eye. Like the perimetric angle, the angular size is measured in the center of the pupil, and it relates the lines from the extreme edges of the test object as they converge at the eye.
*Photometry is the physical science of measuring light. See Chapter 2.

4   Principles of Quantitative Perimetry

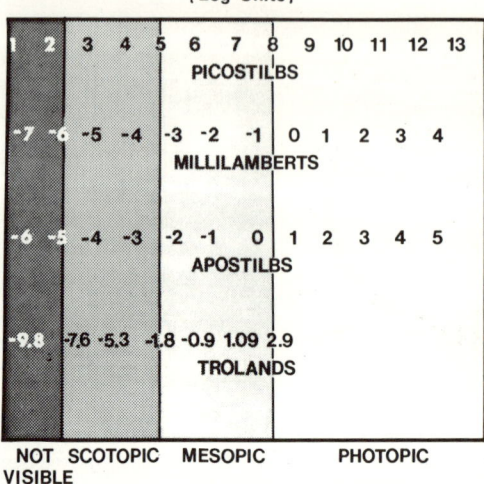

Figure 1-4 Comparative photometric values. Any given intensity of white light may be physically measured on a variety of scales and the effect on the eye at that intensity may also be assayed. This figure shows one aspect by indicating the increasing intensities of light on each of four intensity-measuring scales. For each scale, the intensities are also related to visual function by classifying the intensities as (1) invisible; (2) seen only with well-adapted rods (scotopic); (3) seen by both rods and cones (mesopic); or (4) seen only with cones (photopic). The last scale (Trolands) changes at a different rate when compared with the three physical scales because it is a measure of retinal illuminance, which takes into account the pupil size and the obliquity of light not entering parallel to the optical axis.

When the film of a camera is compared with the retina of the eye, significant exceptions to the analogy should be recognized as well as the elements that are valid. Both film and retina are located at the rear of the respective optical systems; the light does come to focus on each, and both film and retina are changed by light through photochemical processes to "receive" the picture. But beyond these points of similarity are important structural and functional differences.

DIFFERENCES BETWEEN RETINA AND CAMERA FILM

Anatomy

Because the specialized sensory cells in the retina are not homogeneously distributed and their neural connections are not evenly disbursed, the "grain"†

---

†In photography, a film with fine grain is capable of resolving more detail than another film with coarse grain, all other factors being optimum.

of any given retina varies significantly from one zone to another while the grain of a given photographic film is homogeneous, that is, it does not vary from area to area. The grain is finer in the center of the retina, coarser in the retinal periphery. The effect is similar to an exaggeration of the diminished pupil phenomenon, which occurs when light obliquely enters what appears to be an elliptical pupil. Although photographic film has its light-sensitive emulsions on the surface nearest the light, the layer that converts light energy to nerve energy (the receptor layer) is located at the outer surface of the retina. Like a miniature mattress of nerve cells that are collectively transparent, the retina is not affected by light until all its layers have been traversed.

Although anatomists classically divide the retina into 10 layers, only three, those that are comprised of cell bodies, will be described here. A layer of sensory (receptor) cells is external to a layer of interconnecting (bipolar, horizontal, and amacrine) cells which is in turn, external to a layer of transmitting (ganglion) cells (Fig. 1-5).

Polyak has described the form, function, and distribution of receptor cells which collectively number approximately 126,500,000 in each retina.[10] Of these about 110 to 125 million, called rods, function only in dim light. The remaining 6.3 to 6.8 million receptor cells, the cones, are specially adapted for operation under daylight conditions and permit detailed vision and appreciation of colors (see Fig. 1-4). In Figure 1-6, the number of receptor cells of the two types has been plotted by Østerberg as a function of the perimetric angle in degrees.[9] It should be seen in this diagram that the number of cones per square millimeter is

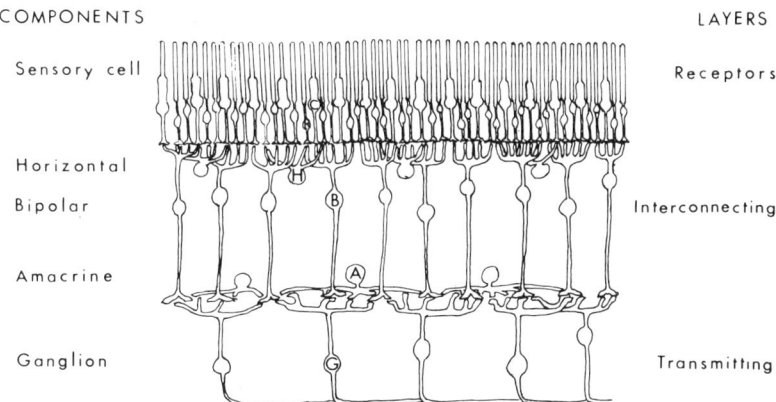

Figure 1-5 Anatomy of the retina. The microscopic anatomy of the retina is simplified in this diagram which is oriented so that light strikes it from *below*, that is, after it has passed into the eye through the pupil. The rods and cones are the sensory cell components and make up the layer of receptors. The horizontal (H), bipolar (B), and amacrine (A) cells comprise the interconnecting layer. The ganglion cells (G) serve as the transmitting layer, for their axons make up the optic nerve.

6   Principles of Quantitative Perimetry

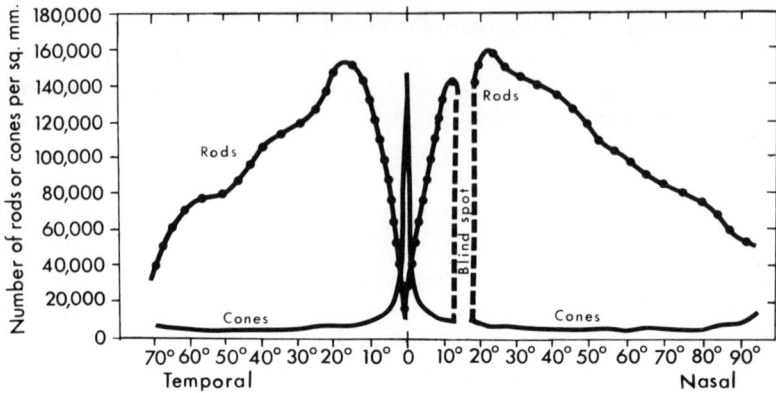

Figure 1-6   Østerberg's curves, showing the density of rods and cones along a horizontal line through the fovea. The density of receptor cells is indicated as the number of each type per square millimeter, and eccentricity from the fovea is expressed in perimetric degrees.

about 145,000 in the fovea,* the retinal area used for fixation of gaze. At an eccentricity or perimetric angle of 10°, the number of cones drops to about 10,000 per square millimeter and never exceeds 8,000 as the count remains relatively stable all the way to the periphery. On the other hand, there are no rods centrally, for the cones are exclusive occupants of the fovea. The number of rods increases to a peak of about 135,000 per square millimeter at approximately 18° from the point of fixation. The rod density then gradually falls off to 115,000 per square millimeter at 35° in the temporal retina and at 50° in the nasal retina. The nonhomogeneous mixture of receptor cells is an important reason for the variable sensitivity or grain of the human retina as contrasted with photographic film.

A second major reason for the inherently variable sensitivity of one retinal zone as compared with another is the changing interconnections, often manifest as a difference in ratios between receptor cells and their ganglion cells. Although the ganglion cells total only 800,000 to slightly more than 1,000,000 cells per eye, or slightly less than 1% of the total number of receptors, they are the only means for transmitting visual information from the eye to the brain.[10] An intermediate number of interconnecting cells are present between the sensory elements and the ganglion cells that represent them. The numbers thus tend to suggest a 10:1 ratio between sensory elements and interconnecting cells and a similar 10:1 ratio between interconnecting cells and ganglion cells, but this

---

*The fovea is the central and most sensitive portion of the zone at the posterior pole of the eye called the macula lutea. The macula is a highly specialized retinal area that is exclusively responsible for visual acuities of 20/70 and more, with foveal function exclusively responsible for acuities of 20/40 or more. See footnote on page 8 for definition of visual acuity.

"average" system may exist, if at all, only in a small part of the retina. That interconnections are not homogeneous in the retina is best illustrated in the fovea where most of the 115,000 cones are served by their own individual bipolar cells and their own individual ganglion cells.[10] In the fovea, the ratio between sensory and transmitting cells approaches 1:1. In the peripheral retina, the ratio must be much more than the average 100:1 in order to make up for the "private line" connections that are so dense in the central field. This disparity in ratios does not have a sharp cutoff but rather a gradual transition from 1:1 centrally to perhaps 200:1 at the periphery. Thus, the central part of the retina is anatomically represented in the brain as individual points while the peripheral retina shows up only as zones.

In summary, the regional retinal differences in density of rods and cones and in the exclusivity of connections that link retinal sensory cells to ganglion cells are the anatomical bases for the markedly different sensitivity in central and peripheral fields. This inherent difference in sensitivity from one part of the retina to another is the major distinction between the retina and the film of a camera where the grain, and thus the sensitivity to equal amounts of light striking it, is homogeneously distributed.

Function

Several measures of visual function parallel the ocular anatomy emphasized above and thus help to reveal the significance of an otherwise obscure structure. Aulhorn's curves (Fig. 1-7) show the average light sense* along a horizontal line through the fovea with a variety of background light intensities.[2] The three lower curves represent visual function in bright light; the two upper curves represent light sense in total or subtotal darkness; and the intermediate curves show function in twilight illuminations. A comparison of Figure 1-6 with Figure 1-7 reveals that cones are associated with vision in bright light and rods with vision in dim illumination. For, when background intensity is high, the shape of the light sense curves shows a peak in the central field and a gradual fall off into the periphery, which is reminiscent of Østerberg's plot of cone distribution. And, when the background light is dim or absent, the light sense improves far more in the midperiphery than it does in the center, similar to Østerberg's plot of rod distribution. Because the two receptor systems are present simultaneously, the central light sense never becomes worse than it is when more background light stimulates the cones exclusively. The rods function exclusively when the background and stimulus values are less than 0.0003 to 0.001 millilamberts.[7]

---

*Light sense is the organism's ability to respond when a change occurs in the light intensity of one area in the visual field as contrasted with that area's background.

8   Principles of Quantitative Perimetry

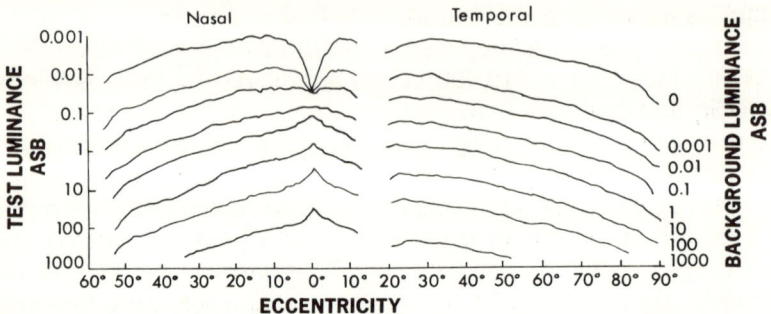

Figure 1-7   Aulhorn's curves of average static perimetric light sense lie along a horizontal line through the point of fixation and the normal blind spot of the right eye. The luminances or intensities of the background light in each of eight adaptation states are respectively indicated in apostilbs (ASB) by the numbers along the right side. The intensity of additional light projected onto the background is on the ordinate scale on the left. (See page 35 for the details on how the curves were determined.)

Because the photopigments of rods are bleached out by high levels of illumination, the cones function exclusively when the background light exceeds 1.0 millilamberts.[7] Both types of receptor cells are said to function simultaneously when the background light is between these two values. Daylight vision (cones only) is termed photopic; visual function at twilight (rods and cones together) is called mesopic; and night vision (rods only) is named scotopic (Fig. 1-4). In photopic conditions, the central area of the retina is more sensitive than its surroundings; in mesopic adaptation, the central area is very similar in sensitivity to the nearby retina; and, in scotopic conditions, the central retina is less sensitive than the area surrounding it.

The analogy between retina and camera film is possible here, though admittedly somewhat weak: rod function resembles "fast" black-and-white film; cone function "slow" color film. The weakness of the analogy is the adaptability of the retina to such a wide range of light values, which is enhanced by the simultaneous overlapping presence of two specialized receptor systems that permit some retinal areas to increase in sensitivity by a factor of 100,000 (Fig. 1-8). If the analogist is stubborn and insists on simulating the sensitivity shifts by changing camera film, the switch to cones ("slow" color film) requires only a few seconds in the eye while use of the rods ("fast" black-and-white film) requires at least 10 minutes for full receptivity to any vestigial light in the dark.

Figure 1-9 shows the visual acuity* of the retina as a function of eccentricity

---

*Visual acuity or form sense is a complex function that requires light sense but also requires the ability to say whether (1) one or two points are present (minimum separable); (2) a line is continuous without any offset (Vernier acuity); or (3) the various geometric patterns represent specific letters,

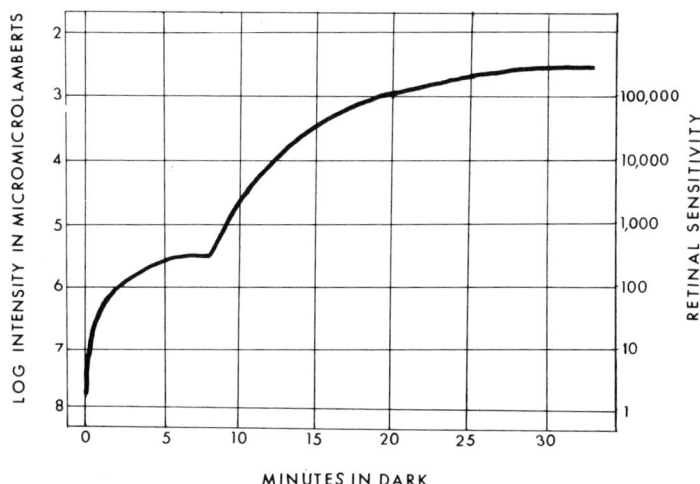

Figure 1-8 Increase in retinal sensitivity with time in the dark. As the eye grows accustomed to darkness, its sensitivity increases as much as six log units or 100,000 times. The eye must be well adapted to bright light just before this test begins by extinguishing all background light. The spot, which is repeatedly tested to find the dimmest visible light, stimulates the rod-rich retina which is 10° from the fovea. The ordinate in this figure ranges from 100 million micromicrolamberts at the baseline to only 100 micromicrolamberts at the top. For comparison with Figure 1-4, this corresponds to a range from one-tenth of a millilambert at the baseline to one ten-millionth of a millilambert at the top (10^9 micromicrolamberts = 1 millilambert).

in degrees from fixation. This curve is plotted in a manner similar to that of the light sense curves. The steep manner in which visual acuity falls (Fig. 1-9) and Østerberg's curve of the cones distribution (Fig. 1-6) resemble one another more closely than either of them resembles the photopic light sense in the three lower curves of Figure 1-7.

In summary, a higher sensitivity during light adaptation to both light and form senses is normally detectable at the center of the field, the area that is used for fixation of gaze. As testing regresses to the periphery of the normal retina, the decrease in sensitivity is not abrupt. But gradually, as the distance from the

---

numbers, or other familiar shapes (Snellen acuity). The usual American designation for clinical visual acuity, a fraction such as 20/40, states the actual test distance in the numerator (e.g., 20 feet). The denominator (40) refers to the smallest size symbol regularly identified by the patient. The sizes of all test symbols on the chart were originally calculated to indicate the distance at which a 20/20 eye could barely distinguish them. The 20/20 eye can read letters at any distance, provided their heights subtend visual angles of 5 minutes of arc and their openings and line thicknesses one minute of arc. Since the acuity measurement is based upon angular size, all symbol dimensions are inversely proportional to the acuities they test, that is, the 20/40 letter is twice as tall as the 20/20 letter.

10   Principles of Quantitative Perimetry

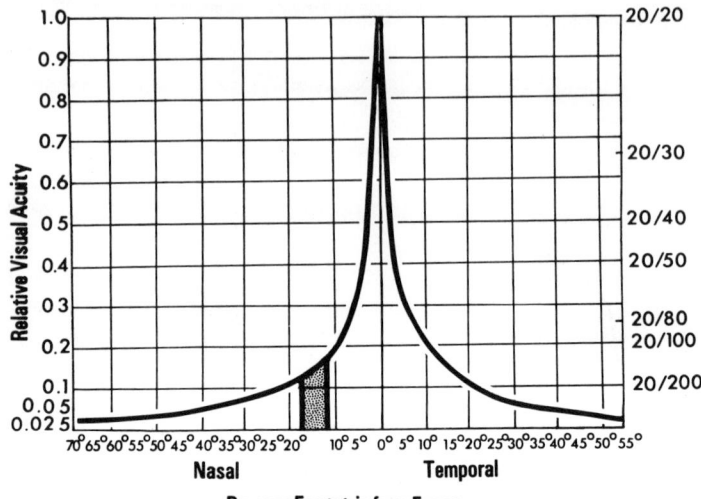

Figure 1-9   Visual acuity as a function of retinal location. The visual acuity, or form sense, is far better in the fovea and its immediate surroundings than in the retinal periphery. Note that the designation for nasal and temporal refers to the horizontal portion of *retina* being stimulated, which is the reverse of the visual field or space where stimulation occurs for light sense or form sense. The right ordinate is the American designation for acuity, as defined in the footnote on pages 8 and 9. The left ordinate, which is the decimal reduction of the acuity fraction, is used in Europe.

fixation area increases, the eye is less and less sensitive. This is another way of saying there is a gradient of sensitivity in the normal, light-adapted retina from the greatest at the center where fixation occurs to least in the extreme periphery where the eye is completely blind.

RELATIVE SENSITIVITIES: SELF-DEMONSTRATIONS

The reader may demonstrate the difference between form sense and light sense to himself by fixating his gaze upon any word in the center of these lines of print and observing his inability to read the words (form sense) at the ends of the same line despite an obvious awareness of their presence (light sense). The light sense, a more primitive function than form sense, must be present for the discernment of form, but conditions that permit detection of a peripheral object's presence often fail to allow identification of its form. In visual field testing, the usual emphasis is testing of light sense rather than form sense.

If the reader has never been the subject of a visual field examination, it is worthwhile to stop here and experience the sharp appearance and disappearance of a tiny test object very near the point of fixation, in this case the hole in a piece of paper. The reader should obtain a piece of typewriter paper, fold it lengthwise twice, then make a hole through all of the layers with a pen or pencil lead about 1" from the end of the 2⅛" by 11" folded strip. The reader should position himself in a modestly illuminated location where he can see a well-illuminated but nonreflecting background, such as the sky or the wall over a table lamp. If the paper is held at arm's length between the reader and the bright background, the hole should appear brighter than the paper itself. The reader should leave the paper at arm's length with the hole visible, then close one eye, fixate his gaze on some point on the bright surface, and move the long edge of the paper so that it lines up with the fixation point. Finally, the reader should slowly move the paper strip back and forth or up and down, leaving the gaze steadily fixed on the same spot on the wall and moving the paper closer or farther from the fixation spot. Although it may be necessary to adjust the size of the hole for background brightness, the reader should be able to find a certain distance from fixation where the hole will suddenly appear as it approaches fixation and disappear as it retreats. No description of the differences that exist is equivalent to this self-demonstration. For, brighter or larger objects are clearly evident beyond the imaginary line where the light-filled hole is suddenly visualized.

A third self-demonstration illustrates how a blind spot may be present in the visual field without the subject's being aware of it. The presence of the optic nerve head, a communication channel with no sensory capability, causes a normal blind spot in each eye. The reader may demonstrate his own blind spots as follows: Hold this page straight out at slightly less than arm's length. Close the left eye and fix the right eye on the + at the left side of the page. After a few minor rotational and distance adjustments, the reader should not see the group of words on the right side of the page. The blind spot of the left eye can be similarly demonstrated with the opposite symbols.

Right eye	Left eye
+	+
Fixation;	**Fixation;**
Left eye	**Right eye**
Blind spot	**Blind spot**

12 Principles of Quantitative Perimetry

LIMIT BETWEEN ZONES OF SENSITIVITY: THE ISOPTER

One tests the visual field clinically in much the same way as the second demonstration, by moving a small test object inward from an unseen area in the periphery until it is barely seen near the point of fixation. The limit of visibility where this small test object can barely be seen is plotted on a piece of paper to create a visual field chart. Conventionally, the visual field of each eye is plotted as the patient sees it. For example, objects seen in the right visual space of the

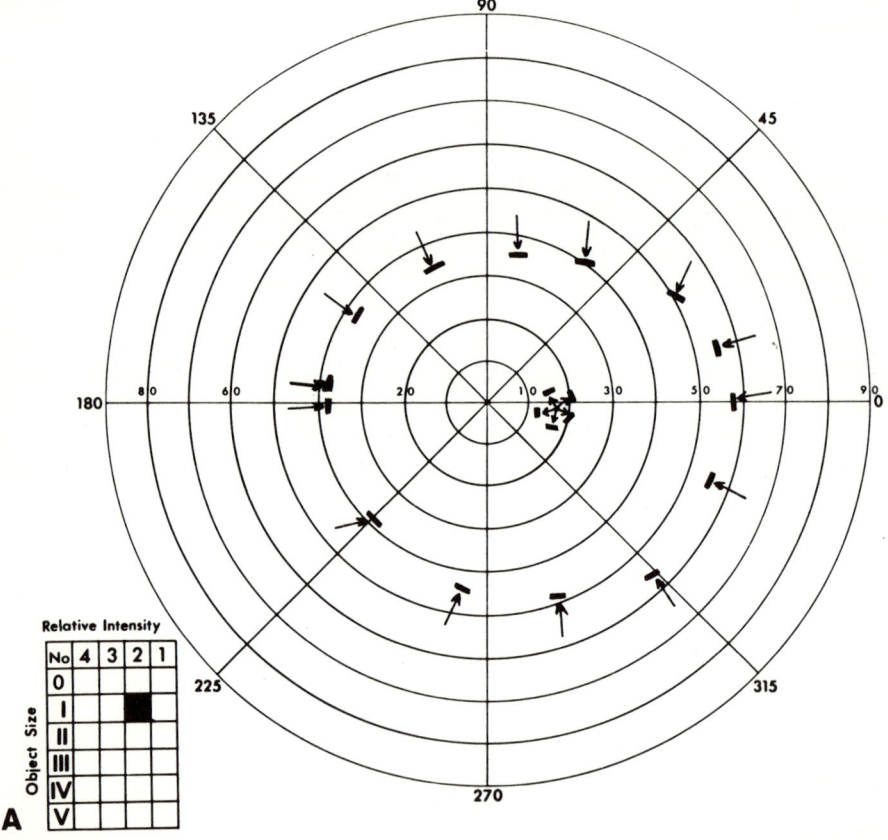

Figure 1-10 A The raw data of one isopter. As the arrows indicate, all points are determined by moving from an invisible zone to the border of the visible area. When the subject reports the sudden appearance of the spot, the examiner marks the chart with a blunt pencil. Enough spots are tested so that the examiner feels confident of the expected response should any remaining gap be tested further.

right eye and in that of the left eye are plotted on the right side of both visual field charts. The limit between the peripheral area where seeing ceases and the inside area where seeing occurs is called an isopter (Fig. 1-10). In the mathematical sense, an isopter is the locus of similar visual threshold determinations, or in the ophthalmological sense, a line joining points of equal sensitivity on a visual field chart. If testing of both periphery and blind spots is performed with the same test object, the limits in the periphery and those surrounding any blind areas inside the visual field are both considered parts of the same isopter. If an examination is limited to one test object, all marks are recorded on the visual field chart in the same color. When enough marks are present so the examiner is virtually certain of the visual field limits in each area, the plotting

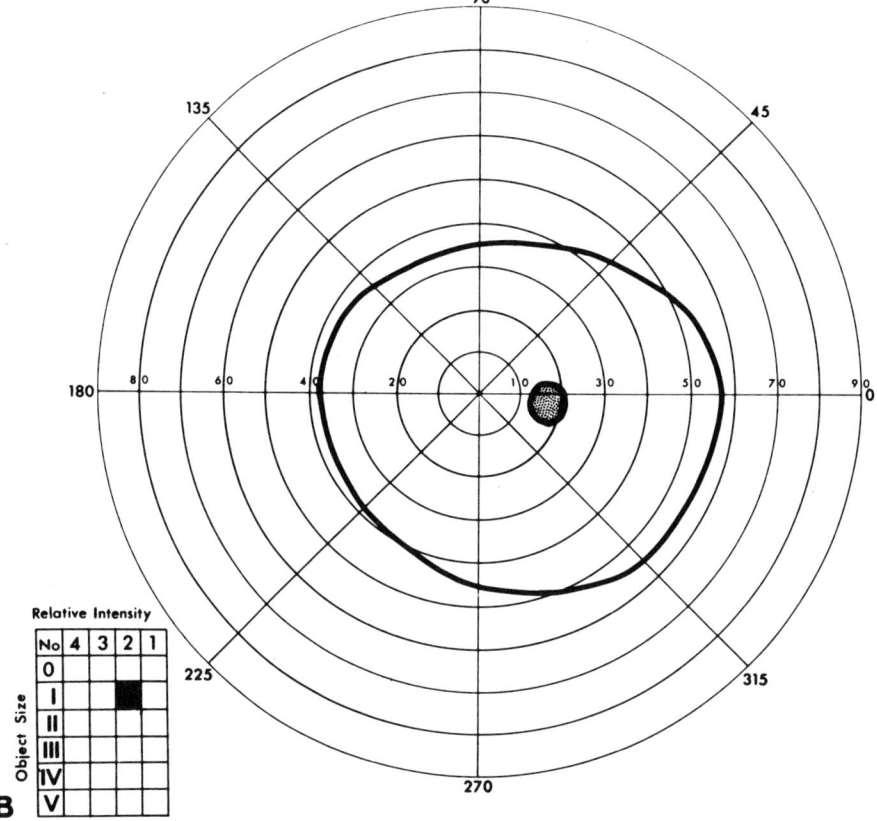

B The plotted isopter. The raw data (blunt pencil marks) are joined by a fine line, the plotted isopter, which represents the perimetrist's opinion regarding the validity of raw data plus the untested gaps between. Note that the line around the blind spot is regarded as part of the same isopter as the peripheral limit, so the same pencil is used to plot both.

14   Principles of Quantitative Perimetry

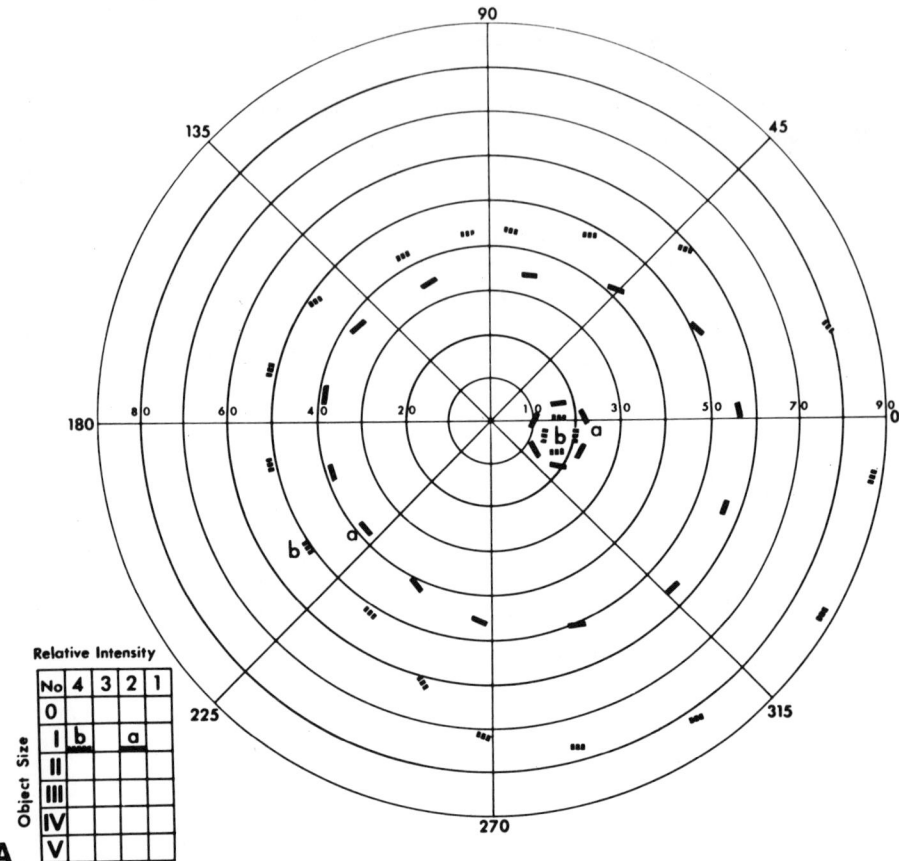

Figure 1-11   A   Raw data for two isopters. The larger isopter with the smaller blind spot resulted from using a test light (b) which was ten times as bright as the one (a) used to outline the initial, smaller isopter. Although all points for one isopter may be obtained before the other starts, the test object should always appear from apparently random (unexpected) directions.

stops. The points are then connected by a line drawn with a finely sharpened pencil that is the same color as the plotted points. This system allows the interpreter to see the perimetrist's opinion regarding the isopter's shape and location (the fine line) and the raw data that led to this conclusion (the original points). If a given isopter is large enough to surround the normal blind spot or any other defects (which would be pathological), the entire isopter that was plotted with the same test object (including the limits of the blind areas and the peripheral limits of visibility) are all charted with the same color pencil.

When larger or brighter test objects are used to test the same visual field, these produce larger isopters. Blind or defective areas within the field either

The Concept of a Visual Field   15

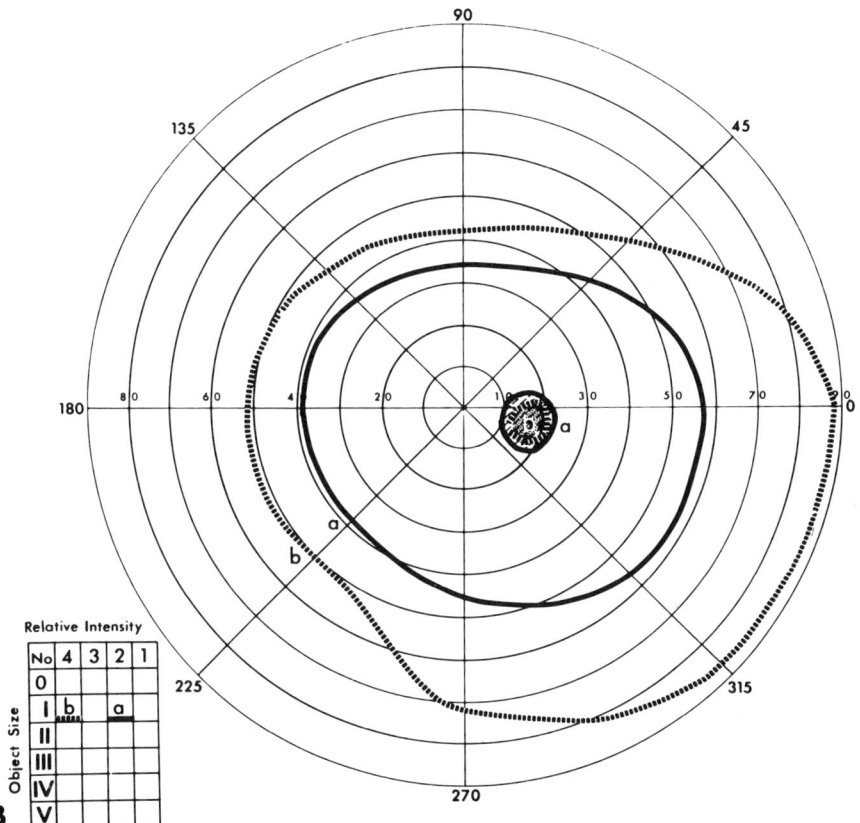

B   Two plotted isopters. The raw data for the smaller isopter are connected with a sharp pencil of the same color. The raw data for the larger isopter are not easily confused with those of the small isopter, for a different color pencil is used to plot them and a sharp pencil of that color is used to join them. A test light of smaller size or dimmer intensity than the first isopter would result in an isopter that is smaller than the originally plotted one.

disappear or appear smaller in size when these defects are plotted with larger or brighter test objects (Fig. 1-11). Isopters are thus recognized as a family of curves, normally ovoid, which describe the variable sensitivity of the eye. The zones of increasing visual sensitivity resemble a family of conoids with their apexes at the pupil and their progressively smaller bases oriented around the optical axis of the eye (Fig. 1-12).*

---

*The optical axis of the eye is the line of sight between the eye and the object of fixation or regard. Light passes along this line from the point in space where gaze is fixated to the fovea at the rear of the eye, via the center of the pupil. The optical axis also represents zero eccentricity, zero perimetric angle, and the direction of gaze.

16   Principles of Quantitative Perimetry

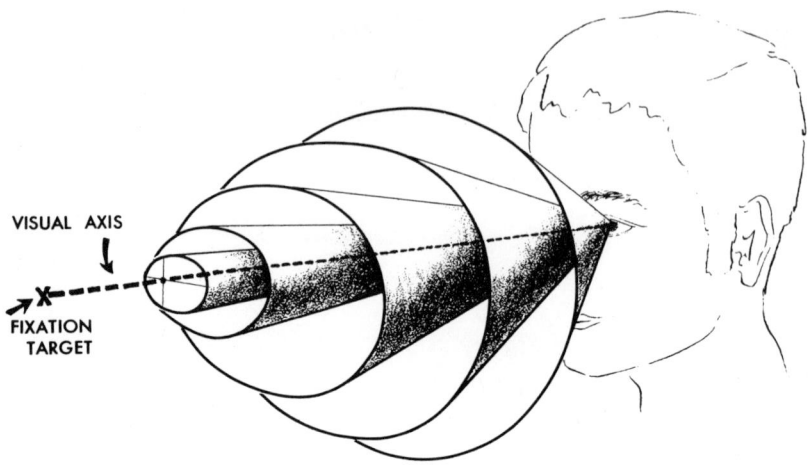

Figure 1-12   Conoids of sensitivity around the visual axis. The visual or optical axis represents the peak of sensitivity in the normal, light-adapted eye. Immediately surrounding this line that connects the pupil with the fixation target is a space where sensitivity is falling from maximum at the visual axis to a slightly lower level at the surface of a narrow-based conoid that limits the space. At any given distance from the eye the sensitivity at the surface of the conoid is equal. Additional conoids of the same type, with progressively wider bases, describe the gradient of decreasing sensitivity as the angle between the visual axis and the conoid surfaces increases. Since the visual axis and the attendant sensitivity conoids change very rapidly with any shift in attention, the observer is not aware of the normal differences in sensitivity except in a test circumstance.

THE IMPORTANCE OF FIXATION: SHARPLY DEFINED ISOPTERS VERSUS SCATTER

Accurate testing of the various zones of sensitivity is limited by the ability of the subject to fixate or hold his gaze steadily in a known orientation. In normal life, the optical axis changes frequently without the subject ever becoming aware of the zones of different sensitivity that rapidly shift along with the direction of gaze. The normal fixation reflex moves the optical axis to coincide with whatever attracts the subject's attention within the visual field. In the testing situation, steady fixation of gaze allows sharp definition of the limits of each sensitivity zone. When fixation is inadequate, the isopter lines become "scatter" zones, which become broader the more the eye moves.

Any test method that encourages steady fixation has an important advantage over other test methods with less adequate control of fixation. The examiner's usual means for encouraging the subject to fixate is to orient him or her verbally and to observe the tested eye to see that it does not visibly wander.

THE PRIMARY STIMULUS VALUES OF A TEST OBJECT: ITS SIZE AND BRIGHTNESS

The range of test objects that are appropriate to probe the variable sensitivities within the visual field of any group of normal and abnormal eyes is so large that differences between test objects are more appropriately created by serial multiplication of sizes and intensities rather than serial additions of any amount. Serial additions of small amounts would require too many isopters for testing defective fields or the normal periphery; large additions would not reveal significant defective patterns in the central field.

On the Goldmann Perimeter, increasing test object intensity is designated by an increase in the arabic number from 1 through 4, and greater test object size is indicated by larger roman numbers from 0 through V. Since any of six sizes may be selected with any of four intensities, a total of twenty-four different combinations is readily available (Table 1-1). Because a single standard

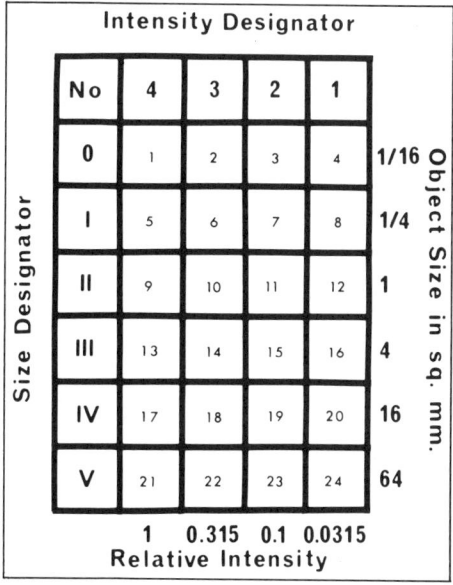

Table 1-1 Twenty-four possible test combinations on the Goldmann Perimeter. The size and intensity or brightness of the test object can be independently selected over a wide range on the Goldmann Perimeter. Using standard intensities only, there are 24 possible combinations of size and intensity. If the background is appropriately calibrated, the relative intensity designated 4 has an added light intensity of 100 millilamberts. Thus, the commonly used test object identified in this table by the number 5 has a projected intensity of 100 millilamberts (4) and an area of ¼ square millimeters (I). The object here labelled 5 is called the I-4-e test, for -e implies the use of no intermediate filters. (See the text and Table 1-3.)

18   Principles of Quantitative Perimetry

change in intensity is regarded approximately the same as a single standard change in size, the roman and arabic designators of any test object may be added together to obtain the "stimulus value" of that test.* Since the smallest, dimmest test object is designated O-1 and the largest, brightest test object is V-4, the stimulus values of these unique minimal and maximal tests are 1 and 9 respectively. The remaining 22 possible combinations provide two to four alternatives for the seven intermediate stimulus values.

Figure 1-13 shows a normal visual field plotted with the nine "standard" isopters: 0-1,† I-1, I-2, I-3, I-4, II-4, III-4, IV-4, and V-4 on the Goldmann Perimeter. On the basis of two considerations, these nine spots are used as standards in preference to the other 15 possible combinations (Table 1-2). First, the smallest test size (0) is prone, as has been shown empirically, to inconclusive results, since, regardless of the intensity used, this test size fails to yield reproducible isopters. The choice of any larger test size avoids this problem. Second, the smaller the test object size, the easier it is to discover and define small blind spots. For this reason, the smaller standard isopters are plotted by varying the intensity while retaining the smallest reliable test size, ¼ sq mm (Size I). After intensity reaches a maximum with the ¼ sq mm test (I-4) it remains at that level so the subsequent test sizes may be as small as possible (II-4, III-4, IV-4, and V-4). Use of the nine standard isopters thus improves reliability and sensitivity and it is also helpful in permitting comparisons of fields tested at different medical centers.

BETWEEN THE STANDARD ISOPTERS: THE INTERMEDIATE TEST OBJECTS

The Goldmann Perimeter has the capacity of mapping four additional "intermediate" isopters between any two adjacent "standard" isopters. As noted above, the added light of the test objects, which outline adjacent standard

---

*Goldmann has shown that a fourfold change in diameter of the test object (16X in area) is equivalent to a tenfold change (one logarithmic unit) in the intensity of the projected light that forms the test spot.[5] Each of the increasing standard sizes on the Goldmann Perimeter (the roman numerals) represents a doubling of the diameter (quadrupling of the area) of the former test. A standard intensity change, represented by a unit change in the arabic numerals (one-half log unit, the square root of ten or 3.16X) is equivalent to this twofold change in test spot diameter. Thus, the standard geometric increase in brightness is obtained by multiplying the former test object's projected intensity by 3.16 or by adding one-half log unit to the log of its previous brightness increment over background. The standard geometric increase in test object size is obtained by multiplying the former test object's diameter by two or its area by four, which is the same as adding 0.6 long units to the log of its former area.

†O-1 is a standard isopter only because it is the minimal stimulus available.

The Concept of a Visual Field   19

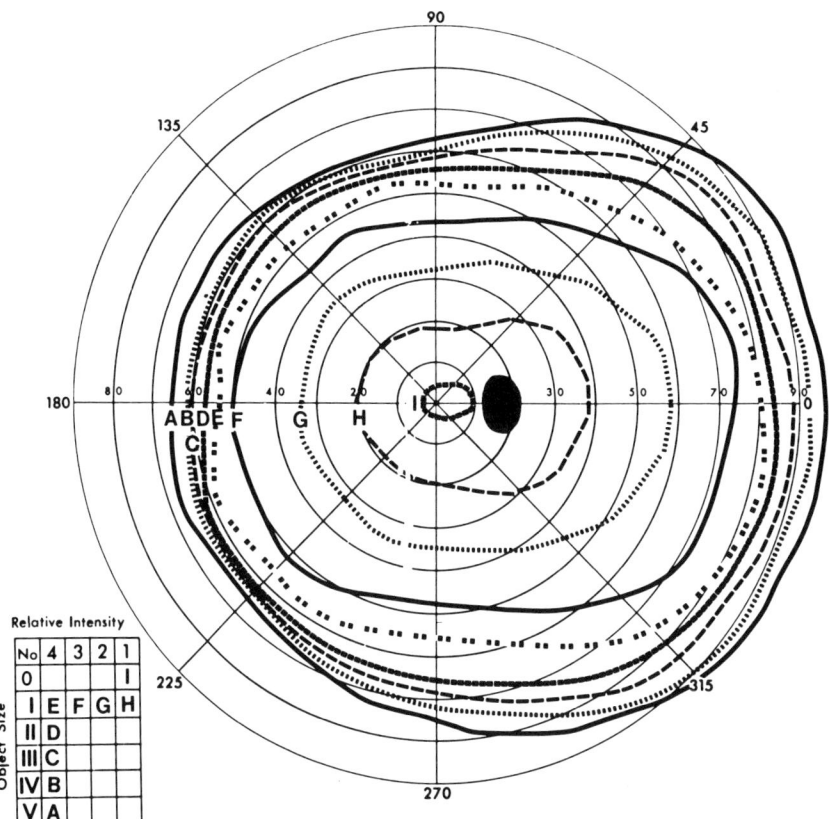

Figure 1-13 The visual field from the right eye of a healthy 28-year-old female using the nine standard isopters on the Goldmann Perimeter. The isopters are labelled from A through I, and they correspond to test objects usually called, respectively: V-4-e, IV-4-e, III-4-e, II-4-e, I-4-e, I-3-e, I-2-e, I-1-e, and 0-1-e.

isopters, differs by a multiplication factor of 3.16, which is an additional 0.5 log unit. The added light of adjacent "intermediate" isopters differs by a multiplication factor of about 1.26, which is equivalent to adding 0.1 log unit.

Since the total light of a projected test object is the sum of the projected light and the light that was already on the background, the sequence of the test objects' total intensities is a geometric progression plus a constant. If, for example, the projected test objects are 1-2-a, 1-2-b, and 1-2-c (see Table 1-3), the added light is respectively 4.0, 5.0, and 6.3 millilamberts. Since the background intensity is typically 3.16 millilamberts, the total intensity of each of these three spots is respectively 7.16, 8.16 and 9.46 millilamberts.

	Intensity Designator			
Size Designator \ **No**	4	3	2	1
0	ESV 4	ESV 3	ESV 2	STD 1
I	STD 5	STD 4	STD 3	STD 2
II	STD 6	ESV 5	ESV 4	ESV 3
III	STD 7	ESV 6	ESV 5	ESV 4
IV	STD 8	ESV 7	ESV 6	ESV 5
V	STD 9	ESV 8	ESV 7	ESV 6

Table 1-2 Nine standard test objects. Because a single change in size is approximately equivalent to a single change in standard intensity on the Goldmann Perimeter, the 24 possible combinations really yield a maximum range of only nine equivalent stimulus values. This table indicates the nine shaded test objects that are "standard" and labels the remaining 15 to show the standards to which they are equivalent. ESV stands for Equivalent Stimulus Value (sum of roman and arabic numerals); STD means Standard. (See the text for an explanation of why the nine standard test objects are preferred over their equivalents.)

Standard Intensity Designator and Multipliers \ **Relative Intensity Designator and Multipliers**	a (×0.40)	b (×0.50)	c (×0.63)	d (×0.79)	e (×1.00)
1 (×0.0316)	1 (0.0125)	2 (0.016)	3 (0.020)	4 (0.025)	5 (0.0316)
2 (×0.10)	6 (0.040)	7 (0.050)	8 (0.063)	9 (0.079)	10 (0.10)
3 (×0.316)	11 (0.125)	12 (0.16)	13 (0.20)	14 (0.25)	15 (0.316)
4 (×1.00)	16 (0.40)	17 (0.50)	18 (0.63)	19 (0.79)	20 (1.00)

Table 1-3 Four standard and 16 intermediate intensities. The intermediate intensities (a through e) differ from their adjacent table members by 0.1 log unit while standard intensities (1 through 4) differ from one another by 0.5 log unit. Standard isopters all use the darker-shaded group of intensities designated -e. Any of the 20 intensities shown could be presented with any of the six test object sizes on the Goldmann Perimeter, but equivalent values make this wide range unnecessary in normal practice.

TRAQUAIR'S ISLAND OF VISION: A THREE-DIMENSIONAL MODEL

If an equal or known difference is established between a series of isopters, as in the choice of Goldmann's standards, an abstract but useful three-dimensional model may be constructed. To make the concept clear, one should envision plotting each of the standard isopters on a separate piece of thick material such as cardboard or plywood. The shapes may then be cut out and the smaller ones, representing the visible limits of dimmer test objects, should be stacked in appropriate orientation on top of those that are made by using larger, brighter test objects until a three-dimensional shape is built (Fig. 1-14). Such a structure was romantically termed the "Island of Vision in a Sea of Blindness" by Traquair who expanded the original ideas of Euclid and Heliodorus and described the variable slope of the island: the peak of sensitivity in the center, and the normal blind spot as a well going all the way to sea level from an area some 15° to the temporal side of the central point, Fixation.[14]

THE HELICOPTER ANALOGY: PERIMETRY

The concept of an island named vision in a sea called blindness has suggested the possibility of mapping the island's topography by flying a helicopter at a specific altitude above sea level in the vicinity of the island (Figure 1-15). Wherever the aircraft comes in contact with the island of vision, a certain color of paint could be applied to mark the island. If one desires much detail about the island's contours, marking at other altitudes could be performed if a different color of paint were available for each altitude chosen. Finally, a helicopter should fly to a location directly above the visual island and make a color photograph to show all the paint marks on the island (Fig. 1-16). In evaluating the resultant picture, the marks made at higher altitudes on the island (near point fixation) surround a smaller area than marks made closer to sea level.

This description of a helicopter mapping the topography of an island is highly analogous to perimetry. Horizontal flying of the aircraft is equivalent to test object movement; contact with the island's surface is signalled by the patient when each test object is first seen. Paint marks on the island are equivalent to the raw data points on the visual field chart. A real or imaginary line joining similarly colored marks represents an isobar on the island's topographic map, an isopter on the visual field chart. Large or bright tests are normally seen far from the fixation point so they are shown at the periphery of the island, where the surface is closer to sea level, and at the periphery of the field chart where the maximum available stimulus value finally separates visible (land) from invisible (water). Presentation of dim or small test objects is equivalent to flying at a

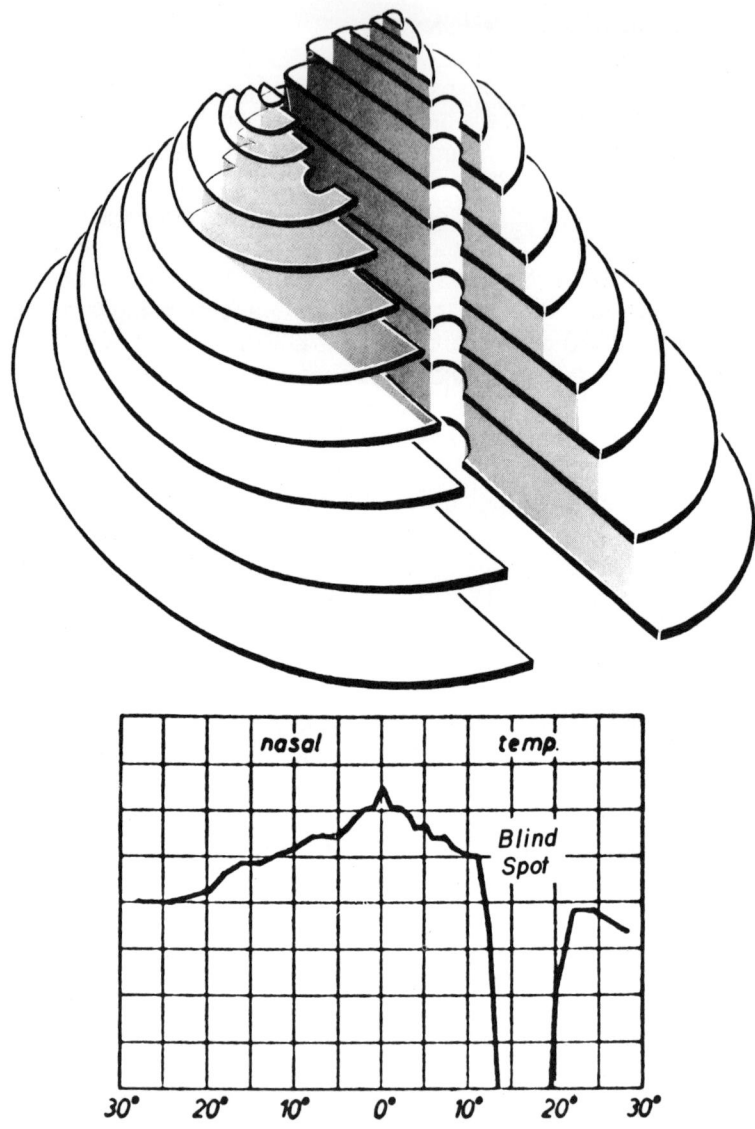

Figure 1-14 Traquair's hill of vision. If pieces of plywood are cut in the shapes of isopters from one visual field and stacked in appropriate positions on top of one another, a view of the resultant model of a hill or island will appear the same as the visual field. A view of the island in profile, or better, of a vertical slice through the center, will appear similar to the light-sense test results that were demonstrated in Figure 1-7. Thus, the hill or island of vision may be sectioned horizontally and visualized from above as isopters, or it may be sectioned vertically through the center and visualized from the side as profiles.

The Concept of a Visual Field   23

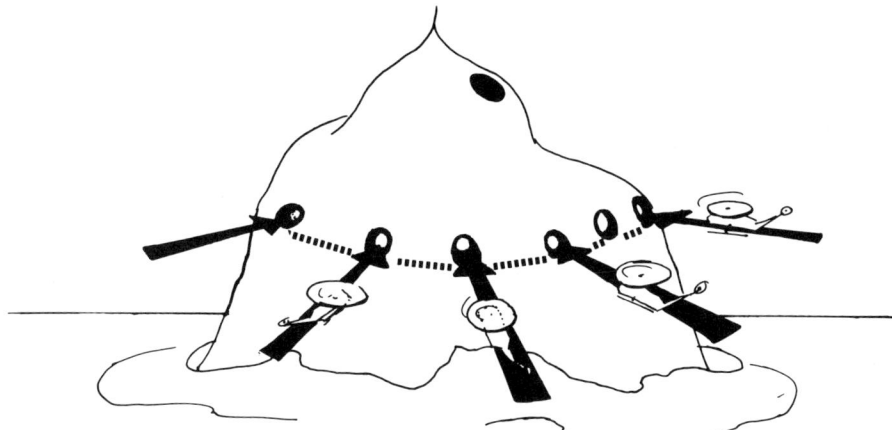

Figure 1-15 A perspective of the perimetry helicopter. As noted in the text, perimetry and mapping an island's topography by helicopter are rather analogous. For orientation, the visual axis of the observer whose visual island is being mapped coincides with a vertical line through the peak of the island. The land corresponds to the space where test objects are seen, with subsurface soil corresponding to easily visible spots and the surface corresponding to barely visible ones. The water level corresponds to the maximum available stimulus level. If the water level can be lowered, more land area might be exposed, just as tests that are larger or brighter than the previously available maximum might plot a larger visual field. The air around and above the island corresponds to invisibility; tests which are too dim or too far from the center of the island cannot be seen. Flying the helicopter at a constant altitude from one spot to another corresponds to movement of a test object in any direction with a constant level of stimulation at the eye.

higher altitude where detection requires more sensitivity, a capability that is present in a progressively smaller zone. Finally, if one flies too high, the island is never contacted, just as a test object that is too small or dim is never seen.

PERIMETRY VERSUS CAMPIMETRY: THE SHAPE OF THE TEST SCREEN

When the visual field is tested on an instrument that is hemispherical or arc-shaped, with the eye located at the instrument's center of curvature, the test objects are a constant distance from the eye. Such an examination, called perimetry, may be compared with an equally valid means of testing the visual field called campimetry.* In campimetry, the testing is conducted on a flat surface, with the eye located a known distance from the screen along a line that is

---

*Campimetry is measuring the campus, a flat place.

24   *Principles of Quantitative Perimetry*

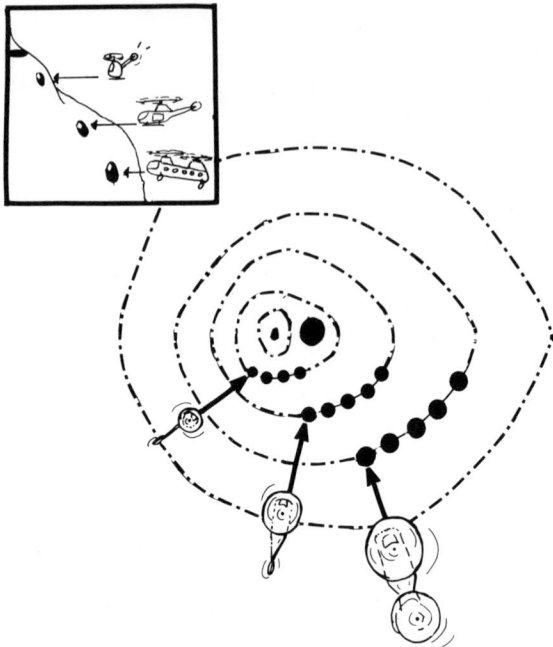

Figure 1-16   Top and side views of three perimetry helicopters. Larger helicopters are required to carry larger test objects; the small helicopters, flying at relatively higher altitudes, carry proportionally smaller or dimmer test objects. The smaller helicopters fly over much of the visual island while maintaining their constant altitudes, and they may not contact the visual island except in its most sensitive zone, a small area surroundng the peak fixation. If they fly too high with too dim a test object, they may not contact the island at all. Each helicopter crew uses a different color of paint to mark the island, providing raw data for the mapmaker's top view of the island so that he can identify the various levels above sea level, or isobars, and distinguish them from one another by color. This system corresponds to collection of raw data from each size–brightness test object with a different colored pencil so the isopter lines can be distinguished. The helicopter can operate on its pontoons in the water and move in to map the absolute edge of the island with the test of maximum available size and brightness. (If maximum-type tests were the only kind used, a boat would serve as well, but you'd give up flying!)

perpendicular to the center of the surface, the fixation point. Although the *distance from eye to fixation point* should remain *constant* during any given test, the *distance between eye and test object* becomes progressively *greater* as the distance between test object and fixation point increases. In campimetry, the increased distance from the test object to the eye means peripherally located test objects of a given finite size stimulate the eye somewhat less than the same size test object in perimetry at that same perimetric angle or eccentricity. Further consideration of the conceptual and quantitative relationships between perimetry and campimetry follows.

The Concept of a Visual Field 25

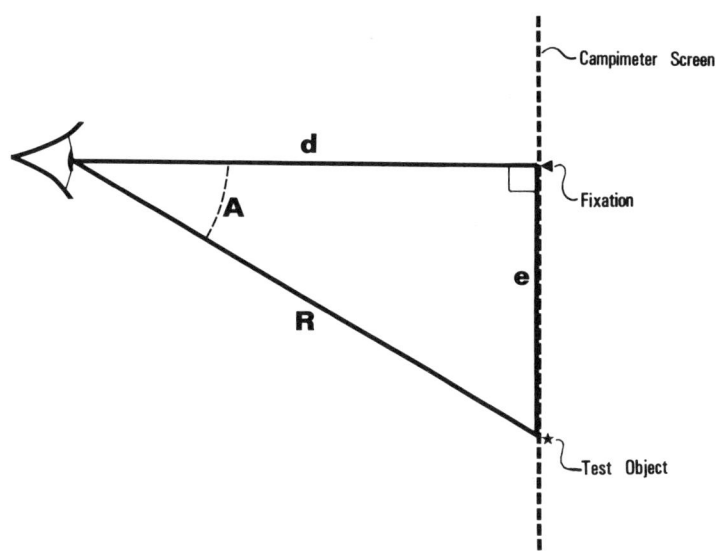

Figure 1-17 Geometry of campimetry: the geometrical considerations. If the eye is at a constant distance d from fixation, a test object at eccentricity e from fixation will be a distance R from the eye. The stimulus value(S) (essentially, the area subtense) may be calculated as follows: $\cos A = d/R$, and thus, $R = d/\cos A$. Since the solid angle (area subtense) of the test object is a/R^2 where a is the apparent surface area, substituting for R, $S = a \cos^2 A/d^2$. But a/d^2 is the stimulus value at fixation (S_f). Thus, $S = S_f \cos^2 A$. If the test object is not spherical but flat, it appears foreshortened so that another $\cos A$ comes into consideration: $a(\text{apparent}) = a(\text{real}) \cos A$. Thus, in this case, $S = S_f \cos^3 A$.

TESTING THE VISUAL FIELD ON A FLAT SCREEN: CAMPIMETRY

Testing the visual field by perimetry yields results that may be compared quantitatively with results obtained during campimetry. In Figure 1-17 an exercise in simple geometry allows the stimulus value of a given test to be expressed as a function of the test value at fixation and of the perimetric angle of the test spot. Figure 1-18 shows how the stimulus value of spherical and flat-surface test objects decrease with increasing eccentricity on a campimeter.

If one prefers to think about the perimetry-campimetry relationship in graphic rather than mathematical terms, Figure 1-19 translates the information of Figure 1-18 to the Island of Vision in the Sea of Blindness. As a given test object approaches the center in campimetry, the stimulus value of the test increases gradually.* Thus, the campimetric approach to the island via helicopter is similar

---

*This is because the eye-to-test-object distance gradually decreases, thus increasing the apparent size of the test object.

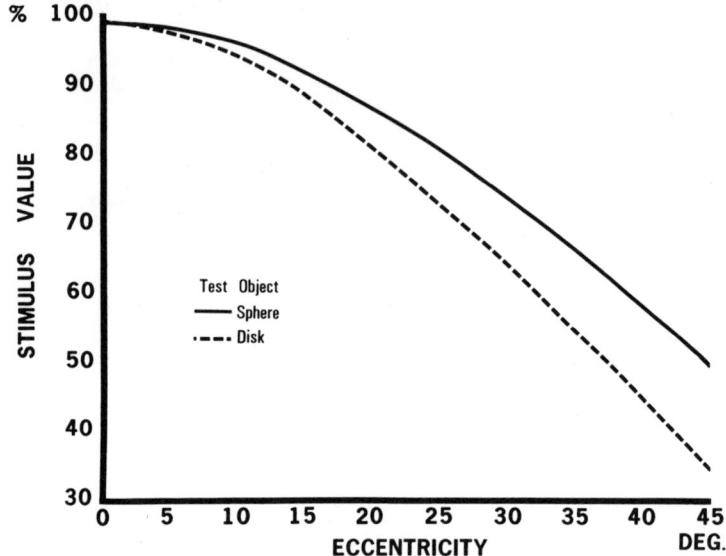

Figure 1-18   A graph of the relative stimulus efficiency of spherical test objects (solid line) and flat test objects (dotted line) in campimetry. Note that at an eccentricity of 45°, the actual stimulus value of a spherical test object is only about 50% of the value of the same test at fixation. The solid curve is a cosine-squared function, whereas the broken curve follows the cube of the cosine. (See also Figure 1-17).

to sliding down the inside of a large shallow salad bowl, for the aircraft must swoop down and inward toward a perpendicular line below the point of fixation. In perimetry the test object remains at the same distance above sea level so the approach is along a horizontal plane. The shape of an isopter from campimetry is equivalent to the shape of an isopter from perimetry when the latter is circular. Retesting with campimetry tends to shorten long oval isopters found with perimetry.

CONCEPTUAL DIFFERENCES IN TEST METHOD: KINETIC VERSUS STATIC

When tests of the visual field are performed on perimeters or campimeters with test objects that move back and forth between nonseeing areas and zones in which they are detected, the technique is termed "kinetic" as opposed to stationary testing, which is called "static." In *kinetic* testing, one attempts to find in the visual field *locations* that are barely sensitive to *preselected test objects*. In *static* testing, one attempts to find in the visual field *sensitivities* of the eye at *preselected locations*. Because these two test methods which give

The Concept of a Visual Field 27

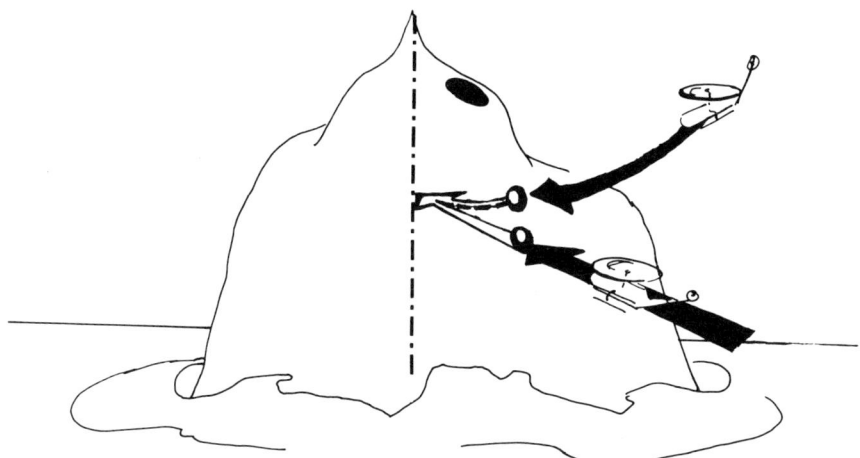

Figure 1-19 A perspective of campimetric and perimetric helicopters. It is rather confusing that the swooping path of the upper campimetric helicopter is an arc in contrast with the straight line which is the path of the lower perimetric helicopter, for campimeters are flat and perimeters are shaped like arcs or hemispheres. This results from the abstract definition of the island where all points are equal in stimulus value if they lie in any given plane parallel to sea level. As indicated in the text and in Figures 1-17 and 1-18, the test objects on a tangent screen or other campimeters have a progressively larger angular size as they approach fixation. The maximum stimulus value of the campimeter test object is chosen in this figure to be equal to the perimetric one when both are at the visual axis. The perimetric helicopter contacts the island more peripherally than the campimetric one since the constant altitude of the perimetric helicopter is lower (the stimulus value is greater) than any part of the campimetric helicopter's path except at fixation.

similar results are inherently different in certain aspects, each is superior to the other in specific instances so that both methods are valuable in measuring the light sense.

THE VISUAL THRESHOLD: STALAGMITE OR STALACTITE?

In perimetry, it is common to compare the three-dimensional curve corresponding to the threshold of vision to "the surface of the visual island," where the hard rock and stone of the island correspond to areas that are seen and the air above the island corresponds to stimuli that are not seen. One could just as easily draw an analogy to a stalagmite, a similarly peaked rocky cone that extends upward from the floor of a cave, often beneath a stalactite. This analogy, however, comes only from the common perimetric convention of plotting thresholds in terms of sensitivities and not in terms of absolute light sense. These two entities are related to each other in that one is the reciprocal of the other. Thus, if one plots the actual brightness of the light that was seen, one would find that the most sensitive parts of the visual field (corresponding to the tip of the stalagmite) are plotted the lowest on the graph, not the highest, as is common in standard perimetric practice. Such a curve would resemble a stalactite, a rocky, icicle-shaped structure hanging from the roof of the cave, far more than a stalagmite. Unfortunately, both presentations of data are in common use today. Sensitivity is important to the clinician, for a lack of sensitivity implies some pathological process, whereas an increase in sensitivity may imply that a previously pathological area is improving. We are accustomed psychologically to seeing good things going up and bad things coming down on graphs; this is true whether we are studying the stock market or a perimetric chart. The experimental psychologist, unencumbered by any need for gratification in the clinical sense, plots his data directly.† If the patient sees a target of a given brightness, that brightness and not its reciprocal serves as the ordinate. In this type of presentation, a stimulus that is "above threshold" is physically plotted above the surface of the stalactite, whereas in the common perimetric plot a similar stimulus would be beneath the surface of the visual island. Conversely, a stimulus that is "sub-threshold" is above the surface of the visual island, and therefore invisible.* In both analogies, the "seen" stimuli correspond to solid rock.

Another difference between the clinical perimetrist and the experimental psychologist is that the clinical perimetrist uses data in a much more simplistic manner. To the clinical perimetrist with an adequate patient, a given test object will either be seen at or inside the isopter, or unseen outside the isopter. To the experimental psychologist, the visual threshold is not a line like the isopter, but a zone of uncertainty of approximately 0.4 log units width[3] in which the subject may or may not respond to the test object. Unfortunately, the experimental psychologist's view more closely corresponds to reality than does the standard perimetric model, and the real visual island, whether measured clinically or experimentally, has an undulating "soft" surface, much like a wheat field. This and other factors that may influence the variable threshold values—often

---

†Although visual experimental psychologists and clinical perimetrists both study the same light sense, the psychological approach requires many presentations in each area—enough to develop statistically valid data. In the interest of obtaining the broad picture in minimal time, the clinical perimetrist accepts one, or at the most two, responses in any single area and ignores much scientifically relevant information (e.g., signal detection theory as opposed to the relatively simple clinical concept of the threshold; forced choice versus "yes-or-no" responses). (See Appendix A and Chapter 2.)

*Although the authors and other clinical perimetrists customarily refer to any object used in a visual field test as a stimulus whether it is seen or not, the experimental psychologist usually applies the term "stimulus" only to a test object that is seen.

BALANCING EFFECTS IN KINETIC TESTING: SUMMATION VERSUS SLOW REACTION TIME

In kinetic perimetry or campimetry, a compensatory balance exists between summation,* which enlarges the field plot, and slow reaction time, which constricts it. The *faster something moves, the larger the area being stimulated by the summation so the more peripherally the test may be seen.* The stimulus value of a moving test is enhanced to include all the interconnected retina which is stimulated within a time period that is reported to be about 500 milliseconds.[2] Yet between the moment when an adequate stimulus is received by the eye, and the report of its presence (the reaction time or latency period), the test object continues to move inward. The visual reaction time varies between 100 and 1500 milliseconds. The *faster the test object moves inward* during this reaction period, the *smaller the field that is registered.* A more slowly moving test object does not stimulate as many receptors within the critical ½ second just prior to ocular reception of an adequate stimulus, so the slow test object penetrates farther than the fast one toward the point of fixation before the signal *starts* along the optic nerve toward the brain. During the reaction time—which is similar whether a test object is moving slowly or rapidly—a test object moving slowly does not travel quite so far as one moving relatively fast before being perceived. As a result of both effects, the recorded locations of both slow and relatively fast stimuli often turn out to be approximately the same (Fig. 1-20). This compensation for inconstant velocity of test movement is very fortunate, for in our relatively crude methods of kinetic visual field testing on manual perimeters, it would be difficult, if not impossible, to eliminate small amounts of variability in the speed of test objects. Although Goldmann has shown experimentally that there is an optimum speed for test object movement,[5] the long duration of reaction times by certain patients requires some flexibility in the velocities of test objects. Of course, the compensation of summation and reaction time is valid

---

*Summation is the ability of the retina to report the presence of a large test object of long-duration, at locations where a smaller test object of short-duration would be invisible, given the same contrast, or intensity relative to the background, in both tests.[2] Summation is related to the simultaneous or near-simultaneous firing of adjacent receptor cells that are appropriately interconnected (see Figure 1-5). Summation is purely "spatial" when stationary tests of enlarging sizes are presented for identical durations or for times in excess of 500 milliseconds. When the size is held constant and the test presentation is varied in duration (up to 500 ms.), the greater visibility of the tests that endure longer is the result of "temporal" summation. Summation that depends on movement within the same time limits to stimulate larger areas of the retina is both "temporal" and "spatial."

30 *Principles of Quantitative Perimetry*

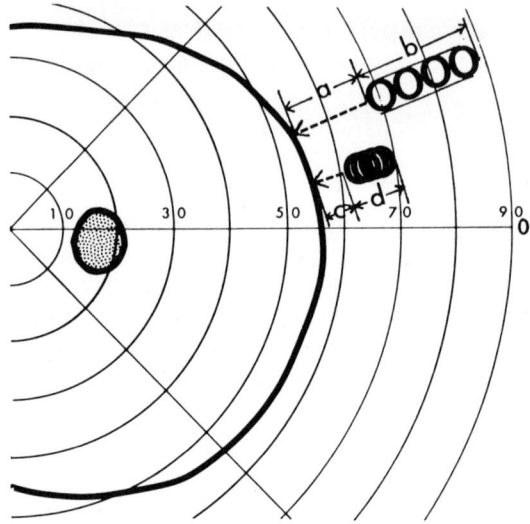

Figure 1-20   Compensating effects of summation and reaction time. The rate of test object movement often yields similar raw isopter data at the same location, whether the test object moves relatively rapidly, as in the path labelled a and b, or more slowly as in the path labelled c and d. Summation occurs during the critical period while the faster test is moving the distance b and while the slower test is moving the distance d. At the moment when the test enters the approximately equal reaction phases, a and c, the stimulus is peripherally "seen" (though not yet perceived) in that the message to the brain has been initiated. Because a larger area is stimulated in b than d, the faster test is "seen" sooner, but because it still moves faster during the similar reaction period, the test moves farther in a than in c. Thus, summation and reaction time tend to compensate one another to yield similar results with tests moving at different rates.

only for a limited range of speeds and reaction times, as indicated below. All the same, this factor has allowed ophthalmologists to obtain reasonably reproducible visual fields since 1856, when the technique was originally introduced to patient care by Albrecht von Graefe as a manual testing technique.[6]

THE INHERENT INACCURACY OF KINETIC TESTING: TEST OBJECT DISPLACEMENT DURING TIME REQUIRED FOR RESPONSE

Despite the compensating effect of temporal and spatial summation, a time lag occurs between the ocular reception of a visual stimulus that is later perceived and the subjective response to that stimulus. Such time lags make the outer plotted limits of any isopter smaller than would be the case if perception were signalled instantly. Similarly, time lags inevitably expand the inner limits of any

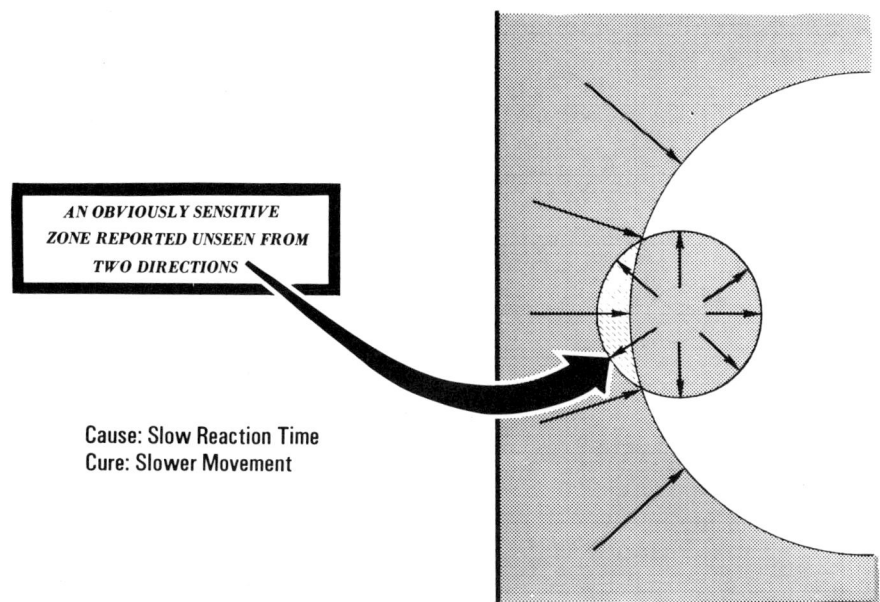

Figure 1-21 The paradox of kinetic campimetry. The inherent flaw of moving or kinetic testing of the visual field is often illustrated by campimetry of the isopter which barely surrounds the normal blind spot. Test objects move inward through the shaded unseen periphery and the unshaded crescent until they are reported. The same test object moves outward through the normal blind spot, across the border where the test was reported coming inward, and again through the unshaded crescent to be reported seen for the first time in an area where the test was not seen coming inward. This doubly unseen crescent is explained by the reaction time zones a and c of Figure 1-20, which represent a significant, though often unrecognized, error that is built into kinetic testing. One can reexamine the area with slower movement or mentally "reverse" the isopter and blind-spot borders a distance that provides a thin margin of visible field, which naturally falls inside the crescent.

blind area artificially. This inaccuracy can go unnoticed most of the time, but when the inner and outer parts of the same isopter are close enough to share points of congruity, one's confidence in the whole testing technique can be shaken. This occurs in many patients during campimetry of the normal blind spot, usually when the peripheral part of the isopter barely fails to surround the blind spot (Fig. 1-21). In this example, peripheral isopter responses are elicited initially as the test moves *inward* from beyond the blind spot. When the test object is then moved *outward* from within the area known to be normally blind, a response is reported after the test object is beyond the intially reported isopter limit, a confusing if not meaningless report. The zone between the two limits is plotted as "not-seen" coming in or going out, yet it is really "seen" from both directions if each of the isopters are corrected by an unknown but individually appropriate distance to compensate for reaction time lag.* Slowing the rate of test object movement can help to eliminate this problem while creating others, such as unsteady fixation, boredom, and fatigue. Some clinicians attempt to solve the problem by oscillation of the test object, but this nonquantitative technique is to be avoided because it cannot be manually reproduced with accuracy and consistency.

AN ANSWER TO VARIABLE REACTION TIMES: STATIC PERIMETRY

The paradox of an area where test objects are at times unseen yet at other times seen can be avoided by static perimetry, for the recorded position of a stationary test object is independent of reaction time. Although it has a specific weakness, the helicopter analogy is again useful (Fig. 1-22). The technique involves flying to one location at a time and then descending vertically until the island of vision is contacted. The locations to be tested are preselected arbitrarily or chosen on the basis of previous testing. The information that must be recorded for each test location is the altitude above sea level whenever a response indicates the island's surface is contacted.

LOCAL ADAPTATION: A LIMITATION OF STATIC TESTING

The weakness of the helicopter analogy in static testing relates to a phenomenon called local retinal adaptation. When any of the retina is exposed to light, whether seen or almost seen, the light energy has a bleaching effect on the photopigments of the retina or, more likely because of its brief duration, a neural effect involving inhibition of certain connecting cells of the retina. When an invisibly dim spot in the field gradually brightens, the retina becomes adapted to the presence of that light, so it requires more light to be seen than would have been the case had the test been presented as flashes of increasing intensity with intervening rest periods. The authors have experimentally presented spots with gradually increasing intensity and observed that the projected light required

---

*The authors regularly advocate moving test objects from nonseeing to seeing areas because fixation and subject concentration are more difficult when movement from seeing to nonseeing is mixed into the test procedure, for many otherwise testable subjects become confused when their tasks are changed. Other authorities advocate testing both seeing to nonseeing and nonseeing to seeing with the same test object to reveal those individuals who are unreliable or have prolonged reaction times.[11]

The Concept of a Visual Field   33

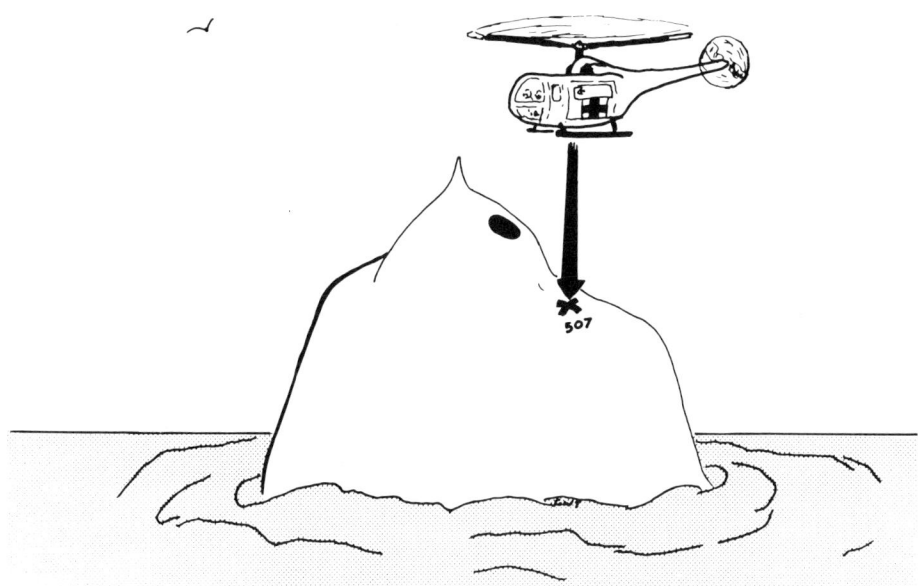

Figure 1-22 Basic principle of static perimetry helicopter. After previous selection of the longitude and latitude of the spot to be tested, the static perimetry helicopter descends directly onto the visual island. The pilot then consults his cockpit altimeter to learn the distance above sea level and enters this number at the appropriate location on his chart of the visual island. This is analogous to preselecting a location in the visual field, gradually increasing the intensity of the test spot there until its presence is reported, and recording the intensity when seen on the visual field chart. (To understand the problem with this oversimplified version, see Figure 1-23 and the text on local adaptation.)

for response is 0.3 log unit more than the same test spot at the same location when it is presented as conventionally described in static perimetry. Rotational movement of the gradually brightening test object about the circumference of a small circle did not significantly alter its threshold, so repetitive motion within a small zone does not avoid local adaptation. If a clinical test utilized the gradually increasing stimulus, the results would probably suffer from scatter because the patients would soon learn they could see much better by constant movement of their eye.

Knowing the limitation posed by local adaptation, we can now correct the helicopter analogy for static perimetry. Flying by instruments, even above clouds, the pilot finds and holds a preselected longitude, latitude, and altitude over the visual island. A bucket is lowered on its supportive cable to one of several special marks and then retracted to see if it has contacted earth (Fig. 1-23). If not, the bucket is allowed to descend again, but the cable length is now

34 *Principles of Quantitative Perimetry*

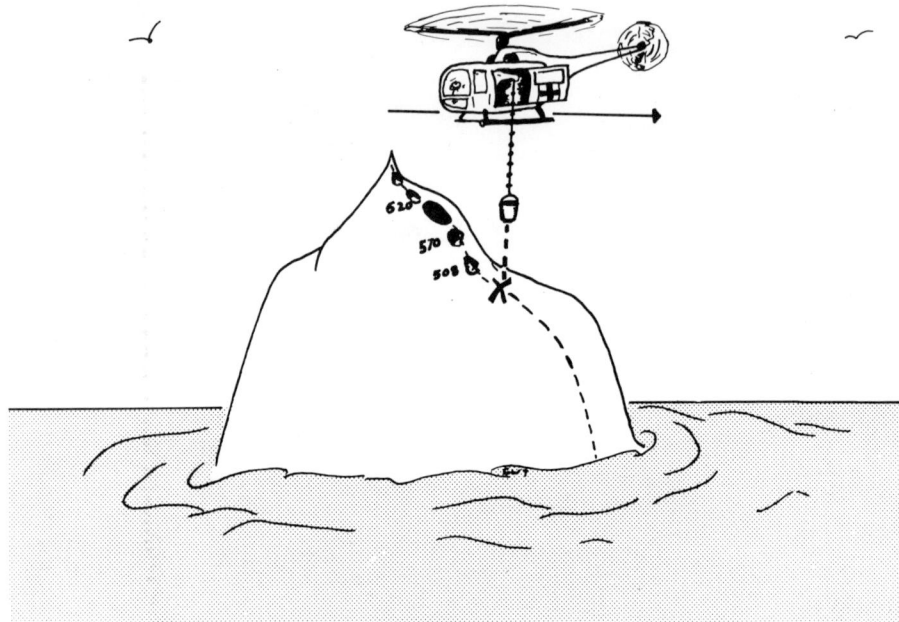

Figure 1-23 The static perimetry helicopter with marked cable and weighted bucket. Because the helicopter can hover at a given location and altitude better than it can repeatedly descend *abruptly* by a *precise* distance, this corrected helicopter analogy for static perimetry differs from that of Figure 1-22 by the additions of a winch, a marked cable, and a weighted bucket. In action, the cable is extended quickly to a given mark, then retracted to see if it contacted the island. If not, the cable is again extended one mark farther than the previous trial to start a new cycle. The sequence ends with retrieval of dirt or water and the recording of the most recent cable extension length for the location. This corresponds to the previous analogy in the preselection of location and vertical probing. The vertical probe here is precise in extent, for the helicopter can hold its altitude well and the winch can be released to the desired mark. The probe is also abrupt, for the weighted bucket is allowed to fall freely to the end of the cable. As noted in the text, the analogous technique of manual static perimetry requires that a flash of light be presented in a certain location, that it be extinguished for two seconds to allow recovery from local adaptation, and that the subsequent flash of light at that location be brighter than the preceding one by an additional 0.1 log unit or 26%.

extended 26% more than the previous trial to the next mark. The cycle of lowering and retracting the bucket continues until earth is touched or until, after the full length of cable is let out, water is scooped up from the Sea of Blindness, an indication that the maximum available stimulus was not seen. Only after the bucket contacts land or water does the pilot chart the amount of unextended cable as a measure of the island's surface altitude at that location, and only then does he move on to the next preselected test site.

STATIC PERIMETRY: HOW IS IT DONE?

Before static perimetry begins, the locations to be tested are selected arbitrarily or, preferably, on the basis of previous testing results. If one idealistically considers testing every available point in the entire visual field of both eyes, the time consumed would be about 240 hours, or six work weeks. Since the number of thresholds to be tested is therefore limited by practical considerations, intelligent choice of a limited number of points is important. Alternatives for choosing the test locations depend upon several factors. If a suspicious area is detected on kinetic testing, a popular static pattern choice, termed a meridian, is a test line that passes through the visual field's center and through the suspicious zone (see central part of Fig. 1-24). In diseases such as glaucoma, static test points are often selected for static screening along the circles located 5°, 10°, and/or 15° from fixation (Fig. 1-25). When an isolated defective area or blind spot is found by kinetic testing of the visual field, the depth of that defect should be established by selecting at least one or two points near the center of the defect for static testing.

Once the locations of proposed static points have been selected, the subject is asked to fixate and respond whenever a stationary test spot is seen. The subject is made aware of the location where the next test object is to appear, and he is alerted prior to the presentation of each stimulus. Each test object is initially presented some three to seven steps (0.1 log unit intervals) dimmer than the expected threshold. If a meridian is to be tested, the first location choice is the central spot where the subject fixates. If the initial presentation of about ½-¾ second goes undetected (as expected), the test spot is extinguished while filter settings are adjusted to increase the intensity of added light by 26% (0.1 log unit). The time consumed in filter change should occupy about two seconds to allow for recovery of local adaptation of the retina, after which a brighter (but probably still unseen) spot is again presented in the same central location. This cycle of test presentation and subsequent filter adjustment continues until the subject responds that he sees the test object. The intensity of the first barely visible spot is then recorded at zero eccentricity on the static perimetry chart. The subject is told or, if necessary shown, the location of the second test position on the meridian, usually one degree from the fixation point, and spots that are dimmer than the expected threshold are again presented in a repetition of the original cycle.

As the spots along a meridian are tested serially, a profile of the visual island develops on the charting paper (upper left portion of Fig. 1-24). The spots are usually presented one degree apart in the central 5°, less frequently the farther the test is presented in the periphery. After one limb of the meridian is completed, the test is presented one degree to the other side of center; the subject is

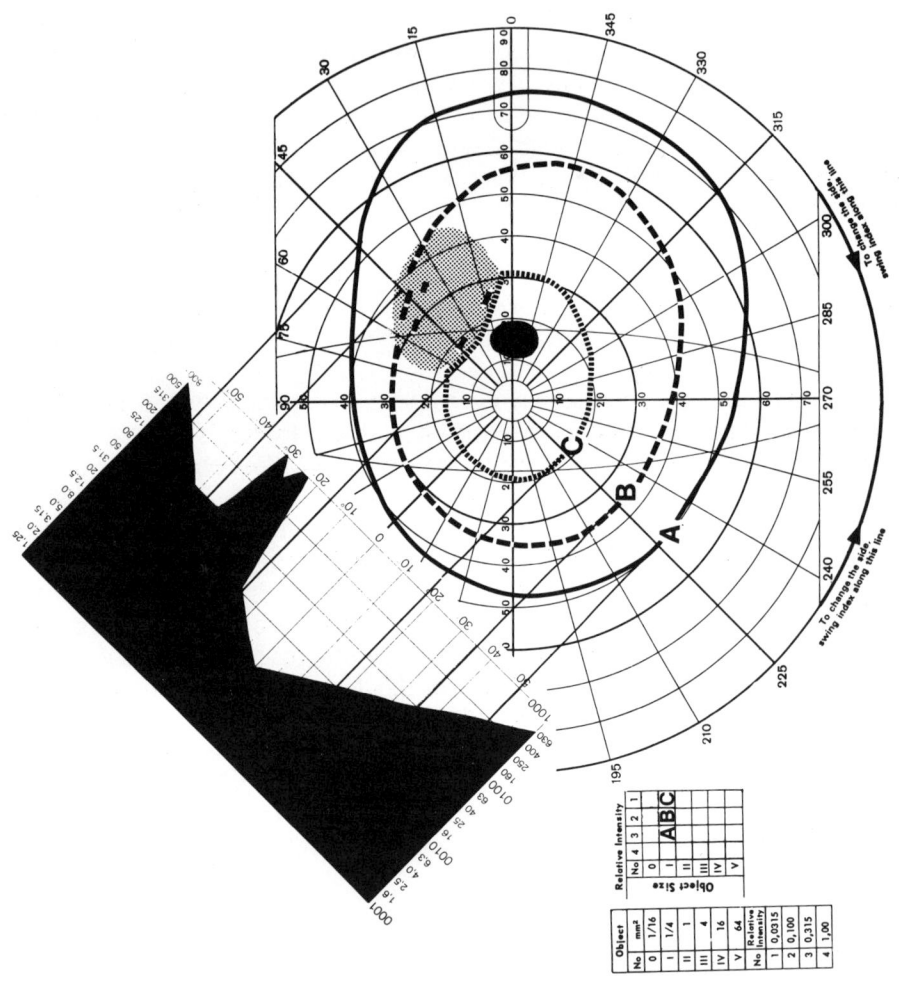

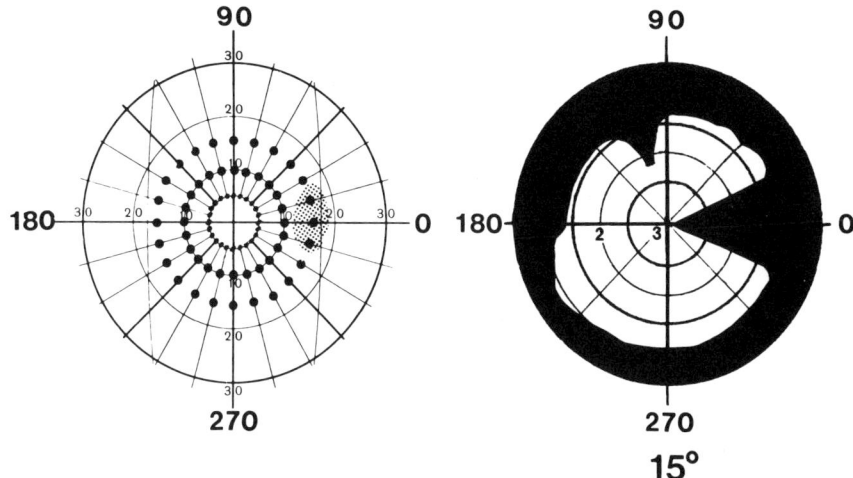

Figure 1-25 Circular static perimetry. The left portion of this figure shows a usual screening pattern of circles at 5°, 10°, and 15° eccentricities, chosen to detect glaucoma. The right portion of the figure shows how results of a circular test pattern are often plotted. The normal blind spot shows an absolute defect (at least 2 log units) as a pie-shaped sector to the right. Two relative defects of 0.3 log unit and 0.7 log unit are also present in the superior nasal quadrant.

alerted more specifically than usual; and the other half of the meridian is tested like the first half.

CLASSES OF VISUAL FIELD DEFECTS: CUTS AND SCOTOMAS

Any defect of the visual field that is plotted with one or more isopters may be classified as a cut or as a scotoma. When a given isopter is indented or constricted in any pattern, the zone between the normal isopter for the test object that was employed and the actual isopter is called a cut or contraction (Fig. 1-26). When a portion of the plotted visual field is defective or blind but *surrounded* by vision (light sense) that is better than the visual function in the defective area, the affected zone is called a scotoma (Fig. 1-27). Depending

---

Figure 1-24 Suspicious kinetic perimetry proved defective by static perimetry. The central portion of this figure is kinetic perimetry of the right eye. The scatter and occasional deep penetration of the raw data for the B isopter plus the slight concavity of the C isopter in the upper temporal quadrant all suggest the intervening presence of a deeper defect. These suspicions are confirmed by static perimetry along the 225°–45° meridian, as shown in the upper left portion of the figure.

38 *Principles of Quantitative Perimetry*

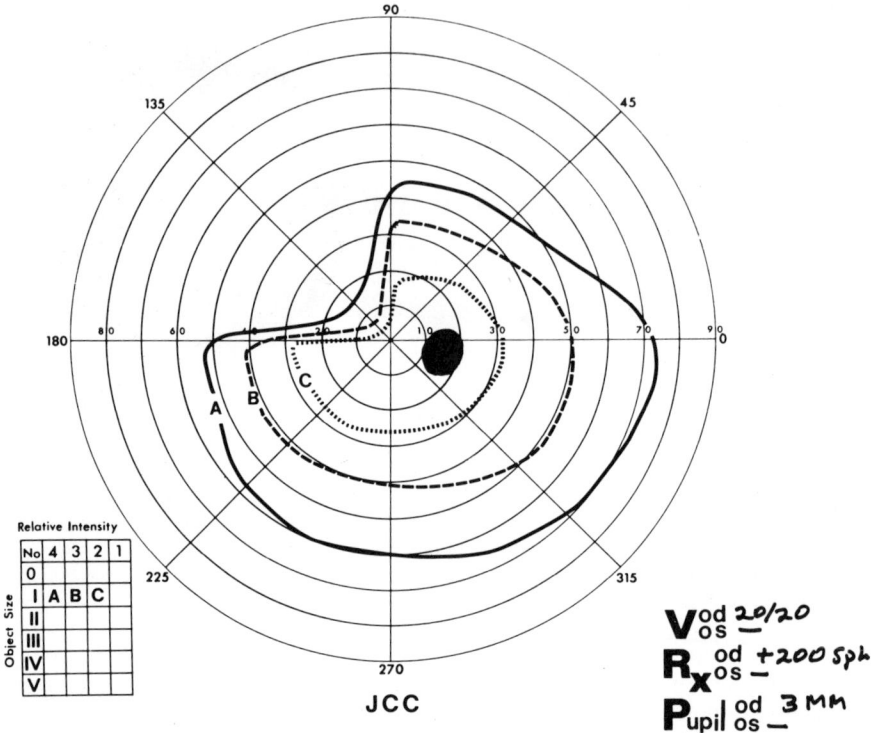

Figure 1-26 A cut or contraction. Because isopters are normally ovoid in shape, it is quite apparent that a defect is present to all three isopters in the upper nasal quadrant. This type of defect typifies the cut or contraction.

upon the test objects used and the type of defect present, a single zone, such as that labelled "X" in Figure 1-28, may be visible to large test objects, a scotoma to medium-sized test objects, and a part of a cut or contraction to smaller test objects. When a test object of *maximum available* stimulus value reveals a cut or scotoma, the defect is termed "absolute". If any available test can be seen within the cut or scotoma, the defect is termed "relative". A test object of large size may overlap the edges of small or even moderate-sized absolute scotomas such as the normal blind spot and may thus make these scotomas appear to be relative rather than absolute. Because a totally blind area with corresponding nil prognosis can be found to show false evidence of function when large-sized tests are used, visual field machines that increase stimulus value by enhancing test object brightness are often preferred.

The Concept of a Visual Field 39

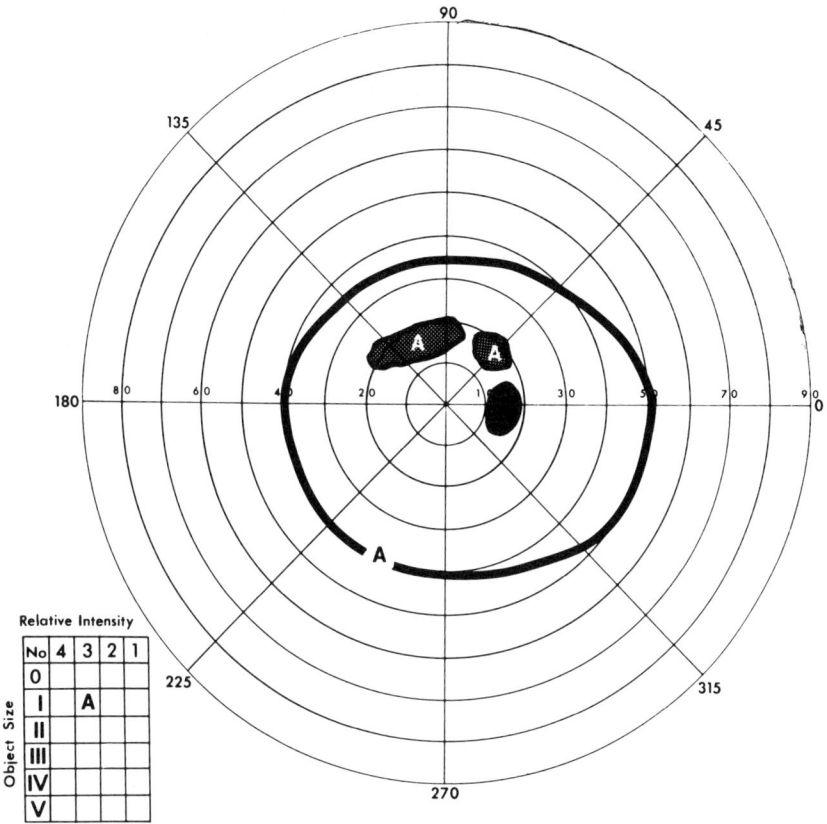

Figure 1-27 The scotoma. Blind spots within the visual field are called scotomas, whether they are abnormal like the examples labelled A in this figure or normal like the ever-present (here unlabelled) blind spot that corresponds to the exit of the optic nerve. Defects may qualify as scotomas whether they are absolute (area not seen with the maximum test object) or relative (area seen with some test objects but not with dimmer ones). Scotomas must be completely surrounded by better light sense than is present within the scotoma or they would be contractions.

TWO TYPES OF HEMIANOPSIA: ETIOLOGIC AND DESCRIPTIVE

Although the word hemianopsia was originally used to describe cases in which both eyes had lost half the visual field as the result of a solitary lesion of the visual pathways, etiologic and descriptive exceptions have led to two different definitions. When a *single* lesion inside the skull causes defects *of any sort* in

40   *Principles of Quantitative Perimetry*

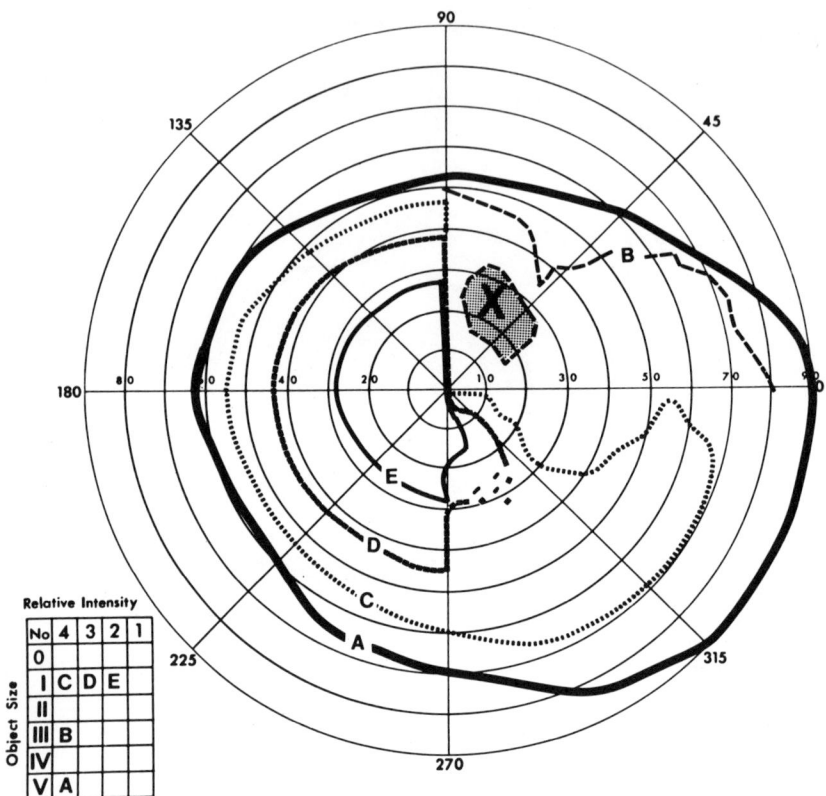

Figure 1-28   A cut, a scotoma, and apparent normality in one area. Depending upon the test object employed, a given zone may vary in its presentation. The area marked X is part of a cut when isopters C, D, and E are considered. It is a scotoma to the B isopter, and it could not be called abnormal when it was probed with the test object that outlined the A isopter.

the visual fields of *both* eyes, the preferred *etiologic* meaning of the term, hemianopsia, is exemplified. When *one or more* lesions of the eyes or optic nerves causes a cut or contraction in any *half of the field* of either or both eyes, the *descriptive* definition of hemianopsia applies, for this Greek word means "half not seen."

Two basic patterns satisfy the preferred or etiologic meaning of hemianopsia, a medical or neurological condition that can only occur where nerve fibers from both eyes in or behind the optic chiasm are near one another (Fig. 1-29). With lesions of the chiasm itself, crossing fibers from the nasal retinas of both eyes are often involved so the typical pattern includes partial or complete loss of the temporal field of both eyes, a condition called *bitemporal hemianopsia* (Fig. 1-30). The degree of involvement is often unequal in field pairs showing bitem-

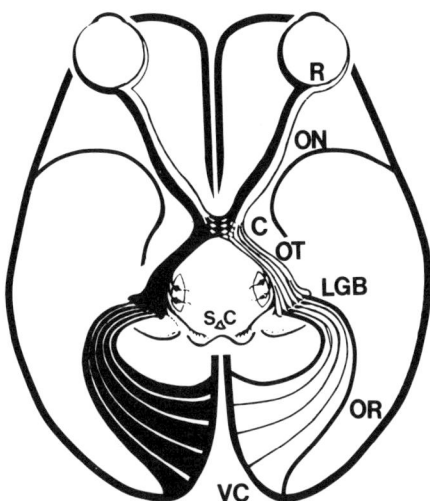

Figure 1-29 The visual pathways. The nerve fibers that subserve the right visual space in both eyes are shown dark on the left side of both retinas (R), to the left of both optic nerves (ON), intermixed in the chiasm (C), and all together in the optic tract (OT), lateral geniculate body (LGB), optic radiations (OR), and visual cortex (VC). Since the fibers from the two eyes are mirror images of one another, it is clear they are never near one another until C through VC. This, then, is the only zone where one lesion can cause defects in both visual fields to produce a true hemianopsia.

poral hemianopsia, with a spectrum that ranges from a temporal defect in one eye and subjective noninvolvement of the other eye (with subtle defects found only through vigorous testing) to total blindness of one eye and variable defects, mostly temporal, in the other.

As indicated in Figure 1-29, the visual fibers representing the right visual space* of both eyes are very near one another from the left side of the chiasm backward through the left side of the brain. When a lesion occurs within the retrochiasmal visual pathway on the left, the right visual field of both eyes becomes impaired, creating a representative of the second basic etiologic pattern, a condition called right *homonymous hemianopsia* (Fig. 1-31). Since the anatomy of the visual system is symmetrical, left homonymous hemianopsias occur with lesions of the right retrochiasmal visual pathways or cortex. When a pair of fields are properly oriented, superimposed and viewed simultaneously by transillumination, homonymous defects involve overlapping parts of both fields.

Although a few descriptive hemianopsias do show eventual evidence of bilateral field loss from single lesions, others cannot qualify as true hemianopsias

---

*The left visual field is projected onto the *right* retina because the optics of the eye invert and reverse the image.

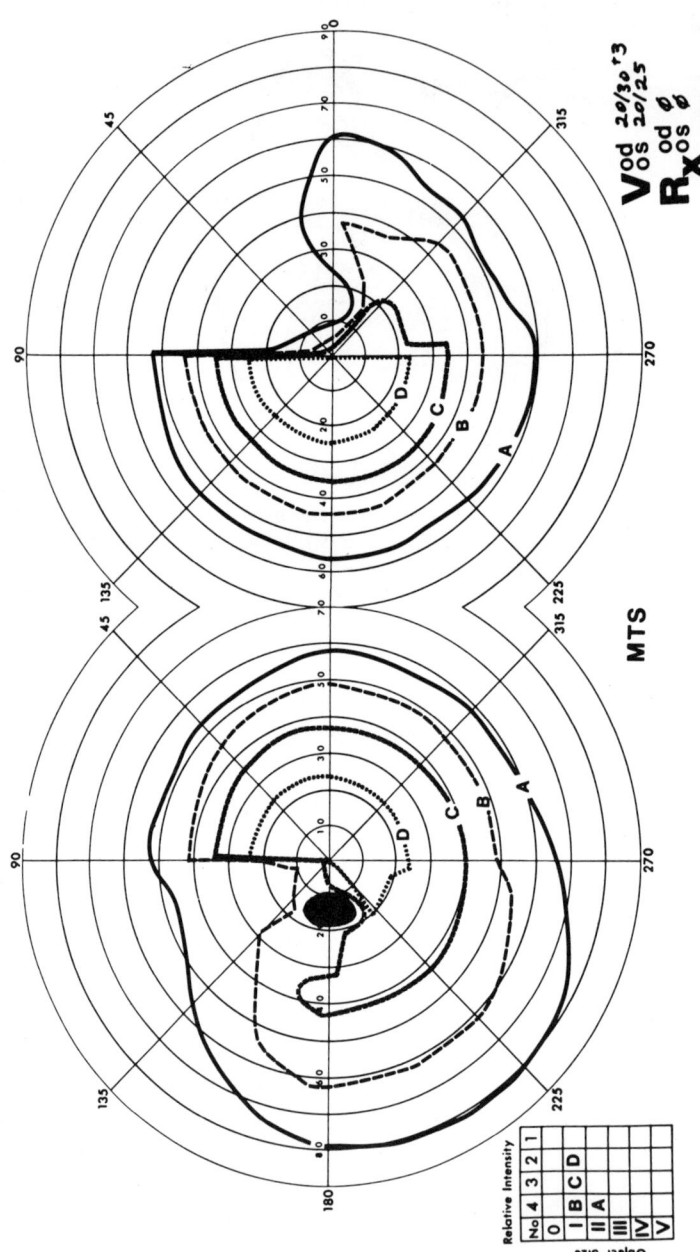

Figure 1-30 Bitemporal hemianopsia. The first of two types of true hemianopsias is exemplified by these fields, which show completely normal nasal fields in each eye and rather unequal but profound losses in the temporal fields of both eyes. The causative lesion could only be located at C in Figure 1-29.

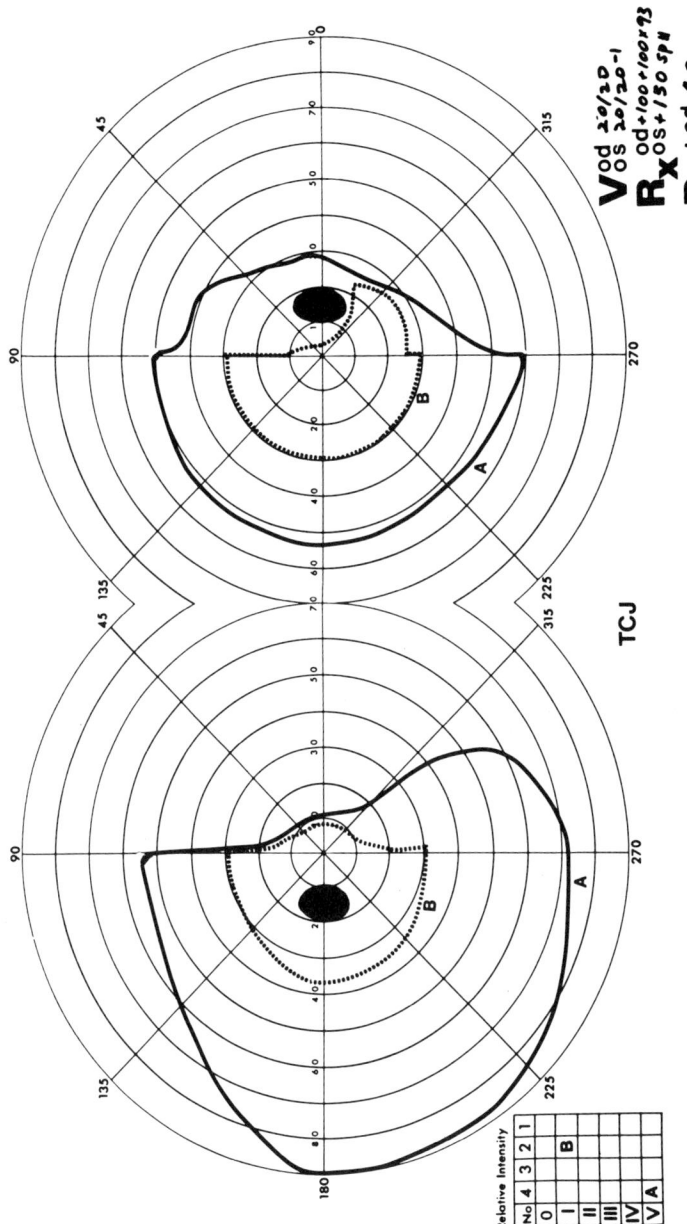

Figure 1-31 Right homonymous hemianopsia. The second of two types of true hemianopsias is shown here. The diagnosis is made by loss of significant temporal field in the right eye and nasal field in the left eye (the right visual space of both eyes), completely sparing the right nasal and left temporal fields. A lesion on the left side behind C in Figure 1-29 is the etiology of this right homonymous hemianopsia.

because their patterns are incompatible with the diagnosis of bitemporal or homonymous hemianopsia. The three types of hemianopsia most commonly cited as *descriptive* are *unilateral, binasal,* and *altitudinal.* All three types require adequate examination of the "uninvolved" field to confirm the descriptive diagnosis. Unilateral hemianopsias (Fig. 1-32) are not known to be unilateral and therefore causally limited to the eye or optic nerve unless a thorough field test of the fellow eye has proved normal. Subjective protestations of noninvolvement should be ignored along with complaints that the second eye sees too poorly to perform a field test (Fig. 1-33). Binasal hemianopsias (Fig. 1-34) all require two lesions of the eyes, the optic nerves, or the lateral chiasm because the uncrossed temporal retinal nerve fibers are never near one another except in intimate association with crossed fibers from the opposite eye. Altitudinal hemianopsias (Fig. 1-35) involve crossed and uncrossed fibers so they are almost always optic nerve lesions. Testing of both eyes assures that the pattern is not a pair of right and left homonymous quadrantanopsias (Fig. 1-36). Quadrantanopsias, as the word implies, are defects in a quarter of the field. The word is used descriptively, but like the example, it can apply to partial homonymous or bitemporal hemianopsias.

CONGRUITY: TO HELP LOCALIZE THE CAUSE OF HOMONYMOUS DEFECTS

Although attempts at using similarities of other field patterns are ill-founded and diagnostically useless, the degree to which a pair of *homonymous* field defects match one another can assist in localizing the cause of the defect. This geometric correspondence of homonymous defects is called congruity, and similar homonymous defects are said to be congruous, whereas dissimilar homonymous defects are called incongruous. The comparison of isopters on superimposed visual field charts is accomplished by transilluminating them and ignoring differences beyond the 62° normal limit of the nasal field.* Since homonymous defects may result from lesions anywhere within the rather substantial space between the chiasm and the occipital cortex, it is fortunate that the nerve fibers

---

*A normal pair of visual fields overlap one another (the binocular field) to the nasal limits of both fields. When all of the uniocularly visible field beyond the 65° limit (the so-called temporal crescent) is exclusively lost, a lesion of the anterior aspect of the visual cortex is often causally implicated—the only retrochiasmal lesion that causes this type of uniocular field defect. Because the other eye is spared, such defects do not technically qualify as true hemianopsias. In most instances, the temporal crescent is lost in the field of the eye that suffers temporal loss in a homonymous hemianopsia. Exclusive sparing of the temporal crescent causally implicates the posterior cortex if a homonymous defect is present. (See Chapter 7 on Interpretation.)

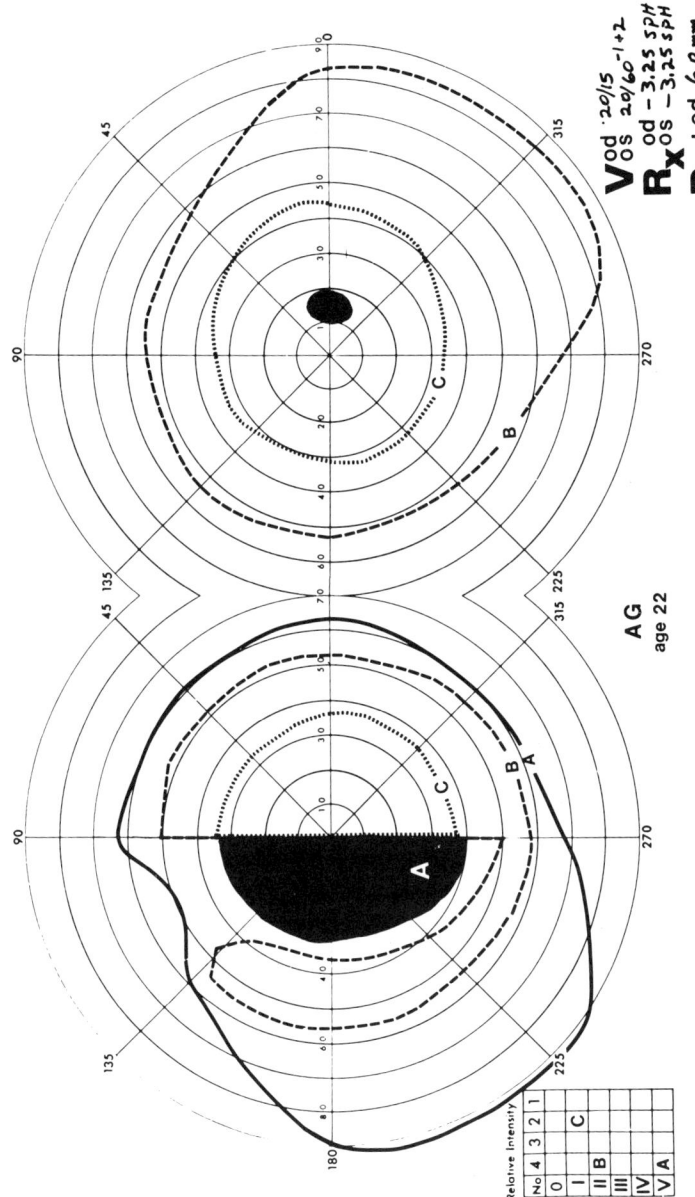

Figure 1-32 Left temporal hemianopsia. The first of three types of descriptive hemianopsias is this unilateral defect. The etiology is optic neuritis, and it is localized in the nasal portion of the left optic nerve (ON in Figure 1-29). Without certainty that the field in the right eye is entirely normal, true hemianopsias of bitemporal and left homonymous types must be suspected. The initial field test on a tangent screen failed to detect any visual function in the central 30° of the left temporal field, but the referring neurologist protested that the field was full to confrontation. This full perimetric visual field proves that both the test and the physician were correct.

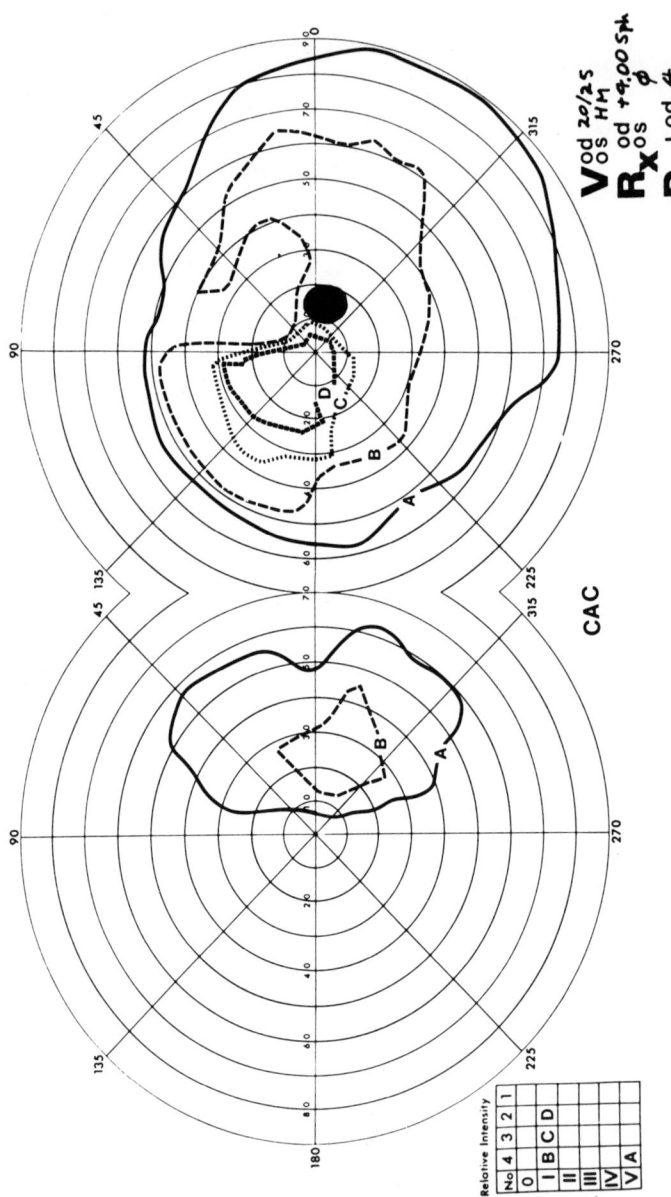

Figure 1-33 Bitemporal hemianopsia with hand motions vision in left eye. These fields illustrate the wisdom of ignoring visual acuity when deciding whether or not visual fields would be of potential benefit. The etiology was a pituitary tumor at the chiasm, more advanced on the left side (C in Figure 1-29). The pattern of loss in the right eye is also typical, for the order of involvement by quadrant is often superotemporal, inferotemporal, inferonasal, and superonasal.

The *true* hemianopsias have a defect in the visual fields of *both* eyes, resulting from a single lesion. As illustrated here and in Figures 1-30 and 1-31, true hemianopsias are either bitemporal or homonymous and always the result of a lesion in or behind the chiasm (C of Figure 1-29). (For a comparison with descriptive hemianopsias, see the text and Figure 1-35.)

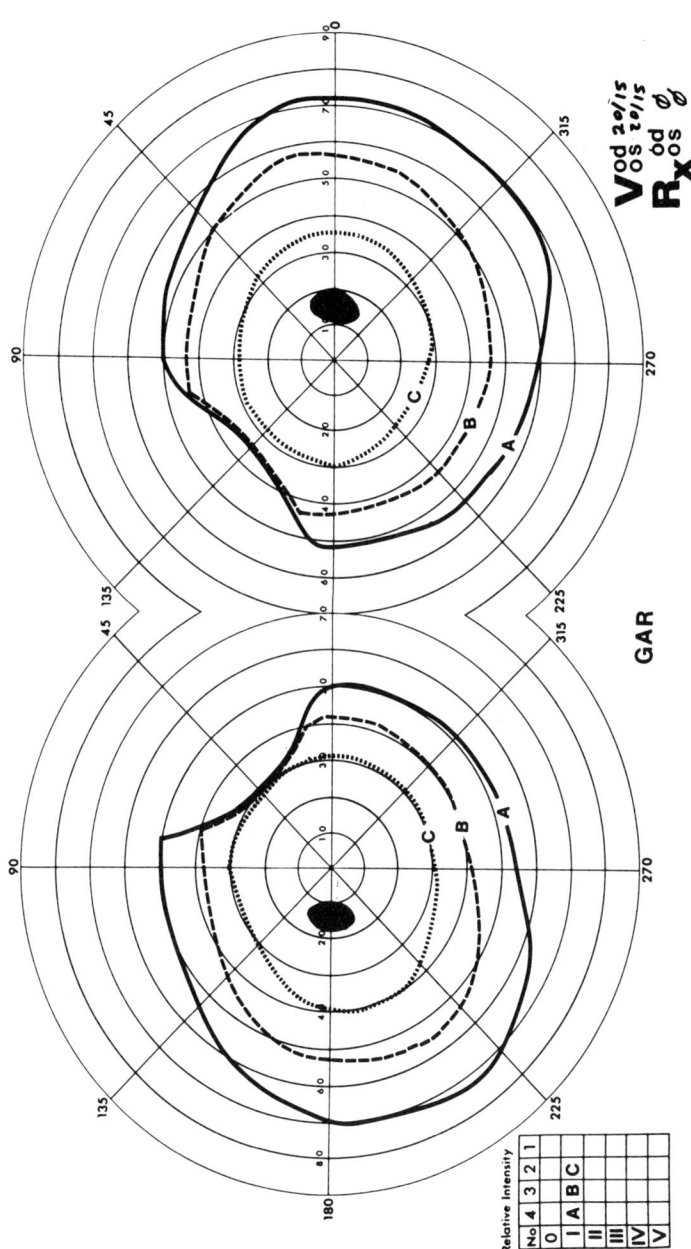

Figure 1-34 Binasal hemianopsia. The second of three types of descriptive hemianopsias is this binasal defect. The shapes of the defects and adjacencies of isopters (see slope on page 52) make a diagnosis of retinoschisis with virtual certainty. The lesions are located in the temporal retinas (R of Figure 1-29) in both eyes. Glaucoma is another common cause of binasal defects, with localization in the optic nerves (ON of Figure 1-29).

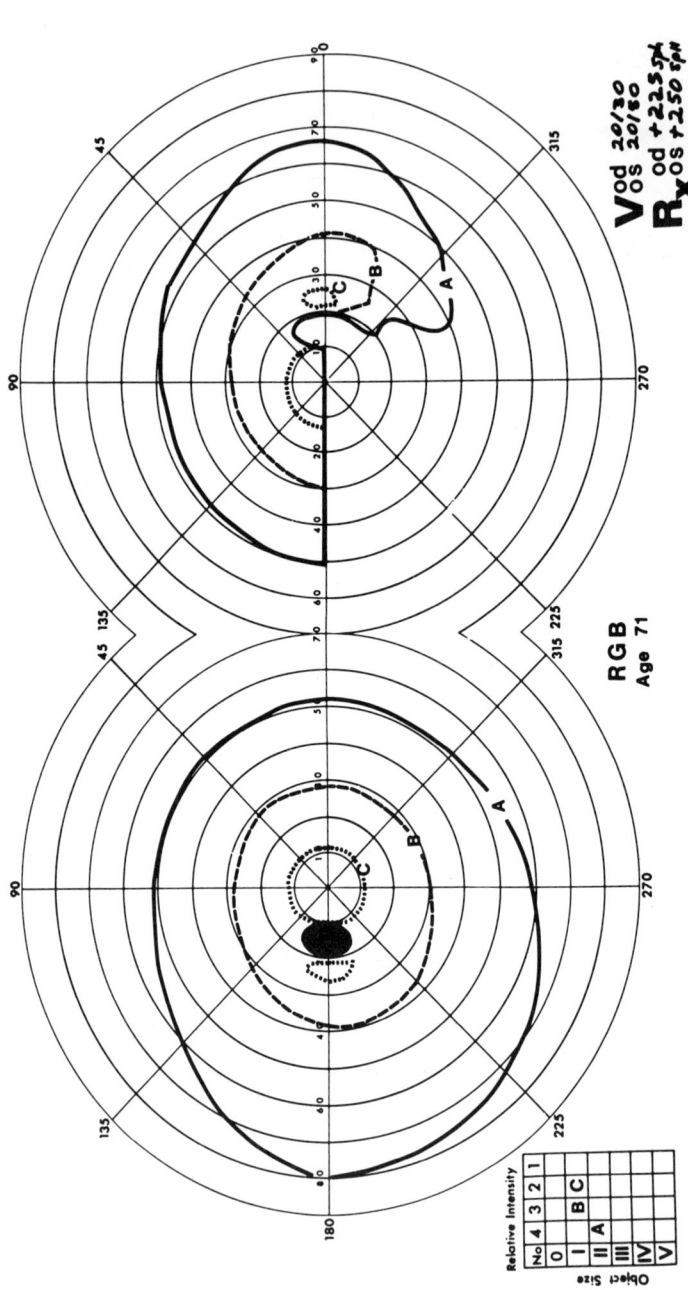

Figure 1-35 Right inferior altitudinal hemianopsia. The third of three types of descriptive hemianopsias is illustrated by the absence of most of the lower half of the visual field of the right eye. This is often due to ischemic optic neuropathy or glaucoma, both of which are localized in the optic nerve (ON of Figure 1-29). A branch occlusion of the central retinal artery can cause a similar defect and is localized in the retina (R of Figure 1-29).

The *descriptive* hemianopsias have a defect in the visual field of one eye if one lesion is present or defects in both fields if two lesions are present. As shown here and in Figures 1-32 and 1-34, the descriptive hemianopsias are *unilateral* (either nasal or temporal), *binasal*, and *altitudinal* (either superior or inferior), and all are the result of lesions in the optic nerve or retina (ON or R of Figure 1-29). (For a comparison with true hemianopsias, see the text and Figure 1-33.)

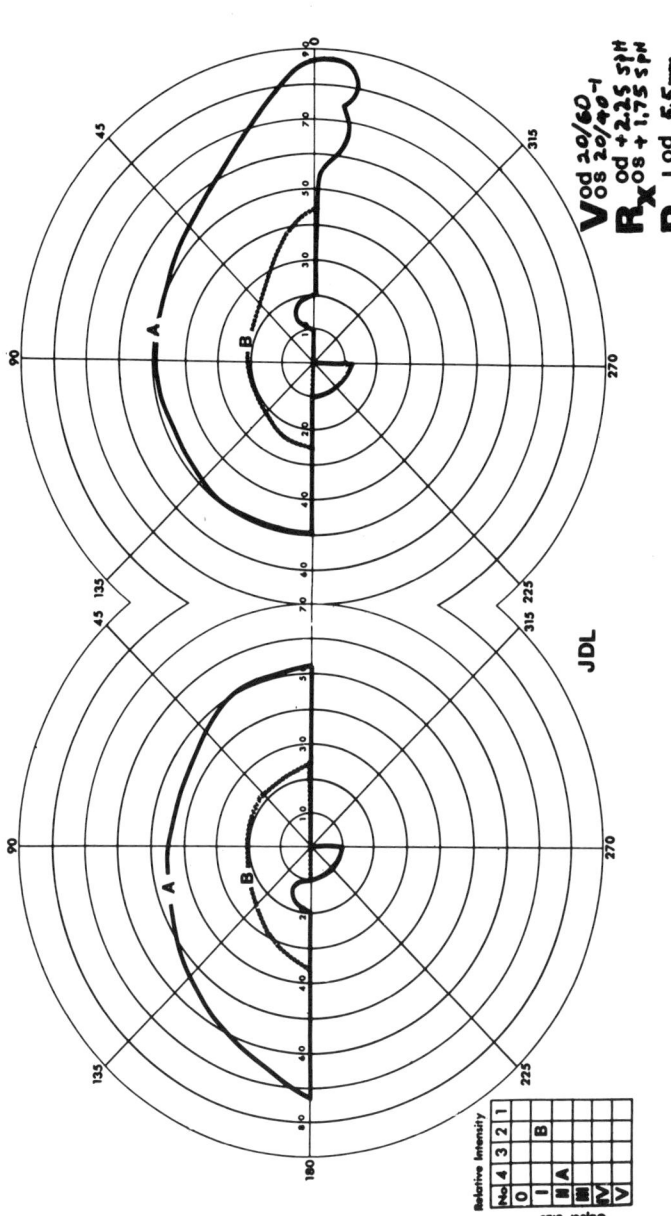

Figure 1-36 Bilateral inferior homonymous quadrantanopsias simulating bilateral inferior altitudinal hemianopsias. The diagnosis and localization of this unusual pattern is made on the bases of history (onset of visual loss in an otherwise healthy young person coincident with massive blood loss and coma), persistently pink (normal) optic nerve heads, and residual function of the left inferior central field of both eyes. The lesions are located in the superior part of the optic radiations (OR) or visual cortex (VC) on both sides of the brain. The left side of the brain is more severely involved, for the right portion of the field defect extends all the way to fixation. (For further explanation, see Chapter 7 on Interpretation.)

These fields are shown here to reemphasize the necessity of testing *both* visual fields, for reliance on what seems a characteristic pattern in the field of only one eye can easily lead the examiner astray.

50   Principles of Quantitative Perimetry

from corresponding retinal points appear to approach one another progressively as they pass to the occipital cortex (Fig. 1-37). This fiber arrangement seems logical because perfectly congruous field defects are usually caused by lesions that are located in or near the visual cortex of the brain (Fig. 1-38); very incongruous homonymous defects are usually caused by optic tract lesions immediately behind the chiasm; and lesions located in the optic radiations cause field defects that are more congruous than defects from tract lesions but less congruous than those resulting from cortical lesions.

Although French recognized that incongruity occurs with lesions of the anterior optic radiations, his series of visual fields, performed after temporal lobe

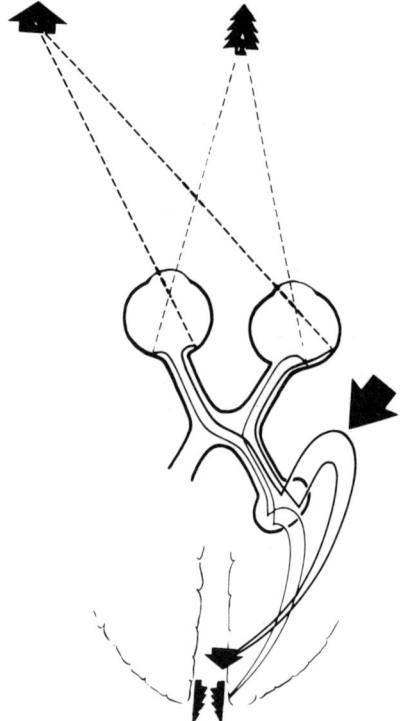

Figure 1-37   The operational model for congruity. Nerve fibers stimulated visually by objects at corresponding points in the visual fields of the two eyes merge by the time they reach the visual cortex (VC of Figure 1-29), for visual field defects caused by lesions in that part of the brain are perfectly superimposable. (See the text on Congruity and Figure 1-38.) When the lesion occurs closer to the eyes, the defects match less accurately, or become incongruous. The illustration implies a progressive approach of fibers from corresponding retinal points to converge at the visual cortex. Whether this is truth or illusion, the mental image of this model serves to predict which defects will be more or less congruous.

The Concept of a Visual Field 51

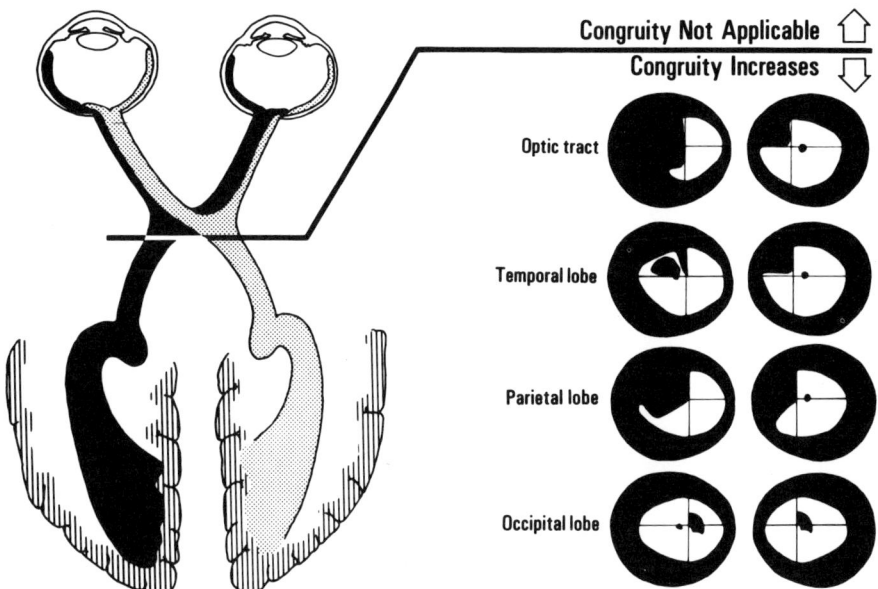

Figure 1-38 Only homonymous lesions show congruity. If the defective isopter lines from the two eyes match one another when their visual field charts are superimposed and observed with strong light behind them, the condition is called congruity. If the lesion involves the optic tracts, lateral geniculate body, optic radiations through the temporal or parietal lobes, or the visual cortex, the degree of congruity increases in the order given, that is, from anterior to posterior. (See Figure 1-29.) Because the intracranial space between chiasm and visual cortex is large, relative congruity can be of significant benefit in localizing the cause of visual field defects in this retrochiasmal region where nearly all visual defects are homonymous hemianopsias. The only field defect of retrochiasmal origin not showing any degree of congruity is the monocular temporal crescent defect described in the footnote on page 44. Congruity is not applicable to field defects resulting from lesions of the retinas, optic nerves, or chiasm since fibers from corresponding retinal points are not at all near one another in these areas. (See Figure 1-37.)

excisions for epilepsy, showed only modest incongruity.[4] This experience led him to conclude that the nerve fibers in the optic radiations are perfectly paired and adjacent to one another from their origin in the lateral geniculate body. He agreed with prevailing opinion that the corresponding fibers are quite separate in the optic tract, but extended his conclusion to attribute all incongruity to the effects of indirect pressure, edema, and inflammation on the optic tract rather than postulating fiber pairs that are still separate in the anterior radiations (Fig. 1-39). Because some of French's "congruous" examples are somewhat incongruous, his theory is not proved, but even if it were, the scheme shown in Figure 1-37 makes the predictive relationship of congruity easy to remember. Since diagnostic benefit is neither expected nor found when other types of field de-

52 Principles of Quantitative Perimetry

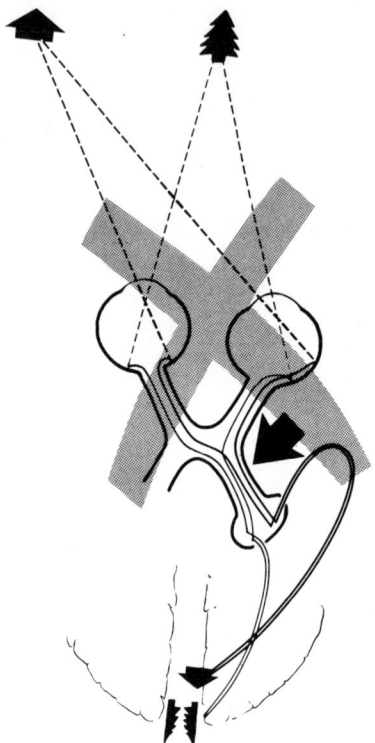

Figure 1-39   A challenge to the basis for congruity. French has excised human temporal lobes for epilepsy and plotted the resultant field defects. Since some of these are perfectly congruous and the others are not very incongruous, he concludes that the basis for all clinical incongruity is pressure or inflammation on the optic tract (large arrow). Unfortunately, this model doesn't make it easy to remember the basis for congruity. Since the published fields by French were only central and, in our opinion, often somewhat incongruous, the authors reject this model at this time. We prefer the one shown in Figure 1-37, where the arrow points to the fiber pairs from corresponding retinal points shown still separate in the optic radiations.

fects are matched for exact superimposition, the qualities of *congruity and incongruity are only applied to the homonymous hemianopsias,* and only then in areas of the field with binocular representation.

SLOPE: A GUIDE TO ACTIVITY AND PROGNOSIS

Within visual field defects, *shallow slope,* represented by definite *separation of standard isopter lines,* signifies *greater activity* of the causative lesion and, if the lesion becomes cured, a *better prognosis* for functional return than when the *slope is steep,* with standard isopter *lines near one another.* Adjacent intermediate isopters are so similar in stimulus value they simulate steep slopes. When nerve tissue in the eye or visual pathway becomes edematous, inflamed, or compressed, the usual result is not blindness, but such tissue does not receive and transmit light sense information so well as healthy tissue. Thus, the nerve tissues immediately adjacent to an active lesion, such as a tumor, abscess, aneurysm, partially ischemic zone, hematoma, contusion, etc., are adversely affected from the functional standpoint by their proximity to the primary lesion. The usual result is a "relative" rather than an "absolute" visual field defect. Tissues that are progressively remote from the lesion become more and more capable of functioning in what is eventually a normal manner. Because the functional changes are not abrupt near the active lesion, the slope of the plotted defect (see Fig. 1-31) is shallow. Should this lesion resolve, the surrounding tissues may regain most, if not all, of their normal function. Thus, defects with shallow slope represent active lesions that, when cured, may show favorable return of function.

When an injury of nerve tissue heals, the damaged zone is replaced by scar that can never function neurally again. The nerve tissue immediately adjacent to a quiet, well-healed scar often functions normally. Thus, the field defect caused by a scar in the visual pathways or a splitting of the retina (see Fig. 1-34) is absolute, and the slope around the defect is quite steep, since nonfunctional tissue—the scar or cyst—is immediately adjacent to normally active nerve tissue, with no intervening buffer zone. This steep-sloped, absolute defect therefore represents an inactive lesion that has an exceedingly poor prognosis for return of function. The abrupt closure of an artery that brings blood to part of the visual system causes steep-sloped field defects if no collateral circulation is available. This "white infarct" of recent onset represents an exception to the activity rule, but the poor prognostic significance of steep slope still holds true even here.

The presence of a steep slope along the vertical meridian (or hemianopsia line) (Fig. 1-28) provides neither prognostic significance nor evidence of inactivity. The physical separation of the fibers from the nasal half of each eye at the chiasm explains the steep slope at the hemianopsia line, for the autonomous projections of the two hemiretinas into chiasm and retrochiasmal pathways cause them to function as independent entities. Each half of the visual island has a gradient of sensitivity on all sides except its junction with the other half of the island, which is an abrupt cliff. If other aspects of the defective pattern are compatible, steep slope along the vertical meridian does lend weight to the possibility (but does not prove) that the defect is a true hemianopsia of either bitemporal or homonymous type.

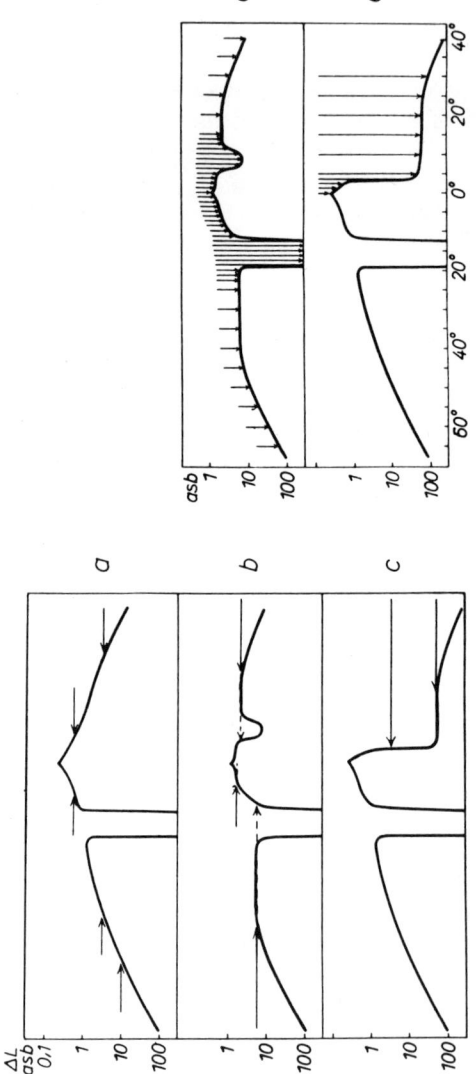

Figure 1-40 Slopes and scotomas are shown better by static than kinetic perimetry. Although the normal visual field with its gradual slope and absence of abnormal scotomas is well outlined by kinetic testing (a), the presence of field defects makes this method less precise than static testing. In (b), the flat temporal slope might yield a response at any point between 40° and 12° if the test object were optimum for testing that zone. Nasally, the best chosen kinetic test might be reported anywhere between 25° and 7°, and it would miss the relative scotoma between 7° and 12°. When the slope is steep, kinetic perimetry usually outlines the defect well with a few well-chosen test objects, but the choice is often arbitrary and may, as in (c), fail to reveal the actual steepness of the slope. Static tests elucidate well the flat slopes and small scotomas in (d) and both kinds of slope in (e). (With permission from Aulhorn and Harms.[1])

KINETIC VERSUS STATIC TESTING: IDEAL RELATIONSHIPS

In cooperative patients, static perimetry is generally more accurate in measuring the depth, slope, and extent of any demonstrated defect, while kinetic perimetry has the advantages of speed of testing, comprehensive coverage of the entire field, and production of recognizable isopter patterns. If kinetic testing were scientifically as controlled as static testing, the speed of test object movement would be regulated for precise knowledge regarding the effects of temporal and spatial summation. The need for control of temporal summation is obviated in static perimetry because the test spots do not move, but the test exposures must exceed one half-second or be precision timed. In scientific kinetic testing, the speed of test object movement should also be proportional to the subject's reaction time. Since reaction time varies markedly from subject to subject, and moderately from moment to moment in a given subject, its repeated measurement is required periodically during the field test.

The direction of movement of kinetic test objects should ideally be perpendicular to the expected isopter if patterns are to be sharp and meaningful. Direction of movement in the normal field is therefore radial, but this is not ideally the case in visual fields with cuts or scotomas. ("Directions of movement" is obviously of no concern when there is no movement, as in static testing.) In the well-intentioned but relatively unreliable subject, fixation is faciliated by test presentations at spatial locations that appear random to the subject, a condition that is easier to achieve in manual kinetic than manual static testing, primarily because record keeping is so difficult in the latter circumstance. Flat-sloped defects are much more difficult to map kinetically than statically (see Fig. 1-40). The delineation of scotomas within the field is easier by static testing than by kinetic, but isopter patterns that show, among their other values, where to test for scotomas are easily produced during kinetic testing and are practically impossible to obtain with static testing. The time required to test a full visual field is much less with kinetic than with static thresholds, but static screening can be both rapid and reasonably efficient.[12]

When a kinetic visual field test reveals areas of uncertainty or suspicion, these areas are ideally tested further in appropriate locations by static testing. The speed and pattern production of kinetic perimetry is thus complemented by the accuracy of static testing. The depth of a scotoma may change without any alteration in the pattern of several isopters surrounding it.

REFERENCES

1. Aulhorn E, Harms H: Early visual field defects in glaucoma. Glaucoma Symp Tutzing Castle 1966. Basel, Karger, 1967, pp 151–186

2. Aulhorn E, Harms H: Visual Perimetry, in: Handbook of Sensory Physiology. New York, Springer-Verlag, 1972, vol 7
3. Bebie H, Fankhauser F, Spahr J: Static perimetry; accuracy and fluctuation. Acta Ophthalmol (Kbh) 54:339, 1976
4. French LA: Studies on the optic radiations—the significance of small field defects in the region of the vertical meridian. J Neurosurg 19:522, 1962
5. Goldmann H: Grundlagen exacter Perimetrie. Ophthalmologica 109:5, 1945
6. Graefe A: Über die Untersuchung des Gesichtsfeldes bei amblyopischen Affectionen. Albrecht von Graefes Arch Klin Ophthalmol 2:258, 1856
7. Jayle GE, Ourgard AG, Baisinger LF, Holmes WJ: Night Vision. Springfield, Illinois, Charles C Thomas, 1959
8. LeGrand Y: Light, Colour and vision, transl. by Hunt RWG, Walsh JWT, Hunt FRW. London, Chapman and Hall, 1957
9. Østerberg G: Topography of the Layer of Rods and Cones in the Human Retina. Acta Ophthalmol suppl (Kbh) 6, 1935
10. Polyak SL: The Retina. Chicago, University of Chicago Press, 1941
11. Reed H, Drance SM: The Essentials of Perimetry—Static and Kinetic. London, Oxford University Press, 1972
12. Rock WJ, Drance SM, Morgan RW: A modification of the Armaly visual field screening technique for glaucoma. Can J Ophthalmol 6:283, 1971
13. Schmidt D, Reuscher A, Kommerell G: Über das nasale Gesichtsfeld bei Strabismus fixus divergens. Albrecht von Graefes Arch Klin Ophthalmol 183:97, 1971
14. Scott GI: Traquair's Clinical Perimetry, ed 7. London, Henry Kimpton, 1957

2
Biophysics, Psychophysics, and the Visual Field

Before putting our helicopter into storage, let us take one final flight. Let us suppose we are flying above a jungle. Below is endless, lush green vegetation. Through this carpet of greenery, there winds a small river, and on it bronzed men fish from dugouts. At cruising altitude the air is cool, crisp, and pleasant. The whole sight is peaceful and bountiful.

But, if we land, say, on that sandbar jutting into the river, we may form a very different opinion of the same jungle. The colorful natives could turn out to be cannibals, the landing site quicksand, and the air oppressively hot, humid, and teeming with mosquitoes. Dangerous animals may appear at any time on any side. At this stage, we may decide it is best to know only the major landmarks—and from aloft. But should we require more specific and detailed information, no alternative remains except to explore the jungle on foot.

Analogously, the first chapter was an overflight. In this chapter we set down on land and penetrate the jungles of physics, anatomical ultrastructure, electrophysiology, and psychology as they are entwined with the visual field. Photometry, optics, and color are discussed in the section on physics. The anatomy and physiology of the retina are covered in some detail from the experimental point of view, and this information is used to amplify and expand observations concerning pertinent psychophysical aspects of humans. Those persons who have no particular interest in these explorations may whirl away to Chapter 3. Others, who wish to be involved deeply in perimetry for whatever reason, or who refuse to do anything until they know why they should, are invited to join our trek. However savage the fauna or treacherous the quicksands, we promise great wonders to be seen.

PHOTOPHYSICS AND PHYSIOLOGICAL OPTICS

Radiometry and Photometry

Although the field of photometry is a body of information that is essential to quantitative perimetry, learning the subject can be confusing unless one undertakes the parallel study of radiometry. The neophyte perimetrist comes away from many of the standard ophthalmological texts with the notion that photometry is some plot designed to distract and to confound. This conclusion is unfortunate because, conceptually, the subjects of radiometry and photometry are relatively simple. Their complexity arises only in the bewildering array of nomenclature that has grown up over the years. In addition, most textbooks available to clinicians ignore completely the more straightforward topic of radiometry because it is not "human-oriented."

Physics of Light

The study of light is essentially the study of energy. It has long been known that light is emitted in indivisibly small packets or *quanta* of energy called photons. These packets have the peculiar property of behaving both as a wave (like the rhythmic rise and fall of the ocean's surface before a steady wind) and as a particle (like the stream of bullets from an automatic weapon). Light is not unique in this regard, for quantum physicists tell us that *all* forms of electromagnetic energy possess both properties, but in some the particle property (e.g., electrons) dominates, while in other forms (e.g., radio waves), the wave property dominates. Light is peculiar in that either of the two properties may assume importance, depending upon the circumstances.

The energy contained in each packet of light is determined by how many times the electrical field of the packet reverses itself each second. The frequency of this reversal is analogous to the 60 Hertz (Hz) electrical current that lights our homes and is so familiar to all of us in our daily lives. The energy and frequency of the light are directly proportional and related by the formula $E = h\nu$,* where E is the energy, h is a proportionality factor called Planck's constant which is needed to make the units match, and ν is the frequency of the light in Hz. In psychophysics, it is not common to specify light by frequency, but by wavelength; fortunately, these are simply interconverted. Since all light

---

*Since many readers may not have a background in physics, it may be well to give some background information at this point. All physical quantities are measured by comparison with standard measures called *units*. Basic units are those for length (meter = m), mass (kilogram = kg) and time

travels at the same speed in a vacuum, the frequency and wavelength are inversely proportional so Planck's equation may also be written $E = hc/\lambda$,* where c is the velocity of light and λ is the wavelength of the light. Therefore, shorter wavelengths of light (e.g., violet and blue) have far more energy per quantum than longer wavelengths of light (e.g., red and yellow). Indeed, 380 nanometers (nm) violet light, which is just on the fringe of the ultraviolet, has twice the energy per quantum as deep red light at 760 nm.

Rate of Energy Transfer

The rate at which a given visible light source emits photons (or quanta) is related to the effectiveness of the source in producing a visual stimulus. If ten million quanta of light are emitted as a short burst in a narrow beam, they will be perceived by an appropriately located observer as a rather bright flash, yet the same number of quanta stand little chance of being seen if they are emitted slowly in all directions. The most important difference between these two situations is the number of quanta emitted per second. Unfortunately, because we have no way of counting individual quanta, we must measure instead the energy transferred by the light (as heat) to a black body† in a given time. This rate of energy transfer P, called *radiant power,* is measured in units of watts.

If we have a small point source that is radiating power uniformly in all directions, at the rate of P watts, one may further characterize the source by defining

---

(second = sec). More complex units exist and are usually given specific names. Thus, a watt, the well-known unit of power, is equal to energy expended in a given time. It may also be written as watt = joule/sec, where the joule, a unit of energy, may be further decomposed into Newton · meter, where the Newton is the unit of force. Since a Newton is a kg · m/sec^2, we finally arrive at the relation watt = kg · m^2/sec^3; the complex unit (watt) is broken into its most basic units (kg, m, sec). Such formulae are called dimensional formulae.

Another convention is to specify division by negative exponents. Thus, $1/X = X^{-1}$. By this convention, the above dimensional formula for watts becomes watts = kg · m^2 · sec^{-3}. The dot between abbreviations in this context signifies multiplication.

Finally, there are a number of terms and constants worth defining: *Planck's* constant, h, is $(6.6252 \pm 0.0002) \times 10^{-27}$ erg·sec. An erg is a small unit of energy, like the joule, but 1 joule = 10^7 erg. The *velocity of light,* c, is $(2.99776 \pm 0.00004) \times 10^{10}$ cm/sec, approximately thirty billion centimeters per second in a vacuum. Multiplying the frequency by the wavelength yields this same value for any color light. A *nanometer* is a measurement of length equal to 10^{-9} meters (one billionth of a meter). It is the same as a millimicron or 10 angstrom units, other terms which may be used to specify wavelengths of light in other texts on the subject. *Hertz* (Hz) is the preferred unit for the old "cycles per second" or "cps."

†A "black body" is a theoretical device that radiates or absorbs heat (or other forms of radiant energy) perfectly.

its *radiant intensity,* J, which is the power per unit solid angle. Radiant intensity has the dimensions of watts per steradian.*

In the case of an extended source, such as a white hot metal plate or a projection screen, one may be interested in how much power a unit area of this source radiates or reflects into space. Power from this type of source is called *radiance,* N. The difference between radiance and radiant intensity is that the latter applies *only* to point sources, whereas radiance applies only to extended sources. The dimensions of radiance are watts per steradian per cm² (watt · ster^{-1} · cm^{-2}).

The amount of energy falling on a given surface area is referred to as *irradiance* (H), and it has the dimensions of watts per square centimeter. We are interested in the irradiance of a surface because if the surface is known to reflect a certain percent of the energy that falls on it, the surface becomes an extended source with its own predictable radiance.

Variable Sensitivity of the Eye to Different Wavelengths of Light

Because the various transmissive media of the eye absorb different wavelengths of light at variable rates and because the rods and cones exhibit unequal sensitivity to various wavelengths of light, the eye's response to light is not equally efficient at all wavelengths. It is wrong, therefore, to assume that a given number of quanta of violet light constitute a more efficient visual stimulus than the same number of quanta of green light even though the former has far more energy per quantum; indeed, the reverse is the case.

A *relative luminosity curve* can be constructed (at least conceptually) by the technique of asking a subject to compare the brightnesses of light patches having different wavelengths and adjusting the radiance of each of these patches until all appear equally bright. The wavelength of the light patch requiring the lowest radiance to appear as bright as the others is regarded as the most

---

*A steradian (ster) is a unit for measuring solid angles. It is defined as analogous to the radian of plane geometry, which is a measure of plane angles. The radian (θ) is defined as the length (L) of arc along the circumference of a circle that is subtended by the angle being measured, divided by the radius (R) of the circle ($\theta = L/R$). Thus, a plane circle contains 2π radians. Similarly, a steradian (ω) is defined as the area (A) on the surface of a sphere subtended by the solid angle being measured, divided by the square of the radius (R) of the sphere ($\omega = A/R^2$). Thus a sphere contains 4π steradians. Since both L and R have dimensions of length, and both A and R^2 have the dimensions of length squared, neither the radian nor the steradian can be subdefined without cancelling their values, so both are dimensionless.

efficient in stimulating a visual response. By comparing the radiance of the most efficient wavelength with the radiance of others when brightnesses are matched, the relative efficiency of all the wavelengths may be calculated. This data is used to plot a relative luminosity curve with ratio values [V (λ)] between 0.0 and 1.0 on the ordinate and wavelengths (λ) of visible light on the abscissa. In practice, this technique is less exact than the more involved methods that are usually employed.[63] In the "standard" light-adapted (i.e., photopic) subject, the curve's peak is at 555 nm. When the subject is dark-adapted (i.e., scotopic), the peak will occur at 510 nm (Fig. 2-1). This shift in the peak of the sensitivity curve when the intensity of surrounding illumination changes from photopic to scotopic levels was first described by Purkinje and bears his name.[76]

In clinical white light perimetry, we are far more interested in the effectiveness of the light that passes from test object to retina than we are in the amount of energy per se that falls on the subject's retina. Perimetry done with ultraviolet light of high energy would be fruitless, for example, since no matter how much ultraviolet light enters the subject's eye, no visual response will occur. In Figure 2-1, one can see that in the photopic state, red light with a wavelength of 650 nm must have 10 times as much energy as green light at 560 nm in order to produce the same degree of visual stimulation. If no allowance is made for this effect, it is confusing to try to compare studies done with light sources of varying

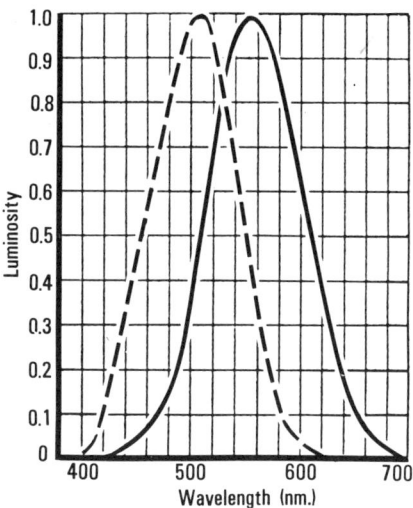

Figure 2-1 Relative luminosity curves. The ordinate is relative Luminosity (V(λ)); the abscissa is wavelength (λ). The solid curve is for photopic vision, the dotted curve for scotopic. Notice the shift of peak of sensitivity toward the blue with dark adaptation. (After Adler.[2])

62   *Principles of Quantitative Perimetry*

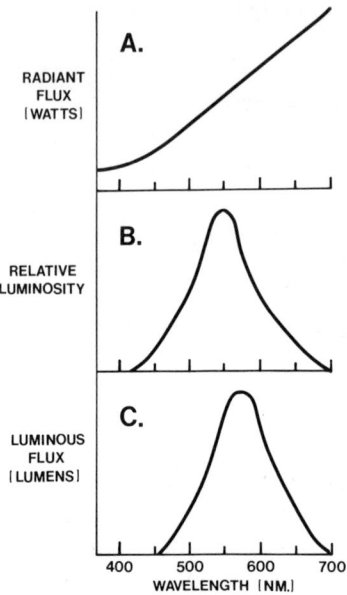

Figure 2-2   Schematic representation of how energy in watts could be converted to luminous flux. Curve A shows radiant flux and curve B shows relative luminosity (V(λ)), each as a function of wavelength. These curves are multiplied together point by point. Each point is also multiplied by a constant, 1/685, to yield a corresponding point on curve C, the luminous flux curve. Thus, we may write $\frac{A(\lambda) \cdot B(\lambda)}{685} = C(\lambda)$

spectral composition.* In human perimetry, therefore, we usually do not employ the terms of radiometry, since they are based strictly on the energy of light. Instead, we employ the terms of photometry based on the *luminous efficiency* of the light.

The luminous (or visual) efficiency of a light source is determined by multiplying point by point the radiometric curve of that particular light (showing its energy level at all parts of the visible spectrum) by the relative luminosity curve of the average human observer and then dividing by 685 to produce a photometric or *luminous flux* curve of the light under study (Fig. 2-2).

---

*Except for lasers, virtually every light consists of a spectrum, with variable contributions to the total energy from several different, if not all visible, wavelengths. The energy level of each wavelength present may be plotted as a *radiometric* or *radiant flux curve.*

Photometry

Although the lumen, a unit of luminous flux, was not originally defined in terms of radiometry, the units of measurement have been translated from photometry to radiometry by measuring a light of only one wavelength in terms of both systems. Since a monochromatic light of 555 nm wavelength was found to emit one lumen at the same time its radiant power was measured at 1/685 of a watt, this proportionality constant must be used in the translation from radiometry to photometry. With the relative luminosity and the proportionality constant considered, lumens mean the same to the photometrist as watts mean to the radiometrist. Indeed, the entire discussion of photometry could parallel the discussion of radiometry. Instead of saying watts for radiant power and abbreviating it with a P, one can say lumens for luminous flux and abbreviate it with an F. Similarly, radiant intensity (J) of a point source and watts per steradian can be understood as luminous intensity (I) of a point source and lumens per steradian. Irradiance (H), the power falling on an area (measured as watts per cm^2), can become illuminance (E), which has the dimensions of lumens per square centimeter. Radiance (N), the power per unit solid angle per unit area of an extended source, can become brightness or *luminance* (B)*, the number of lumens per steradian per unit area of a source. This approach allows anyone with a basic knowledge of mathematics to understand how each of the units relates to one another in a straightforward fashion. Unfortunately, units of measurement evolved in several different systems before communications developed fully among scientists in adjacent fields.

The early standards for luminous intensity varied between fragile glass lamps, which were forever out of calibration (The International Candle), and an actual candle flame (The German Hefner Candle), which was just as unsatisfactory. The C.I.E. (Commission Internationale d'Eclairage) adopted the New Candle in 1939. This was defined by stating that a blackbody radiator at the solidification temperature of platinum has a luminance of 60 new candles/cm^2. The new candle was subsequently renamed *Candela* in 1948.

Mercifully, only one unit of luminous flux evolved, the lumen. By definition, a source, the intensity of which is one candela, emits one lumen per steradian, so

---

*Many workers, including physicists and optical engineers, tend to use the terms luminance and brightness as completely interchangeable and equivalent terms. Thus, the standard mathematical symbol for luminance is B, suggesting brightness. On the other hand, most persons involved in psychophysical investigations such as perimetric research refer to the objectively measured physical quantity as luminance and reserve the terms brightness and subjective brightness to describe the subjective sensation evoked in the observer by a target of a given luminance under the experimental conditions.

the lumen is equal to one candela · steradian. Since illumination involves area receiving light, multiple units arose. Thus the lux, the phot, and the foot-candle are equal, respectively, to one lumen/m², 1 lumen/cm², and 1 lumen/ft². The meter-candle is the illumination produced by one candle one meter from a screen, which luckily turns out to be equal to 1 lux.

The subject of luminance is more confused. Luminance is basically intensity per unit area of source, but there are two avenues of approach to the problem. First, one simply measures the light output to derive the luminous intensity of the source had it been a point. Dividing the luminous intensity (i.e., candelas or lumens/ster) by the actual area of the source, one derives the luminance as stilbs or nits, which are respectively candelas/cm² and candelas/m². In English units, the candela/ft² and candela/in² are sometimes used. A second approach is based on the illumination of a completely reflecting perfect diffuser that obeys Lambert's law (see below). If such a surface receives an illumination of 1 phot, the resultant luminance of the surface is one *equivalent phot* or *Lambert*. Similarly, one may define an equivalent lux (or apostilb) and an equivalent foot-candle (or foot-Lambert).

The second system differs slightly from the first in that more emphasis is placed on the spatial distribution of the radiation from the illuminated (secondary) source.* Thus, because a Lambertian surface spreads its radiation over a hemisphere in accordance with Lambert's law, it is necessary to introduce the factor $1/\pi$. As a result, a perfectly reflecting Lambertian surface, which receives illumination of one lumen to each cm², has an emittance† of 1 lumen/cm² of source and a luminance of $1/\pi$ candela/cm².‡

For practical purposes, however, the perimetrist is mainly concerned with the brightness or the luminance (B) of the background and objects. Classically, in Europe the apostilb was the most commonly used unit, whereas in the United States of America the millilambert found favor. These terms are easily related in that one millilambert equals ten apostilbs. More recently, the C.I.E. standard, the nit (one candela · m⁻²), is replacing these units in international usage. These units of measure are compared with the other radiometric and photometric terms in Table 2-1, and their values are compared in Tables 2-2 and 2-3.

---

*Primary sources of radiation emit energy because of their excitation, usually a function of temperature. Although secondary sources are never points, these reflecting surfaces behave like primary sources in most other ways. The only surfaces that reflect as much directed intensity as they receive are mirrors.

†Luminous emittance is total, multidirectional luminous flux per unit area of source, (lumens/cm², for example) whereas luminance is luminous intensity per unit area of source measured (lumens [ster · cm²] or candela/cm²). Luminous emittance is not often used.

‡Although half a hemisphere contains two π steradians, the fact that intensity is multiplied by the cosine of the angle from the normal of a Lambertian surface introduces the factor 1/2 when one integrates over the sphere to get luminous flux. Thus, the factor $1/\pi$ is correct.

RADIOMETRIC				PHOTOMETRIC			
Name	Symbol	Description	Units	Name	Symbol	Description	Units
1. Radiant Power	P	Rate of Transfer of Power	Watts	1. Luminous Flux	F	Radiant power corrected for visual efficiency	Lumen
2. Radiant Intensity	J	Power per unit solid angle from a point source	W/Ster	2. Luminous Intensity	I	Lumens per steradian from a point source	Lumens/Ster Candela, Carcel, Hefner, "Old Candle"
3. Radiance	N	Power per unit solid angle per unit area of an extended source	W/Ster·cm^2	3. Brightness (Luminance)	B	Lumens per steradian per unit area from an extended source	Lumens/Ster·cm^2, Candela/m^2 (Nit), Stilb, Lambert, Foot-Lambert, Millilambert, Apostilb
4. Irradiance	H	Power per unit area incident on a surface	Watts/cm^2	4. Illuminance (Illumination)	E	Lumens per unit area incident on a surface	Lumen/cm^2 (Phot), Lux, Foot-Candle

Table 2-1 Radiometric and photometric quantities.

From \ To	Stilb (Candela/cm^2)	Nit (Candela/m^2)	Candela ft^2	Candela in^2	Lambert	Millilambert	Apostilb	Foot-Lambert
Stilb (Candela/cm^2)	1	10000	929	6.45	3.142	3142	31420	2919
Nit (Candela/m^2)	0.0001	1	0.0929	0.000645	0.0003142	0.3142	3.142	0.2919
Candela/foot^2	0.001076	10.764	1	0.00694	0.00338	3.382	33.82	3.142
Candela/inch^2	0.155	1550	144	1	0.487	487	4870	452.4
Lambert (Equivalent Phot)	0.3183	3183	295.7	2.054	1	1000	10000	929.1
Millilambert	0.0003183	3.183	0.2957	0.002054	0.001	1	10	0.9291
Apostilb (Blondel, Equivalent lux)	0.00003183	.3183	0.02957	0.0002054	0.0001	0.1	1	0.09291
Foot-Lambert (Equivalent foot-Candle)	0.0003426	3.426	0.3183	0.00221	0.001076	1.076	10.76	1

Table 2-2 Interconversion of units of luminance.

To From	Lux	Phot	Milliphot	Foot-Candle
Lux (Meter-Candle, Lumen/m^2)	1	0.0001	0.1	0.0929
Phot (Lumen/cm^2)	10000	1	1000	929
Milliphot	10	0.001	1	.929
Foot-Candle (Lumen/ft^2)	10.764	0.0010764	1.0764	1

Table 2-3   Interconversion of units of illumination.

Reflectance

The subject of reflectance is obviously relevant to the perimetrist, for in most clinical forms of perimetry, the stimulus source is light reflected from a solid object or a spot of projected light reflected from a screen. Both the test object and the light spot on the screen become secondary extended sources of light, and as such, one is interested in their luminance (brightness). For a screen that diffuses light perfectly, Lambert's law holds: that is, the intensity of the radiation reflected from a small area of the surface is maximal perpendicular to the surface and decreases as the cosine of the angle of incidence to the surface. This is the same thing as saying that the luminance (or radiance) of the surface remains constant at all angles, because with increasingly oblique view the projected area, or the object's apparent size, decreases by the same mathematical function as the intensity. If the radiation were absolutely constant at all angles, the object would appear to become brighter as one viewed it obliquely. The luminance remains constant because it is the ratio of intensity to area. Although the luminance of a perfect Lambertian reflector is constant with respect to angle of view, many available test screens do not fit this definition; so they vary from ideal (Lambertian) behavior.

The most obvious example of a non-Lambertian surface is a mirror. Some test objects used with tangent screens do not have a diffuse reflecting surface but are made of glass that has a definite shine. Such beads are non-Lambertian, for they change their stimulus value as a function of screen position. In deciding which test system to use both scientifically and clinically, this effect should be considered along with the greater difficulty of providing precisely uniform illumination on a flat screen* and with the factor that makes

---

*A Lambertian concave spherical surface will be uniformly illuminated by light reflected around its surface although the source of illumination falls only on a restricted area. This principal is used in a variety of instruments, notably the *Integrating* or *Ulbricht* sphere. Practical examples include most bowl perimeters such as the Goldmann and the Tübinger.

perimetry differ from campimetry (i.e., the solid angle subtended by the test object varying predictably with screen position).

On a diffuse reflector, the fraction of incident light that is reflected is referred to as the *albedo* (from the Latin word for white) or *reflectance* of the surface. A reflector that diffuses perfectly would reflect 100% of the light that falls on it and have an albedo of 1.0. Most white screens, such as the Goldmann Perimeter, are about 70% efficient, so they are said to have an albedo of 0.7. In the case of a Lambertian reflector, the luminance of a test spot produced by a light with a given illuminance may be calculated simply by multiplying the illuminance by the albedo. However, screens may become dirty, may have a nonlinear reflectivity across the visual spectrum, or may change their spectral reflectivity characteristics with aging. Also, the spectral characteristics of the light source may change with the age of a bulb, and thus, unless one has uncommonly accurate information regarding these variables, calculation of the luminance of a test object by knowing the amount of light falling on a screen is not very practical. It is best to consider screens and test objects merely as secondary sources of radiation and to measure the light returning from them to the observer with a light meter. An obvious corollary is that anything (such as dirt) which changes subsequently or locally the albedo of the screen or of the test object, changes correspondingly the stimulus value of the test.

Effects of Changes in Pupillary Size

The effectiveness of the pupil in allowing light to pass to the periphery of the retina is somewhat diminished at more oblique angles. Because of the optical properties of the cornea, the available area of the pupil decreases more slowly than the cosine of the angle of eccentricity.[57,83] The decrease in pupillary area is offset because summation is to some extent better in peripheral than in central retina. Since this effect cannot be modified by the perimetrist and remains constant from test to test, it is unimportant. A quantitative consideration of the issue has shown how light originating behind the iris plane may enter the pupil and defined the theoretical limit of the temporal visual field at 110°, a level actually achieved clinically in a few individuals.[63]

To the perimetrist, the effect of the pupil on the resolving power of the eye is more important than the way it theoretically limits the extent of the visual field. In any optical system, image quality ultimately reflects the sum of the effects of refraction and diffraction. The first effect is the relative ability of the lens to focus light, where the second is represented by "scattering" of light by edges within the optical system. Refractive effects may either improve or degrade image quality, while diffractive effects always degrade the image. The degrading refractive influences, such as lens aberrations and shallow depth of field, are worse with large pupillary apertures, while the reverse is true of the diffractive effects. If one starts with a very large pupil diameter and slowly decreases the size to 2.5 mm, one finds the image on the retina with a given set of optics gradually improves, because the smaller pupil size decreases the effect of the lens aberrations or small defects in focus similar to "stopping down" a camera. However, light is diffracted by the edge of the pupil, and as the pupil drops below about 2.4 mm in diameter, the diffraction effect becomes significant. In fact, with very small pupils, diffraction is the limiting factor for resolution.[16] The eye's optimal optical performance thus occurs at a pupil size of 2.4 mm.

With decreasing pupil size, the illumination of the retina also falls. The illumination of the retina is roughly proportional to the square of the diameter of the pupil or its area, and a change from a pupil that has a diameter of 4.75 mm to one that has a diameter of 1.5 mm decreases the illumination of the retina by approximately 1 log unit, which may be enough to shift from photopic to mesopic or from mesopic to scotopic light adaptation. If pupil size falls much below 2.4 mm, the combination of decreased resolving power along with changes in the adaptive state of the retina can significantly alter the shape of the visual field.

Brightness of the Retinal Image

Finally, it is important to note that image brightness is independent of the distance of the object from the eye, provided that one views an extended source. This is not true of point sources of light, nor of finite extended sources far enough from the eye to be considered as a point source (e.g., a star). Basically, this is because the retinal image size will decrease as the square of the distance from the eye, as does the luminous flux, so the net result is a constant illuminance of the retina (lumens·m^{-2}), provided the area of the pupil remains constant. The exact relationship becomes $E = 0.36\ TBA_p$* (Eq. 2-1) where E is illuminance of the retina, B is luminance of the source object, T is transmissivity of the optical media, and A_p is area of the pupil. (Note that size of the object and object distance play no role in this equation.)

---

*Equation 2-1 may be derived as follows: Let As, Ar, and Ap be the areas of the source, the retinal image, and the pupil respectively; η_a and η_v, the index of refraction of air and vitreous respectively; d, the distance of the source; and f, the focal length of the eye. Now, because in differing refractive media the vergence must be multiplied by the index of refraction of the media and because some vertical solid angles are equal, we may write:

$$\frac{Ar\eta_v^2}{f^2} = \frac{As\eta_a^2}{d^2} \tag{F-1}$$

The luminous flux at the pupil is

$$F = \frac{B\ Ap}{d^2}\ As$$

(continued)

Trolands and Other Scary Things

A point of real concern to all workers in the field of visual physiology is how much light actually reaches the retina. From Equation 2-1, it is seen that the product of target luminance and pupillary area (B·A) would provide a convenient measure of *retinal* illumination, provided one disregards the factors of the constant and media clarity. Troland first proposed this in 1922 and named the unit the *photon,* an unfortunate choice since it relates only indirectly to the quantum unit of radiation. This name was later changed to *Troland* by the Optical Society of America. The Troland corresponds to a luminance of one candela per square meter (or nit) seen through a pupil of one square millimeter in area.[63]

Unfortunately, the Troland suffers from two problems; hazy media and the Stiles-Crawford effect. A prediction of the influence of cloudy media, which filters and scatters the light reaching the retina, necessitates an accurate measurement of the effects of the irregular clouding caused by cataract, vitreous opacities, and corneal problems. Such measurements are extremely difficult.

A more predictable problem is the Stiles-Crawford effect. This phenomenon occurs because the photoreceptors are somewhat directional, and they are most sensitive to light directed along their long axis. Thus, light entering the center of the pupil elicits a larger visual response than light entering the pupil more eccentrically.* By lengthy mathematical calculations, it is possible to discount this phenomenon and arrive at a figure for the effective Troland. The efficiency of an eccentric point is related to the center by η, the *coefficient* of relative directional efficiency. Various empirical formulae have been prepared to relate R (the pupillary radius) and η. Stiles and Crawford have suggested $\eta =$ Exp (-2.3 Kr^2)† where K = 0.5 for white light, but varies with wavelength.

The illuminance of the retina is

$$E = \frac{TF}{Ar} = \frac{TB \, Ap \, As}{d^2 \, Ar} \qquad (F-2)$$

But from equation (F-1) we may substitute into F-2 for Ar, thus

$$E = \frac{TB \, Ap}{f^2} \left(\frac{\eta_v}{\eta_a}\right)^2 \qquad (F-3)$$

Substituting numerical values for η^v, η^a, and f into Equation F-3 reduces to Equation 2-1.

*Although it is generally important that light enter the optical center of the lens, the point of entry for maximum efficiency in some observers may be very eccentric in the pupil, or the location of this point may actually be some function of brightness or time in other subjects. The reasons for this variation are obscure.

†The term Exp relates to a power of the transcendental constant, e (= 2.71821828 . . .). Thus, Exp (x) = e^x.

Another formula is $\eta = 1 - 0.85 R^2 + 0.002 R^4$. The net effect of all this is that the effective pupillary area (Ae) is now $Ae = 2\pi \int_0^R \eta r\, dr$. By substituting the above values for n and evaluating this integral, and finally substituting into the definition of Troland, we obtain the following definitions of *effective Trolands:*

$$E_{(T)} = \frac{\pi B}{2.3K} [1 - \mathrm{Exp}\,(-2.3\, KR^2)]$$

or

$$E_{(T)} = \pi BR^2 \,(1 - 0.425 R^2 + 0.00067\, R^4)$$

The basic difference between a Troland and an effective Troland is that the former is a measure of how much light reaches the retina, whereas the latter provides an index of how effective the light will be in producing a visual response.

Another unit, sometimes used in animal experiments where the retina is exposed and illuminated directly, is *incident photon flux,* where the actual number of photons likely to be absorbed per second per receptor is calculated. This may be done by knowing the power output of the light source as a function of wavelength, the absorptiveness of the rod and cone photopigments (which may be obtained from the Dartnall nomograms[65]) and the size of the receptor. The units will thus be of the form "quanta·sec^{-1} · rod^{-1}" or "quanta·sec^{-1} · cone^{-1}" since the diameter of the rods and cones varies. These units are numerically huge, rarely falling toward zero log units, which would correspond to one quanta · sec^{-1} · receptor^{-1}, and are frequently in the range of five to nine log units. Many of the graphs appearing in the section on physiology are calibrated in terms of incident photon fluxes, but in the clinical literature this term is almost never used.

The Stimulus Problem in Color Perimetry

The sensation of color is one of those subjective sensations that no one is able to define adequately, yet everyone seems to know exactly what it is. Our major interest in this section will be the properties of colored light that may make it useful for the perimetrist. We will discuss as well the pitfalls that can trap the perimetrist who chooses to use colored stimuli.

Light of different wavelengths produces sensations of different color. Thus, light with a wavelength of 430 nanometers (nm) is violet; 460 nm corresponds to blue; 529 nm, green; 575 nm, yellow; 600 nm, orange; and 650 nm, red. Obviously, the intermediate wavelengths produce intermediate colors usually described as though they were mixtures of the other colors. Monochromatic light appears to be undiluted, while the addition of white light tends to make the color appear washed out, or *desaturated.* Thus, colored light is traditionally described

72 Principles of Quantitative Perimetry

by three terms: hue (wavelength); saturation (purity); and brightness (radiance).

It is a well-established fact that the hue of any color may be matched by a mixture of two or more other colors, so-called metameric matching. The implication of this fact to the perimetrist is immediate and obvious: the light radiating from the surfaces of test objects and appearing as a given color to the eye may not have the same spectral composition and thus, may have very different stimulus values. It is largely for this reason that classical color perimetry has represented such a nightmare for the perimetrist in his efforts to standardize it accurately. If one wishes to do accurate quantitative color perimetry, one must use monochromatic light.

Radiometry Versus Photometry with Monochromatic Light

The units of brightness of monochromatic light deserve some comment. As we recall from the section on radiometry and photometry, photometric units are nothing more than radiometric units that have been corrected for the sensitivity of the human eye to the spectral composition of the light being used. Since perimetry is nothing more than a determination of the sensitivity of the eye to light, perimetry utilizing monochromatic light is nothing more than determination of the sensitivity of the eye to a given wavelength of light. Photometric units are not only unnecessary with monochromatic perimetry, but the double conversion can become a source of error. Thus, many reputable observers in the field of color perimetry[5] do not use terms such as apostilbs or millilamberts, which are common with white light perimetry, but instead utilize the radiometric term of watts per square centimeter.

Monochromatic Perimetry

Perimetric studies with monochromatic light have been carried out in the past by Wentworth and more recently by Nolte. Although both studied the dark-adapted eye, Nolte extended his studies to the light-adapted eye, and his data are presented in Figures 2-3 and 2-4. Also, Wentworth projected light directly into the subjects' eyes while Nolte utilized a more conventional perimetric technique, and his studies are therefore a bit more comparable to a clinically useful technique. The photopic curves are more or less parallel to each other, but they are at different heights, corresponding to the relatively different sensitivities of the retina for different wavelengths. One noteworthy point is that the red light (Fig. 2-3, bottom curve in the bottom panel) has a much sharper central peak than the other colors. In the mesopic range (middle panel) there is a good deal of flattening of the upper curves, whereas the red curve still shows some peak. In total dark adaptation (upper panel), all colors except red show a relative

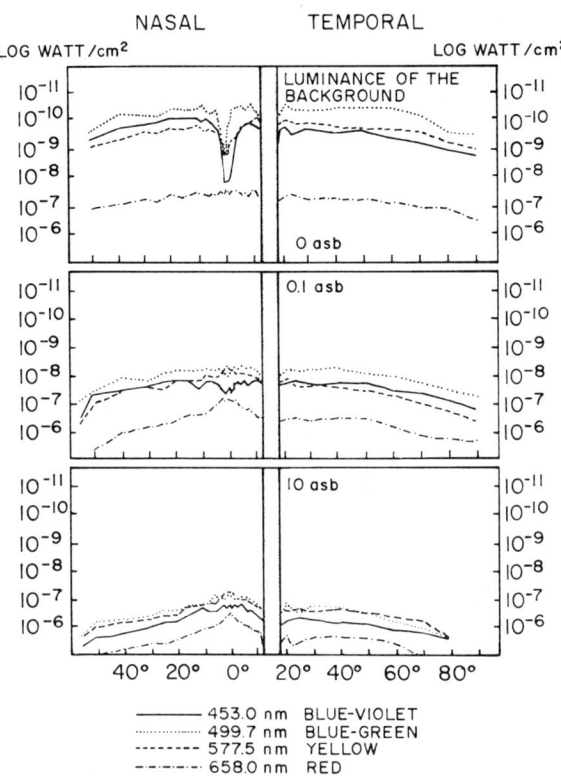

Figure 2-3 Monochromatic threshold data. Color perimetry with four different hues of monochromatic light on white background at three different levels of dark adaptation. Top curve, total dark adaptation (background 0 asb); middle curve, mesopic adaptation (background 0.1 asb); and lower curve, photopic adaptation (background 10 asb). Note that test spot "brightness" (ordinate) is given as a radiance (watts/cm^2). Note also that the sensitivity to red never increases as much as does the shorter wavelength with dark adaptation. (See also Fig. 2-4.) (Redrawn after Nolte, as quoted by Aulhorn and Harms.[5])

central scotoma. The curve for red, although greatly depressed peripherally relative to the others, is perfectly flat across the entire field. Although green shows some central scotoma, it is less marked than the others, whereas violet and blue show the deepest central scotomas. This work implies that red light is primarily a stimulus to cone function, whereas the other wavelengths of light stimulate the rods to a greater or lesser degree. This fact is underscored in Figure 2-4 where sensitivity curves for the central 10° are plotted at seven different wavelengths in three different states of dark adaptation. It is important to note that with dark adaptation, the shorter wavelengths increase in sensitivity far more than the longer wavelengths, although some increase in sensitivity is

74   Principles of Quantitative Perimetry

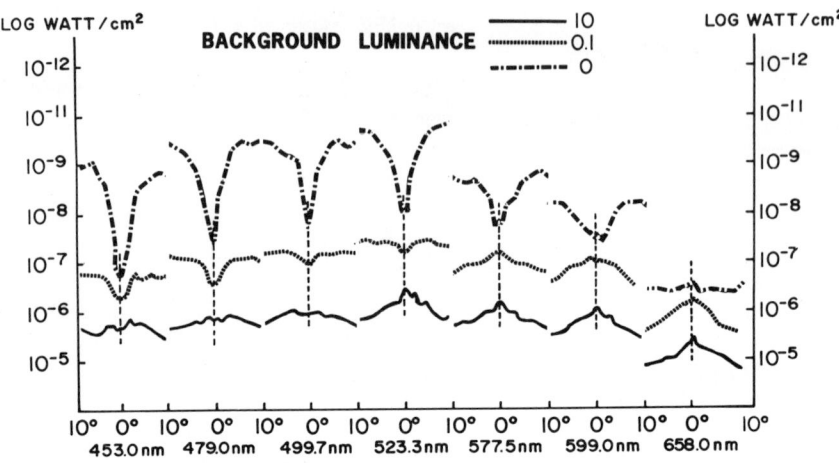

Figure 2-4   Effect of wavelength and background luminance on central monochromatic thresholds. Perimetry of the central 10° as in Figure 2–3 at seven different wavelengths of monochromatic light (red at the right, violet at the left). Two points are particularly noteworthy: sensitivity to red increases only slightly with dark adaptation; and, with scotopic vision, a relative central scotoma never develops to red light. On the other hand, the scotopic relative central scotoma becomes increasingly prominent with decreasing wavelengths. (Redrawn after Nolte, as quoted by Aulhorn and Harms.[5])

noted regardless of wavelength. Thus, dark adaptation is not only a change in sensitivity to light, but a change in the spectral sensitivity curve. This results in a shift of the curve toward the blue end of the spectrum, with the most sensitive wavelength dropping from 555 nm to about 510 nm. (For the Purkinje shift, see Fig. 2-1.) Teleologically, this makes some sense, since nightlight contains relatively more blue than daylight.

Color Perimetry in the Clinic

Clinically, the use of colored test perimetry is, at the least, controversial. The theoretical argument for its use is that disease alters the spectral sensitivity curve in one way or another. Although several authors[6] have suggested that colored perimetry is only a means of producing a less intense stimulus than with achromatic perimetry, others[9,37,44,91,92] have suggested that it adds important information to that obtained by conventional perimetric techniques. The conventional clinical use of color will be discussed in a subsequent chapter. This latter hypothesis has not been truly confirmed because of the impossibility of comparing the results of perimetry by standard chromatic techniques from one laboratory to another. Until recently, the equipment has been bulky, expensive, and only a few stimulus gradations were available for color perimetry. An exact picture of the rather complex shape of the visual island was not, therefore, readily obtainable. Nevertheless, workers using strict monochromatic red light from a laser[9] have indicated that a red light may indeed be more useful than white light in diseases involving the chiasm. Other workers[44] have reported that narrow-band blue test spots on a yellow background are a very sensitive technique for plotting macular lesions, particularly those due to central serous retinopathy. All such studies need to be amplified and confirmed. Thus, color perimetry gives some promise of being useful as a clinical tool but, at the same time, remains somewhat controversial.

ELECTRON MICROSCOPY OF THE RETINA

The Anatomical Organization of the Retina

Our knowledge of the neural organization of the human retina has been expanded since the advent of the electron microscope. Although the basic retinal histology has long been known, the recent electron microscopic studies by Dowling and Boycott[26] have shed new light on retinal anatomy and provided us with the basis for a deeper understanding of certain electrophysiological and psychophysical observations.

Of the ten retinal layers usually described in anatomical texts, only five are pertinent to this discussion.

The cell bodies of the retinal neurons are found in three of these layers (outer nuclear, inner nuclear, and ganglion cell) whereas most synapses occur within two interposed synaptic layers, called respectively the outer and inner plexiform layers. According to classic lines, only three types of cells synaptically interact in each plexiform layer. Thus, in the outer plexiform layer, where the first information transfer occurs, we have synaptic contact between receptor cells, bipolar cells and horizontal cells.* In the inner plexiform layer, there is synaptic contact between bipolar cells, ganglion cells, and amacrine cells. Recent studies have disclosed additional cell types and interconnections. In some species of fish and monkey, Dowling and Ehinger[27] have described interplexiform cells that arise in the inner plexiform layer; they apparently receive their input from amacrine cells. The interplexiform cells apparently synapse in the outer plexiform layer on horizontal and perhaps bipolar cells (Fig. 2-5). Although the normal flow of information through the retina is from outside in, that is from receptor to ganglion cell, this recent description of interplexiform cells raises the possibility of feedback from the inner to the outer plexiform layer. Other authors have reported

---

*Horizontal and amacrine cells are classically considered to be horizontal association cells that transmit information sideways, or parallel, to the surface of the retina.

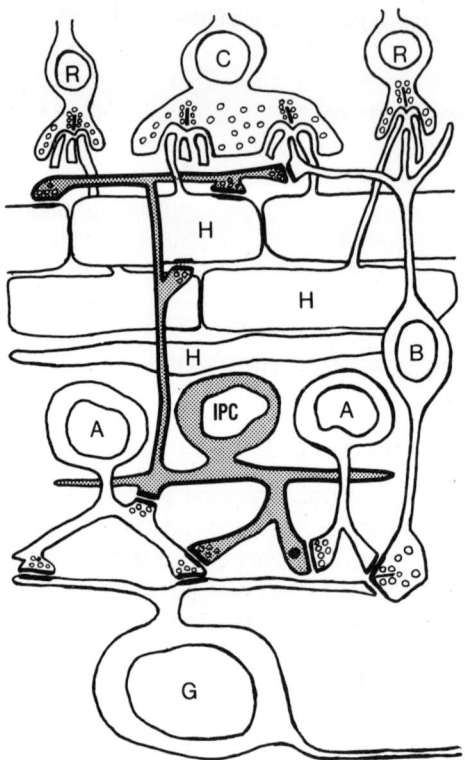

Figure 2-5 Summary diagram of the synaptic connections of an interplexiform cell (IPC) of the goldfish. These cells receive synaptic input from the amacrine cells (A) in the inner plexiform layer. They may in turn synapse back onto the amacrine cells but never the ganglion cells (G). The IPC sends a process into the outer plexiform layer that may contact the perikarya of the external layer of horizontal cells (H) or the bipolar cell (B) dendrites. Synaptic contact between the IPC and the rods (R), the cones (C), or the more internal layers of horizontal cells (H) has not been reported. (Redrawn after Dowling and Ehinger.[27])

similar cells in additional species,[20,62] but the existence of the interplexiform cell in humans, though considered likely, has not yet been demonstrated.

Locations and Types of Retinal Synapses

There are three types of synapse found in vertebrate retinas: the ribbon, the conventional and the gap junction synapses. These synapses may be differentiated on the basis of morphology observable with the electron microscope (Fig. 2-6). Although the first two types are found in both plexiform layers, the gap junction is confined to the outer plexiform layer.

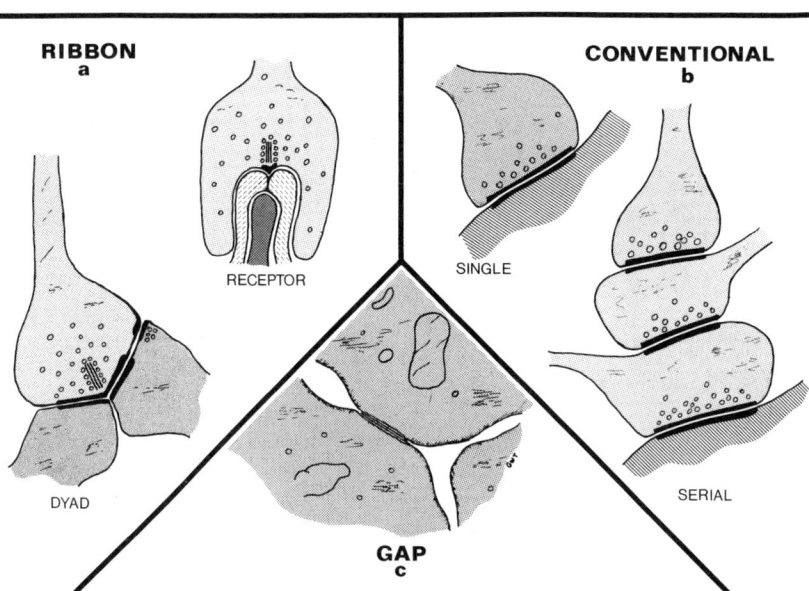

Figure 2-6 Retinal synapses. Summary diagram of the synaptic configurations found in the retina. Ribbon synapses (a) are of two types: the *receptor* type of the outer plexiform in which dendrites from two horizontal cells (light shading) enfold a dendrite from a bipolar cell (dark shading); and the *dyadic* type of the inner plexiform, formed between bipolars (light) and ganglion cells or amacrine cells (dark shading). Amacrine cells may synapse back onto the bipolar cell in a different part of the dyad, as shown in the upper right postsynaptic element. Conventional synapses (b) also may be of two types: *single,* which resemble those found elsewhere in the nervous system, and *serial,* in which multiple synaptic butons synapse one on another. The serial arrangement is most typical of amacrine cells. The gap junction (c) is found only between receptors (only cones in man) and has no synaptic vesicles. This is a "tight" approximation of the cell membrane thought to allow passage of electric potential from cell to cell.

The first type of synapse to be discussed is the *ribbon synapse.* Ribbon synapses are characterized by an electron-dense bar in the presynaptic cytoplasm surrounded by a ring of vesicles. The bar itself is usually oriented precisely at a right angle to the adjacent cell membrane. Two or more postsynaptic elements are always present. The ribbon synapse is confined exclusively to receptor terminals in the outer plexiform layer and to bipolar terminals in the inner plexiform layer, although the morphology varies between the two layers. For example, in the receptor cell ribbon synapse, there are invaginations in receptor terminals with a precise arrangement of three postsynaptic elements. Two processes are deeply inserted in either side of the synaptic ribbon and a third lies centrally and more superficially (Fig. 2-6a). The two lateral processes are always from horizontal cells, whereas the central, more superficial one is from a bipolar cell. Each of these three processes are thought to receive input from the receptor cell.

The ribbon synapse formed by the bipolar terminals is somewhat different from that of the receptor terminals. In all species studied, only two postsynaptic elements are associated with this synapse as opposed to three in the outer plexiform layer. Also, the postsynaptic elements are not invaginated into the presynaptic cell as occurs in the receptor ribbon synapse. Dowling has termed this synaptic arrangement a *dyad*. These postsynaptic elements may be any combination of ganglion cell dendrites or amacrine cell processes.

The *conventional* synapse is the second major synaptic type found in both plexiform layers of the retina.[15,26] It is similar morphologically to synaptic contacts found elsewhere in the nervous system and is characterized by an aggregation of synaptic vesicles close to the presynaptic membrane. The presynaptic and postsynaptic membranes are thickened in the region of the synapse. Unlike the ribbon synapses, only one postsynaptic element is found at these contacts. Like the ribbon synapse, however, the conventional synapse is found in both the inner and outer plexiform layers, and only certain cell types participate in their formation. In the outer plexiform layer, horizontal and interplexiform cells are the most frequent presynaptic elements for this type of synapse, while the amacrine cells are usually the responsible parties in the inner plexiform. Dowling has described conventional synapses onto the proximal processes and perikarya of amacrine cells made by centrifugal fibers in the border region between the inner plexiform and inner nuclear layers of the pigeon retina.[25] These are small in number in comparison with the number of amacrine cell synapses that are present. These centrifugal fibers are intriguing since they suggest physiologically the central control of peripheral visual processing.

Many variations in the exact pattern of conventional synaptic contact exist in both plexiform layers. In the outer plexiform, the best-studied cell is the horizontal cell. These cells may either synapse with bipolars near the ribbon synapse, or they may send out specific cell processes to contact the bipolars conventionally. Since horizontal cells have never been observed to make presynaptic contact with a receptor terminal, it is assumed that horizontal cells are only responsible for lateral interactions through their effect on the bipolar cell dendrites. The effect of the horizontal cells is probably mediated via conventional synaptic activity, but some authorities suggest that horizontal cells may somehow control the flow of transmitter substance to the bipolars at the receptor ribbon synapse, or even somehow provide "feedback" to the receptor cells themselves.[15,25,93] Uncommonly, a conventional synapse is made between the receptor cell (usually a cone) and a bipolar cell without other postsynaptic elements being present. Bipolars that take part in such synapses do not partake in receptor-bipolar ribbon synapses and are termed *flat bipolars*. They are probably the same cell as the *brush bipolar* of the light microscopist.

In the outer plexiform layer, the amacrine cells make abundant conventional synapses in all species and have been observed synapsing back onto the bipolar terminals, onto ganglion cell dendrites, onto interplexiform cells, and onto other amacrine cell processes. Since the amacrines do synapse with both the bipolar and the ganglion cells (Fig. 2-7), the signal path is occasionally changed to receptor-bipolar-amacrine-ganglion cell instead of the normal receptor-bipolar-ganglion cell as is usually described.

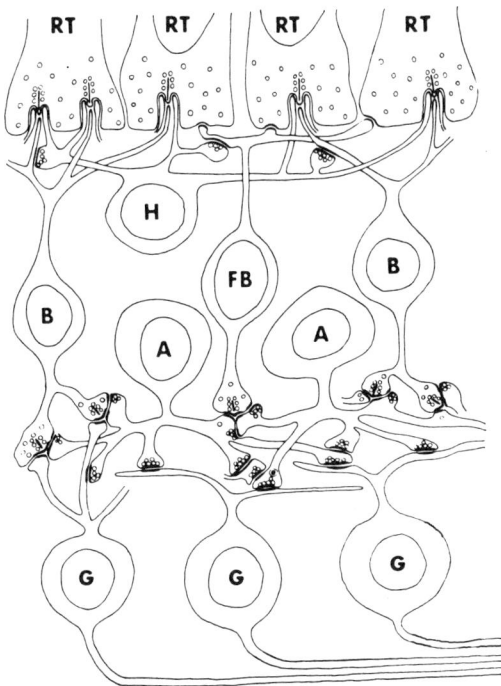

Figure 2-7 A "wiring diagram" of the retina summarizing the synaptic contacts found in vertebrate retinas. In the outer plexiform layer, bipolar (B) and horizontal (H) cells send processes into *invaginations* of the receptor terminals (RT) to form ribbon synapses. Flat bipolar cells (FB) make superficial contact with some receptor terminals. Horizontal cells may form conventional synapses with the bipolar dendrites (and occasionally onto other horizontal cells, not illustrated). In the inner plexiform layer, the bipolar cells form ribbon synapses (dyads) with the amacrine (A) and ganglion (G) cells. The bipolar terminals may either contact an amacrine and a ganglion cell (shown on left), two amacrine cells (shown on right), or two ganglion cells (not illustrated, rare). The amacrine cells may form synapses with other amacrine cells (as in the serial synapse, center) or ganglion cells or even synapse back onto the bipolar cell at the dyad. Thus, two signal paths, receptor-bipolar-ganglion and receptor-bipolar-amacrine-ganglion, are possible. (From Dowling.[25])

Special arrangements abound in the inner plexiform layer with regard to the conventional synapse. In one such, amacrine cells that partake of dyads may be seen to synapse directly back onto the bipolar terminal, an arrangement that suggests presynaptic inhibition. In other arrangements, an amacrine process may synapse on an adjacent amacrine process that in turn synapses with a third element, an arrangement termed the *serial synapse* (Fig. 2-6, 2-7). The third element of the serial synapse may be a ganglion cell dendrite, a bipolar terminal, or even another amacrine cell. Obviously, this arrangement suggests a wide variety of local signal modification by the amacrine cells, and comparative studies bear out this supposition. Those species that are exquisitely well adapted for motion sensitivity have a greater number of amacrine cells than those species with less motion sensitivity.

The final type of synapse is the *gap junction,* also called a "tight junction." This consists of the close approximation of the cell membranes of adjacent neurons, actually fusing into a single multilayered membrane at the site of the synapse. (Fig. 2-6c) This fusion allows for the passive spread of potential from cell to cell without the necessity of transmitter substance. Accordingly, no presynaptic or postsynaptic vesicles are seen. The gap junction has been reported to play various roles in a variety of species,[32,100] but in man it provides only receptor-to-receptor couplings, which presumably function as a part of some sensitivity control. This role has been demonstrated in man between two cone pedicles* and between a rod and a cone, but not between two rods.[51]

ELECTROPHYSIOLOGY OF THE RETINA

Intracellular Recordings

Potentials recorded intracellularly from the retina are remarkable in several ways. First of all, the receptors, horizontal and bipolar cells (i.e., the distal cells of the visual pathway) do not show "all-or-none" spike impulse activity so characteristic of nervous tissue elsewhere in the body. Instead, these cells respond with slow "graded" potentials (i.e., electrical activity that is proportional to the strength of light stimuli). In contrast, the more proximal amacrine and ganglion cells do show that transient spike potentials are superimposed upon slower potentials.[25]

Another finding of considerable interest is that all receptor cells and most of the other distal cells of the retina respond to light with a hyperpolarizing poten-

---

*A pedicle is the part of the cone that forms synapses with the bipolar and horizontal cells. The pedicle of a cone is far larger than the corresponding portion of a rod.

tial. That is, the potential between the inside and the outside of the cell increases in magnitude. This is surprising, for elsewhere in the nervous system, hyperpolarization is associated either with inhibition or rest, whereas depolarization is associated with activity. Stated in a different way, when light is at a minimum, the vertebrate receptor cell is maximally active, or "on" full blast; as light increases, the same cell becomes hyperpolarized and turns "off," thus releasing *less* transmitter substance to affect the cells downstream from the flow of activity. This may be verified by observing the effect of magnesium ion on the retina. Magnesium ion is well known, from studies on other neural tissue, to stabilize cell membranes, thus preventing the action of transmitter substance. These studies do confirm that receptor cells release transmitter substance maximally in darkness.

Information may be transferred from the receptors to the horizontal and bipolar and then onward since these cells all respond with graded potentials; hence a potential change in either direction is capable of signaling a corresponding change in activity. Indeed, this system of graded potentials allows a more precisely accurate interpretation of retinal activity by the distal cells than would be possible by a system based on variations in firing rates, which is the kind of neural response found typically elsewhere in the body. Information cannot be transferred over long distances, however, by this technique. Consequently, the ganglion cells respond with a depolarizing spike potential, like the activity of conventional neurons in the nervous system.

Most of our knowledge of the intracellular activity of the various retinal elements is the result of work on the mud puppy *(Necturus maculosus)*, a vertebrate noted for the large size of its retinal cells.[25,73,93,95] In most other animals, extensive intracellular recording has not been possible from these cells because of their small size. Despite this technical problem, several recordings have been made from most of the retinal neurons in a number of other species, and in each cell type, the results have been consistently similar to those of comparable mud puppy cells. For this reason, the patterns of electrical activity in the various retinal cells of Necturus are considered by most workers in the field to be valid throughout the vertebrates.

The Center-Surround

As one might expect with the rich lateral interconnections anatomically described in the preceding section, all ganglion cells of the retina do not behave in the same way, yet each of them is influenced by light falling on different portions of the specific retinal zone in which it is contained. Indeed, ganglion cells may be divided into three types on the basis of their response to a small spot of light that explores the retina at various distances from the cell body. The first type, called the "on" cell, increases its discharge when the cell itself or its immediate vicinity (the *center*) is illuminated by a spot of light. The second type ceases activity altogether when the center is illuminated; it is called the *"off"* cell.[61] (A third type, called *"on-off"*, is sensitive only to motion or changing illumination and is discussed in the next section.)

When the illuminating spot is applied at eccentricities slightly beyond the center, (i.e., to the *surround*), the effect elicited in the first two ganglion cell types is the opposite from that seen when the spot lies exclusively over any part of the homogeneously sensitive center. Thus, "on" cells are turned off by illumination in the surrounding area, and "off" cells are turned on by light directed at the surround. (See Fig 2-8.) As the spot moves yet further from a retinal gan-

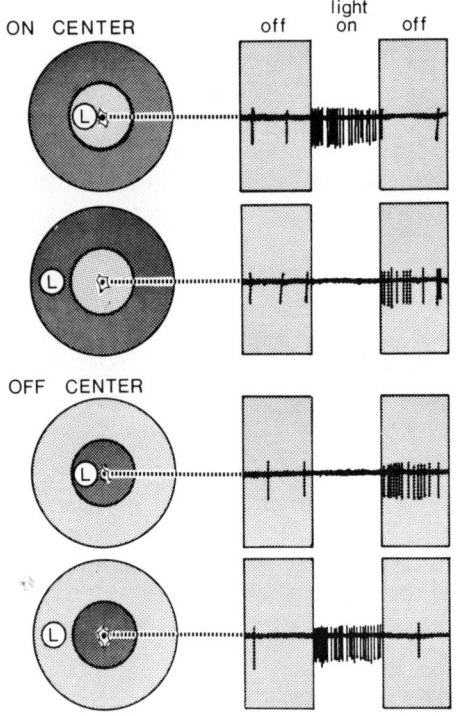

Figure 2-8 Center-surround organization. Two possible organizations, the "on-center" (top) and the "off-center" (bottom) are shown. In the "on-center" receptive field, a light (L) falling on the center (see first diagram) causes the ganglion cell being recorded to increase its firing rate when the light is on. When the light falls on the surround (second diagram), the light causes inhibition of spontaneous firing. This behavior is reversed in the "off-center" field (bottom two diagrams); light in the center inhibits firing, whereas in the surround it promotes an increased rate of discharge. Note that both types of fields are organized approximately as two concentric circles, the size of which is a function of retinal location and dark–light adaptation, with the largest fields in the dark-adapted periphery and the smallest fields in the light-adapted center.

glion cell, it ceases to have any effect on the discharge pattern of that cell. The entire area in which a retinal ganglion cell may be affected in some manner by a spot of light is referred to as the cell's *receptive field,* and the above-described arrangement of that field is generally referred to as "*center-surround*" organization. The fields of "on" cells are generally referred to as "on-center" receptive fields. Occasionally a zone at the margin between the center and its surround gives an "on-off" response in cells that have either "on" or "off" centers. Wiesel[99] notes that in the cat, fields tend to be quite small near the fovea, "about 0.25 mm," whereas they may grow to approximately 2 mm toward the periphery.* Also, receptive field size is partially dependent on the level of background illumination.

In summary, the receptive field may be considered for the moment as a roughly circular area that includes two topographically concentric and functionally antagonistic zones where stimulation of a point in one zone excites or inhibits the firing of the cell and stimulation of a point in the other zone has the opposite effect. Changing such variables as background illumination or activity in the surround may change the size of the field, but an "on-center" field may not be converted to an "off-center" field, nor conversely.

Simple Versus Complex Receptive Fields

Receptive fields such as those just described are found in the monkey and cat and are termed "simple," since they may be satisfactorily mapped using static spots of light. A third type of receptive field has been found in other species by Hartline,[49,50] who has described frog ganglion cells that respond only to movement of the stimulus spot. Other workers have borne out his findings and agreed to the term of "on-off" ganglion cells in this "complex" type of receptive field.[7,8,74,94] On-off ganglion cells respond best (though not exclusively) to spots or edges of light that are moving in a specific direction. Strangely enough, a shadow moving through the field is just as effective in stimulating these cells as the movement of a light spot itself. When stimulated with static spots of light, on-off ganglion cells respond with transient bursts of impulses at both the onset and cessation of the light-spot presentation. Although on-off ganglion cells do not appear to have an inhibitory surround in the same sense as cells that have simple receptive fields, Werblin and Copenhagan have shown that movement or a flashing light in the surround can inhibit the on-off ganglion cell.[95] Because lateral inhibition of the on-off ganglion cells and the activity of amacrine cells are identical in time course and amplitude, mediation of this control is attributed to the amacrine cells.

---

*Since the optic nerve head measures about 1.5 mm and causes a physiological scotoma of about 7.5°, one can say in humans that 1 mm on the retina represents about 5° in the visual field.

Comparative Electrophysiology

Although it has not been possible to test directly the center-surround organization in the human, Enoch et al[30,31] have described a perimetric test utilizing a modified Goldmann Perimeter in which a small, flashing spot of light is superimposed on a larger spot of variable size and intensity. The size of the second spot is varied, and its intensity is adjusted until subjective perception of the small, flashing central spot is just inhibited. Further increasing of the size of the second spot results initially in a decrease in the intensity necessary to prevent the small, flashing central spot from being seen (the "summation arm"), but when the size of the surrounding spot surpasses a certain area, the intensity of the surround must again increase (the "inhibitory arm") in order to maintain the inhibition. This has been interpreted as testing the center-surround properties of the human retina, with the "summation arm" corresponding to the stimulation of the receptive-field center and the "inhibitory arm" corresponding to stimulation of the surround. Preliminary mathematical modeling of this phenomenon by Tate and Aulhorn based on the findings of Werblin et al in the mud puppy lend credence to this assumption. The phenomenon has been widely researched by Westheimer[96,97,98] and by Teller et al[85,86,87,88,89] and the interested reader should refer to their works.

Receptive-Field Organization of Various Retinal Cells

Although the receptive-field organization was studied initially in ganglion cells only, each cell type from the various layers of the retina has now been evaluated in the same way by intracellular recording while the illumination was varied both centrally and in a surrounding annulus. The organization of each cell type's receptive field will be described in the order the cells occur in the visual pathway (i.e., receptor, horizontal, bipolar, amacrine, and ganglion cells).

Receptor Cells

Unlike the more proximal cells, both types of receptor cells (i.e., rods and cones) respond well to central illumination, but poorly to any sort of illumination in the surround. In addition, the functional characteristics of the rods and the cones differ sharply from one another. The rods have their maximum electrical response to stimulation by light spots after total dark adaptation. As the background illumination is increased, rods gradually saturate or become so hyperpolarized they cannot respond by further hyperpolarization. Thus, with bright background luminances, the rods are in a state of total saturation and contribute little to the electrical output of the retina as a whole. Cones, however, do not

Biophysics, Psychophysics, and the Visual Field   85

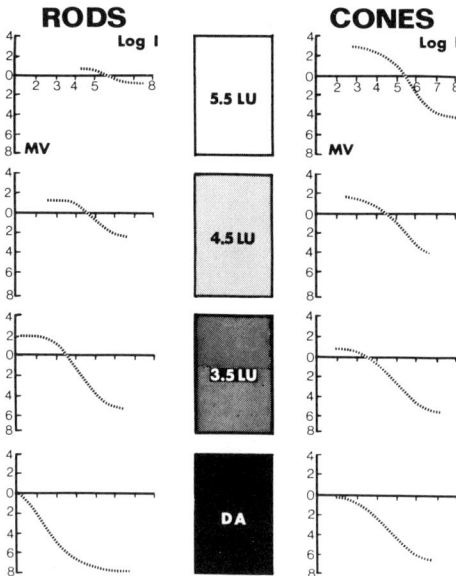

Figure 2-9   A comparison of the stimulus-response (or operating) curves of the rods and cones with different degrees of dark-adaptation, ranging from completely dark-adapted (DA) (bottom) to 5.5 log units (LU) incident photons absorbed by the receptor per second (top). Note that with increasingly bright backgrounds, not only does the response curve shift along the ordinate in both cases but the magnitude of the rods' response is also diminished by bright backgrounds, whereas that of the cones is not. Data were obtained by the method of substitution thresholds; thus, the response is zero with equal test and background brightnesses. The abscissa is the test luminance in log absorbed photons. The ordinate is the cell response in millivolts. A hyperpolarizing response occurs below the abscissa. (Drawn from the data of Norman and Werblin.[73])

saturate but rather show a shift of their operating curve* along the background intensity axis, leaving the form of the curve substantially unchanged (Fig. 2-9). Once the background luminance is bright enough to cause negligible rod contribution to the operating curve of the receptors, the output from the cones in the receptive layer is roughly a linear function of the stimulus brightness versus the background brightness (Fig. 2-10). Thus, the cone response is linear over a wide range of adapting luminances, while the rod response is nonlinear.

In some species, there is definite spread of potential from receptor to receptor, possibly by gap junctions,[32] and some authors have postulated the spread of potential between receptor cells by feedback from horizontal cells.[15]

---

*As the term is used in this discussion, the operating curve of a cell is a plot of the electrical potential across the cell wall versus the stimulus strength (i.e., the brightness of the stimulating light).

86 *Principles of Quantitative Perimetry*

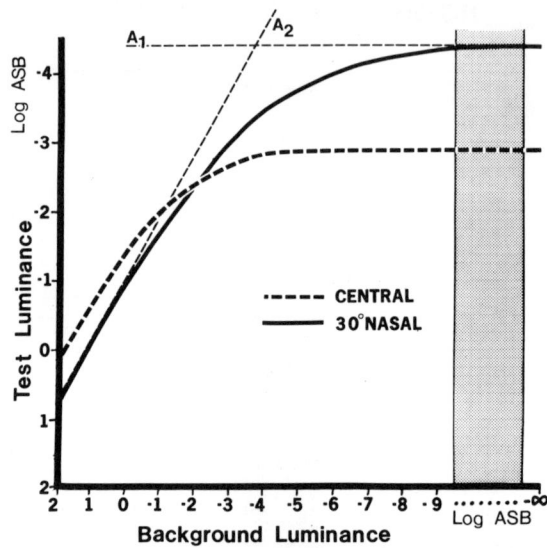

Figure 2-10 Plot of log increment threshold as a function of log background intensity. At very low background luminances, the curves tend to parallel the abscissa (asymptote A_1), while at high background luminances, the curves approach the abscissa with a slope of one (asymptote A_2). This may be restated by saying that the curve in the photopic region approaches a state where contrast sensitivity ($\Delta L/L$) remains constant, whereas in the scotopic state, increment sensitivity (ΔL) remains constant. Note also that this transition occurs at higher background luminances centrally than peripherally. Thus, if a perimetric device is to be made maximally resistant to small changes in background luminance, testing should be confined to the photopic region or the deep scotopic. (After Aulhorn and Harms.[5])

Horizontal Cells

Horizontal cells respond with large hyperpolarizing potentials when any of the associated retina is stimulated by added light; when the light is reduced, the cells are depolarized. No antagonistic center-surround pattern is seen with these cells, for response to the illumination of the center is additive to that of the surround. The horizontal cell essentially operates much like a cone, shifting its operating point as the input is changed. The horizontal cell promptly hyperpolarizes to a new potential when stimulated with brighter light, essentially maintaining this potential as long as the stimulus is present and dropping the potential to its original resting level promptly after the stimulus conditions return to their previous status (Fig. 2-11). When the stimulus is a decrease in light intensity, the time course of the horizontal cells' depolarizing reponse is similar to that of the hyperpolarizing response.

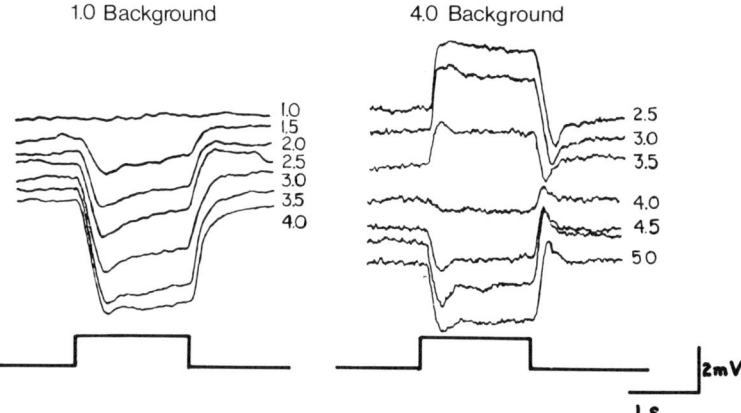

Figure 2-11 Horizontal cell responses to substitution stimuli against a background of 1.0 and 4.0 log unit absorbed photons per receptor. Note that about 200–300 msec are required to reach full potential. The stimulus value is given beside the corresponding tracing. Stimuli dimmer than the background show a depolarization; stimuli brighter than the background show a hyperpolarization. All responses against 1.0 background (left) are hyperpolarizing. A small response with a stimulus of 4.0 is seen against a background of 4.0 as the result of imprecise calibration. Two responses at 4.5 stimulus are also recorded, accounting for the extra trace seen on this figure. (With permission from Werblin.[93])

Bipolar Cells

Antagonistic center-surround organization of both on-center and off-center types first appears in the visual pathway at the level of the bipolar cells. The bipolar cells may be divided into two physiological types, those that respond to center illumination with hyperpolarizing potentials, and those that respond with depolarizing potentials. The potential produced by activity in the center is antagonized or reduced with either type of bipolar cell by illumination of the full field or of any area immediately surrounding the center. Illumination in the surround cannot change a hyperpolarizing bipolar cell into a depolarizing bipolar cell, and activity must be present in the center in order to see the effect of the surround. Also, the two types of bipolar cells help to explain the difference between on-center and off-center ganglion cells in the simple receptive fields. Hyperpolarizing bipolars are associated with on-center receptive fields (and "on" type ganglion cells) while depolarizing bipolars are associated with off-center fields (and "off" type ganglion cells).

The story of the origin of the inhibitory effect of the surround is told by Figures 2-11, 2-12, and 2-13. Figure 2-12 shows a *depolarizing* bipolar cell at three levels of background intensity and at test intensities spanning about 3 log units. The responses can be divided into three phases: an initial reponse that is

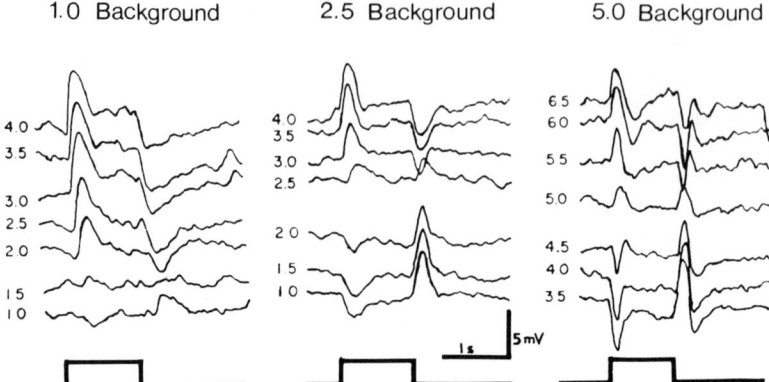

Figure 2-12 Depolarizing cell response to substitution stimuli with backgrounds of 1.0, 2.5, and 5.0 log units absorbed photons per receptor. Stimulus value appears beside each tracing. Note that the sustained phase of the response decreases with higher background potentials, with two "overshoots" at "on" and "off," each overshoot occupying about 250 msec. Note also that only small "off" overshoots are seen at low background levels; thus, the inhibition of the sustained bipolar response is graded and has a time course similar to that seen in horizontal cell activity. (With permission from Werblin.[93])

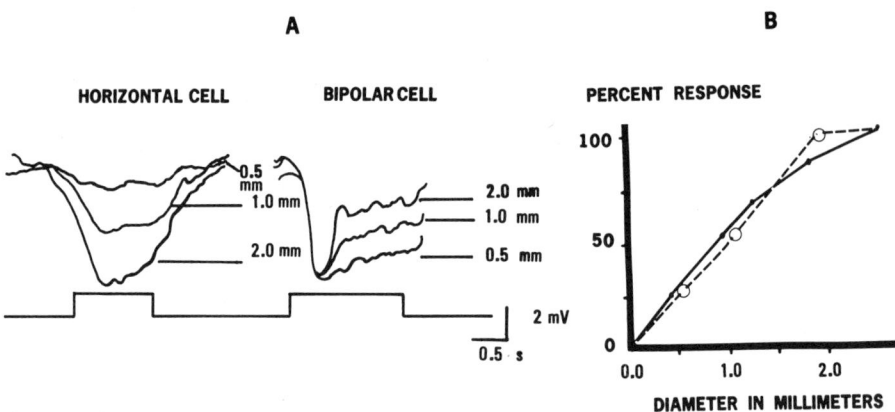

Figure 2-13 **A** Change in magnitude of response with different sizes of test disks of light centered on the receptive fields of horizontal and bipolar cells. The disks were of constant intensity and variable radius. Larger disks increased the response of horizontal cells and increased the inhibition of bipolar cells. **B** Graph of percent of maximum response in a horizontal cell and percent of maximum decrement of response in a hyperpolarizing bipolar cell as a function of disk size. Each has identical values, and both are represented by the open circles and the dotted line. The solid line is the predicted values of the response weighted by the function $W(x) = Ae^{-4x}$, where A is an arbitrary constant and x is the radius of the disk in millimeters. (Redrawn from Werblin.[93])

roughly proportional to stimulus strength; a sustained response that decreases with increasing background luminance; and an "off" response that is enhanced by higher background intensities. The bipolar's initial and off responses each last for around 250 milliseconds, approximately the time required for the horizontal cell to peak and to return to baseline respectively. The sustained response lasts as long as the test spot is on; its magnitiude is an inhibited version of the initial response. At low background levels (e.g., 1.0 log units, Fig. 2-12, left), inhibition of the sustained response amounts to only 50% or so of the initial response, but at higher background levels of illumination, (e.g., 5.0 log units; Fig. 2-12, right) the entire sustained response may be obliterated by inhibition. Moreover, a step increase that doubles the background illumination during the sustained phase causes an increased inhibition of the bipolars (see Fig. 2-14) at the same time it causes an increase in the activity of the horizontal cells.

The overshoot at the end of the test corresponds to holdover horizontal activity at a time in which the return to baseline levels of the excitatory input to the bipolars precedes that of the inhibitory input from the horizontal by some 200 to 300 milliseconds. Thus, the inhibition corresponds fairly well to horizontal cell activity in magnitude and time course.

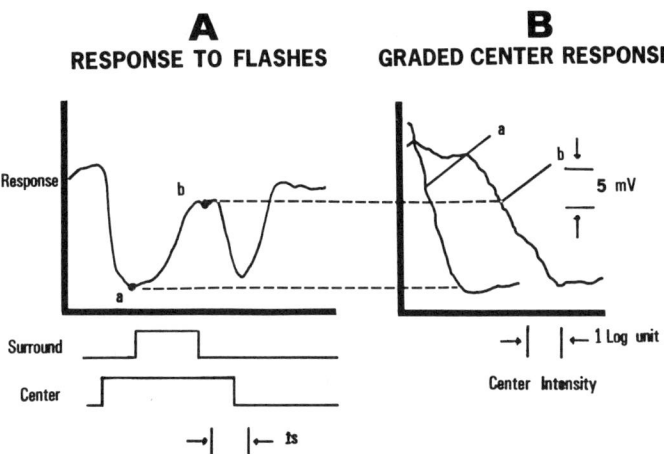

Figure 2-14   **A**   Response to flashes. Time course of response of a hyperpolarizing bipolar to a center flash followed by an additional surround flash. The surround flash antagonizes the center response (a) so that the initial hyperpolarization is diminished (b) and the membrane potential is driven back toward its dark level.   **B**   Graded center response. Intensity response curves for the center of the bipolar cell receptive field in the dark (a) and with a fixed-intensity annulus (b). The brightness of the center spot was varied to produce these curves. Note the effect of the annulus was simply to shift the curve approximately 1 log unit to the right. (Redrawn from Werblin.[93])

More evidence incriminating the horizontal cells is seen in Figure 2-13. In this figure, the size of the test spot varied while the background remained dark and the test spot luminance was held constant. The response of both the horizontal cells and the bipolar cells is seen to vary in proportion to spot size, with the horizontal cell becoming progressively more hyperpolarized and the sustained phase of the bipolar response becoming more inhibited. Figure 2-13B shows a plot of this inhibition (as percent of maximums) and horizontal cell activity (open circles) which may be seen to coincide exactly. Moreover, these data fit very well the theoretical curve Ae^{-4x} (black dots) where x is spot radius and A is arbitrary constant. Several authors have shown that this function describes exactly horizontal cell activity as a function of distance from the center of the receptive field.[94] Thus, the evidence incriminating the horizontal cell in the production of the center-surround seems damning; no other cell has electrophysiological properties that match nearly so well.

Earlier workers felt the lateral inhibition of the center-surround serves to enhance contrast only by inhibiting neighboring cells, but current evidence is that lateral inhibition also performs its function in a much more subtle way, namely, by optimizing bipolar cell performance. And lateral inhibition performs this function even against a contourless background.[93] The story of how this is done tells the true worth of this mechanism to the eye.

The experimental facts that form the stage upon which the story unfolds are illustrated in Figures 2-14, 2-15, and 2-16. In Figure 2-14, the left curve illustrates an inhibition of a sustained bipolar response by a temporary increase in illumination of the surround while the right half of the figure shows bipolar operating curves at both levels of surround illumination. This is seen better in Figure 2-15A, where the predominant effect of purely surround illumination is to shift the curve to the right without diminishing its amplitude. Thus, a similar curve is retraced, but at higher test luminances. Additional background illumination only in the center (thus driving the receptors that in turn drive the bipolar under test) does not shift the curve, but merely compresses its magnitude (Fig. 2-15B) as the bipolar is driven into saturation. The combined effect of center and surround illumination are favorable, however; the bipolar not only has its operating range shifted in the direction of the higher test intensities, but the bipolar comes somewhat out of saturation (Fig. 2-15C). Thus, horizontal cell activity is important for sensitivity control.

Figure 2-16 shows the value of small shifts of the operating curve to the right or left in increasing the sensitivity of the eye to a flickering signal. In Figure 2-16A and B, the flicker is adjusted so that it oscillates about the midpoint of the operating curve without the surround. When the surround flash occurs, the amplitude of the bipolar cell response to the flicker is dampened to about half, since the operating curve shifts to the right, thus moving the flicker onto the shoulder of the curve. The reverse situation is seen in Figure 2-16 C & D. Thus,

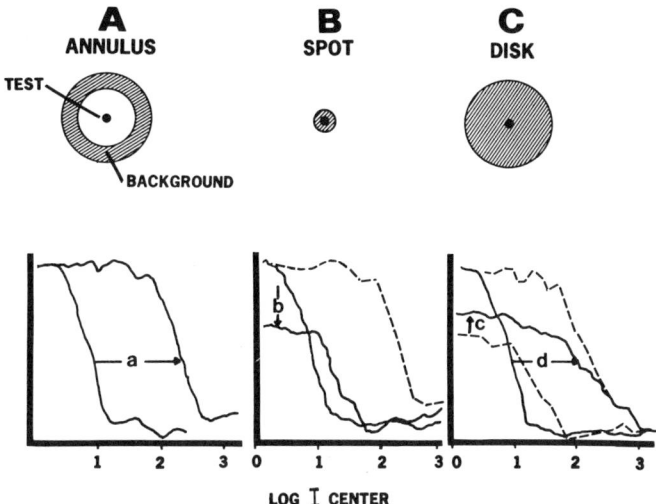

Figure 2-15 The combined effects of center and surround background on the form of the bipolar cell operating curves. **A** The surround causes the operating curve to shift parallel to itself toward the right, as indicated by arrow a. **B** The presence of an additional center spot causes the cell to hyperpolarize along its original curve, partially saturating the cell and compressing its operating curve as represented by arrow b. **C** This demonstrates the effect of expanding the background spot to include both center and surround. The effect of the center is antagonized (arrow c) and the curve is shifted to the right (arrow d). (Redrawn from Werblin.[93])

the horizontal-cell interaction increases the sensitivity by inhibiting its input, a necessity since a glance at Figure 2-15 shows that the operating curve of the bipolar spans only about 2.5 to 3.0 log units at most, whereas the receptors cover about 7 log units.

The data of Figure 2-16 also have an interesting clinical correlation. Workers in flicker fusion perimetry have noted that with *large* flickering targets, the center often appears to be fused, while the periphery appears to flicker.[67] Here, the target corresponds to the situation illustrated in Figure 2-16A & B. The edge of the target covers receptive fields still on curve A, but the center of the target (since the target is large enough to cover several receptive fields) is on curve B, and thus appears fused.

Amacrine Cells

Amacrine cells (Fig. 2-17) are the first cells of the visual pathway to exhibit transient (as opposed to sustained) slow potentials, the first to show spike activity, and the first in which activity is always associated with a depolarization. In amacrines, transient depolarizations are observed both at the onset and at

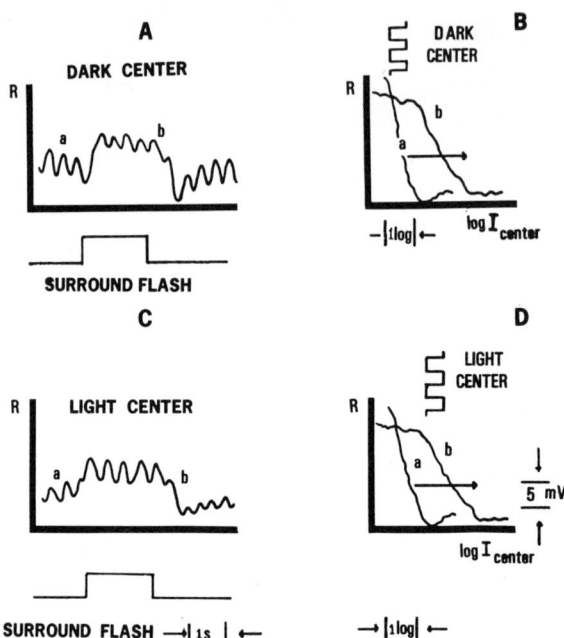

Figure 2-16 Sensitization and desensitization by annular surround backgrounds. A and C show time course of response to a flickering test against a dark background (A) and with a light central background (C). B and D show the effects of background on flicker, interpreted as intensity-response data. In A and B, the flicker (square wave at top of figure) is aligned along curve a, so when the surround shifts the curve to position b, the flicker amplitude is diminished. This is because the flicker now moves the potential along the shoulder of curve b rather than the steeply sloped portion of the curve. In C and D, the flicker is initially aligned with curve b, so enhancement of the flicker results from the addition of the surround. (Redrawn from Werblin.[93])

the cessation of illumination anywhere within their receptive fields.* Depending upon their size, these transient potentials may give rise to several (usually two or less) spike potentials.

These spikes are not thought necessary for impulse transmission since the blocking of spike activity in the dragon fly by use of tetrodotoxin does not prohibit the appearance of a postsynaptic potential in the ganglion cells.

The transient "on" and "off" response of the amacrine cell is somewhat enigmatic. How the sustained responses of the bipolar, horizontal, and receptor cells are converted into transient responses by amacrine cells is not yet proved

---

*The position of the illumination and other factors, however, may cause the relative size of these "on" and "off" responses to vary somewhat.

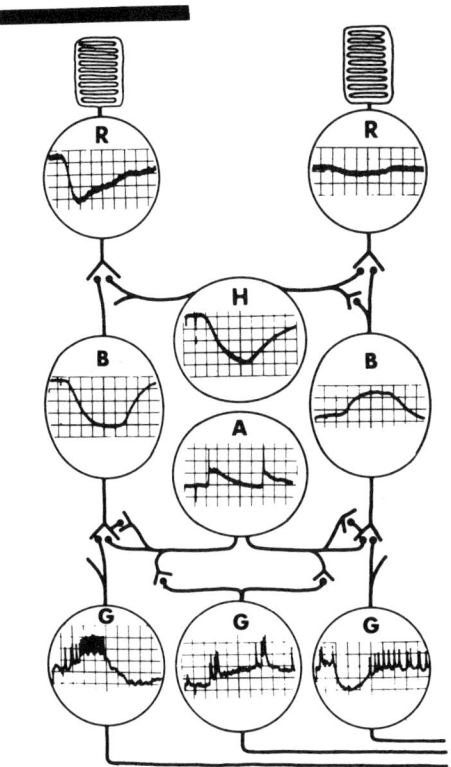

Figure 2-17 Summary diagram of the correlation between the synaptic interconnections and the intracellularly recorded neuronal responses in the mud puppy. (See also Fig. 2–7 for morphology.) The experimental condition depicted here is a bright flash of light on the left receptor (R) with a lower background level falling on both receptors. [The presence of background illumination is necessary to demonstrate the antagonism of the horizontal cell (H) on the right bipolar cell (B).] The left bipolar shows a strong hyperpolarizing response from input from the receptor, as does the horizontal cell. The hoizontal cell successfully antagonizes the weaker input from the right receptor, and the right bipolar shows a depolarization. This picture would be reversed in the case of a depolarizing bipolar cell. The amacrine cell (A) is shown receiving input from the bipolars and synapsing onto the central ganglion cell (G), which is a simplification of the actual myriad of synaptic arrangements. The amacrine cells fire at the onset and cessation of a spot of light within their receptive field. Note that two small depolarizing slow potentials are seen, accompanied by spiking on the rising phase. Three types of ganglion-cell responses are illustrated. "On" activity (left), with spiking during the stimulus, is due to the contact through direct bipolar–ganglion interaction. "Off" activity (right) may be due to input from the surround or from a depolarizing bipolar. "On-off" activity (center) is due to amacrine–bipolar interaction and is found largely in motion-sensitive ganglion cells with complex receptive fields. (With permission from Dowling.[25])

exactly, although this conversion is thought to be involved with the synaptic morphology of the amacrines. As we indicated earlier (Fig. 2-7), amacrine cells often immediately synapse back onto the presynaptic element. This anatomical connection may serve as the mediator of presynaptic inhibition, for picrotoxin does abolish the transient response of the amacrine cell and convert it into a sustained response. The fact that picrotoxin is known to eliminate presynaptic inhibition is not conclusive, however, for the drug has other effects on the nervous system.

Like the cones and bipolar cells, the amacrine cells show a smooth response curve that spans about one log unit of intensity. This curve shifts along the intensity axis as a function of background intensity. The behavior of the amacrine can also be modified to a large extent by other conditions of the surround. Movement, for example, is especially effective in eliciting a response. A moving "windmill" pattern of light spinning about the amacrine cell causes a sustained level of depolarization. Central test spots that are static, however, still elicit a transient depolarization at "on" and "off." Flashing annuli of light also depolarize the response of amacrine cells to change in the periphery of the visual field and carry lateral antagonistic signals to the ganglion cells.[95]

Ganglion Cells

The ganglion cell is the first cell in the visual pathway in which spike potentials are unquestionably necessary for the cell's function. These cells exhibit numerous spikes riding on transient depolarizing potentials, and the number of spikes fired is closely related to the degree of depolarization. Unlike the remaining cell types of the retina, the ganglion cells are thus much more similar to the other cells of the nervous system.

Ganglion cell response can be roughly divided into three types. One resembles an amacrine cell in that transient spiking occurs at the onset and cessation of stimulation. The other two mimic a bipolar cell with spiking either during the "on" or the "off" phase. Because this behavior seems to correlate well with the cell's anatomy, it suggests those gangion cells that show "on-off" activity are very likely receiving most of their input directly from amacrines, while those that show "on" or "off" activity are synapsing with either hyperpolarizing or depolarizing bipolar cells respectively. The "on-off" ganglion cell is affected by light and especially by movement in the surround (Figs. 2-18, 2-19). Both the "on" and the "off" ganglion cells show a shift in their operating curves parallel to their original waves with an illuminated surround, but movement in the surround has no effect (Fig. 2-20). The receptive field of the "on" or "off" ganglion cell seems to be determined exclusively by the bipolar field; the receptive field of the "on-off" ganglion cell is further modified by amacrine cell interaction.[95] Thus,

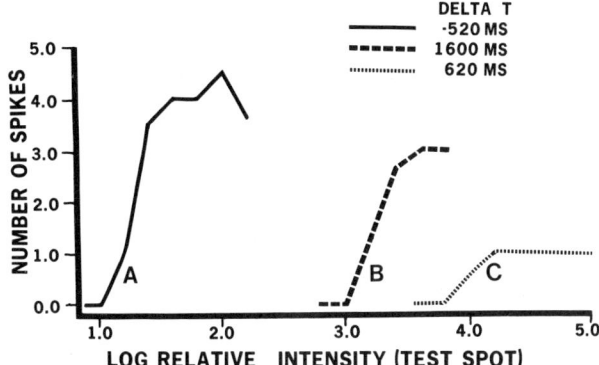

Figure 2-18 Effect of a flash of light peripherally on the operating curves of an "on-off" ganglion cell. A was plotted 520 msec before the peripheral flash, B at 1.6 sec after the flash, and C at 620 msec after. Note that a test spot 4 log units brighter was required to elicit a response at C as compared to A. Recovery has already begun at C. Maximum inhibition occurs 250 msec after the flash but is unmeasurable. The ordinate is the number of spikes and the abscissa is the log intensity of the test spot. (Redrawn from Werblin and Copenhagen.[95])

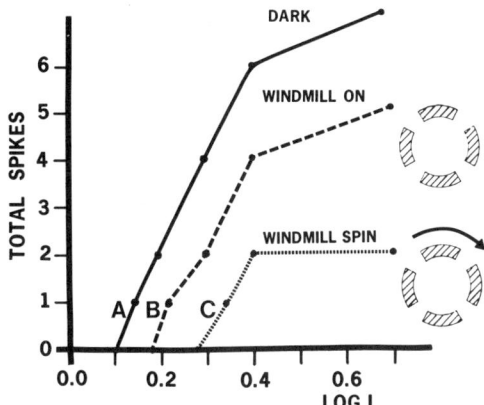

Figure 2-19 Effect of movement in the surround on the "on-off" ganglion cell. A "windmill" pattern consisting of a circular annulus with alternating illuminated and dark segments (as illustrated) provided motion in the surround. Operating curves were determined under dark conditions both with the windmill illuminated but stationary and with the windmill illuminated and rotating. Some inhibition occurs with unchanging illumination of the surround, but movement in the surround is most effective in producing inhibition. The ordinate is the number of spikes fired, and the abscissa is the log intensity in absorbed photons/receptor. (Redrawn from Werblin and Copenhagen.[95])

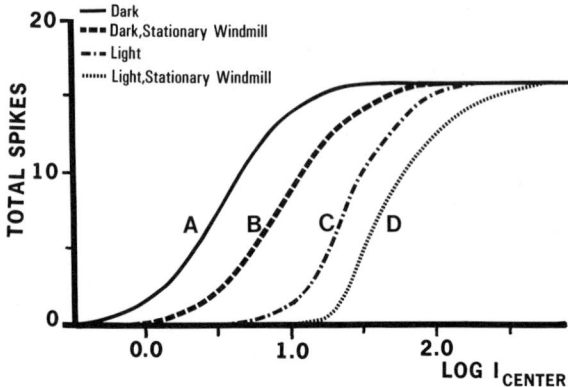

Figure 2-20   Intensity response curve for an "on"-type ganglion cell. The abscissa and ordinate are the same as in Figure 2–19. Curve A was plotted with dark adaptation, curve B, with a dark background plus a stationary windmill, curve C with a light background, curve D with a light background and a stationary windmill. Rotation of the windmill in curves B and D did not have an effect, so no data for movement alone is plotted. Thus the "on" (and the "off") cells are affected by light, but not movement, in the surround. (Redrawn from Werblin and Copenhagen.[95])

some ganglion cells are very sensitive to motion whereas others are not, a finding in keeping with previously discussed division of receptive fields into simple and complex types.

Summary of Electrophysiology

One may summarize the physiology so far by stating that the receptor cells have relatively small receptive fields and react only to central light. They may or may not have feedback from the horizontal cells. Horizontal cells, on the other hand, receive input over a wide area, and are apparently driven directly by the receptor cell. Their response is sustained for the duration of the stimulus. Likewise, the bipolar cells receive input directly from receptors and respond with a graded, sustained potential, which is antagonized by horizontal cell activity. The simple center-surround organization is the function of the horizontal cell. The horizontal-bipolar organization serves to maximize the sensitivity of the bipolar.

Amacrine cells appear to be involved in motion detection, and are responsible for directional sensitivity in those species with complex receptive fields. Certainly, the center-surround activity of simple receptive fields cannot be explained by amacrines since this center-surround antagonism is sustained over the duration of the stimulus whereas amacrines show only transient potentials at the onset and at the cessation of the stimulus. Motion sensitive ganglion cells appear to receive mainly amacrine input, but exactly how they interact has not

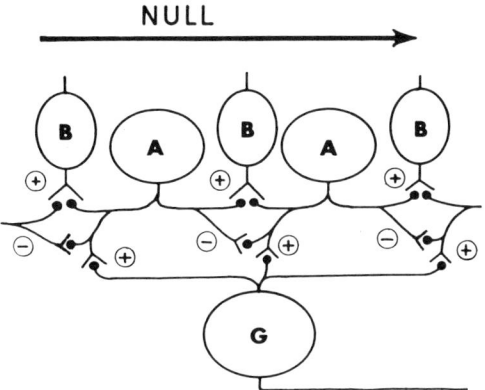

Figure 2-21 A proposed scheme of how directionally selective ganglion cell activity could be mediated by synaptic activity if bipolars (B) terminate mainly on amacrine cells (A), and the synapsing ganglion cell receives input from only amacrine cells. A spot moving in the direction of the null arrow will cause no response, since the amacrine cell "upstream" presynaptically inhibits "downstream" cells at the serial synapses. A spot moving in the other direction will be seen. Circled pluses indicate facilitation; circled minuses indicate inhibition. (With permission from Dowling.[25])

yet been shown. One hypothetical scheme is shown in Figure 2-21. The transient nature of the amacrine cell response, however, is well suited to explain the similar responses to a bright spot moving on a dark background and a dark spot moving on a light background. The presence of serial synaptic organization from the outer plexiform layer affords the opportunity for complex facilitory or inhibitory interactions among bipolar, amacrine, and ganglion cells. Thus, it may be said that the outer plexiform layer is concerned with static and spatial aspects of retinal physiology whereas the inner plexiform layer is more concerned with the dynamic and temporal aspects of retinal function.

One may utilize the operating curves for each cell type to derive the input-output curve for the retina as was done by Werblin and Copenhagan.[95] Examples of the responses and relationships of each cell to the other are illustrated in Figure 2-17.

The Control of Retinal Sensitivity

The title of this section, "The Control of Retinal Sensitivity," was deliberately chosen to avoid the word adaptation. Although we will discuss the physiological bases of adaptive processes, first let us turn briefly to the electrophysiological happenings that form the basis of the psychophysical events. In describing retinal events, we will not spend much time with data that are subjectively acquired, that is, data as influenced by such factors as responses from the higher centers or the observer's psychological state. However incomplete our knowledge concerning the adaptive processes may still be, we hope to refocus our current knowledge so that the reader may "see the light" a little easier for himself.

A dark-adapted rod is a magnificently efficient mechanism for the detection of light. Its efficiency occasionally permits it to react to the absorption of one quantum of light, thereby reaching the theoretically maximum possible sensitivity.[75] The coincident absorption of from six to eight quanta of light by a rod results in the appreciation of a visual sensation by most observers approximately 55% of the time.* This figure is not 100% because of statistical variations in the number of quanta of light that are emitted from a source at such low illuminances. One should recall, however, that the function of the eye is to see detail and not merely to inform one that darkness is total or that light is present in some degree. Six quanta of light may be significantly different from none, a totally dark background, but when one considers the vast number of quanta being emitted from light sources in the photopic range, six quanta are far less than the statistically significant variance in the output of bright light sources. Therefore, if the eye is to discriminate accurately among objects under normal lighting conditions, the eye must not respond to a difference in brightness that is constant in terms of quanta across the entire visual range but to a brightness difference that is somehow proportional to current brightness. The success with which the eye is capable of performing this task is truly magnificent, for the operational range of the eye spans some ten log units of brightness.

Perhaps the first thought that comes to mind when the subject of variation in retinal sensitivity is discussed is bleaching of the retinal photopigments. To be sure, bleaching of the retinal photopigments does occur and each time a photon is absorbed by a rod, one molecule of pigment is apparently bleached. Under conditions of fairly bright illumination, bleaching serves as an efficient means of diminishing light sensitivity of the eye, since bleached photopigments are unable to absorb photons and thus unable to cause energy to be imparted to the photoreceptor. A significant amount of photopigment bleaching does not occur, however, until a substantial adapting intensity is reached. For example, Dowling noted in rats that the increment threshold† for the electroretinogram rises linearly after the adapting intensities exceed the absolute ERG threshold by 0.5

---

*About 80 quanta are required at the cornea for threshold stimulation of a rod because many photons are lost by reflection and absorption in the media and a few pass through the rods without absorption by rhodopsin. Threshold stimulation of a cone requires direct absorption of 38 to 40 quanta at the receptor, or 490 to 800 quanta at the cornea.[10]

†An increment threshold is a value obtained by *adding* small increments of stimulus (here, brightness) to a background stimulus. Perimetry is typically done in this manner. A *substitution* threshold depends upon the opposite procedure in which the background and test stimuli replace one another and are never present at the same time.

log units.[24] In these same experiments, no measurable fraction of the total rhodopsin is bleached until the adapting intensities exceed the ERG threshold by five log units (Fig. 2-22). Thus, photopigment bleaching does not appear to play a part in the process of light adaptation until substantial intensities are reached. Essentially the same result was obtained by Normann and Werblin in Necturus.[73] In summary, adaptation consists of two processes, one photochemical and the other neural. Neural adaptation is characterized by rapid onset at low light levels while photochemical processes occur more slowly at illumination levels that approach the photopic range.

It has also been suggested that "signal pooling" by the rods is significant in the adaptation process. This idea was initially postulated by Rushton[78] and demonstrated in the toad by Fain.[32] Basically, when a photon is received by one

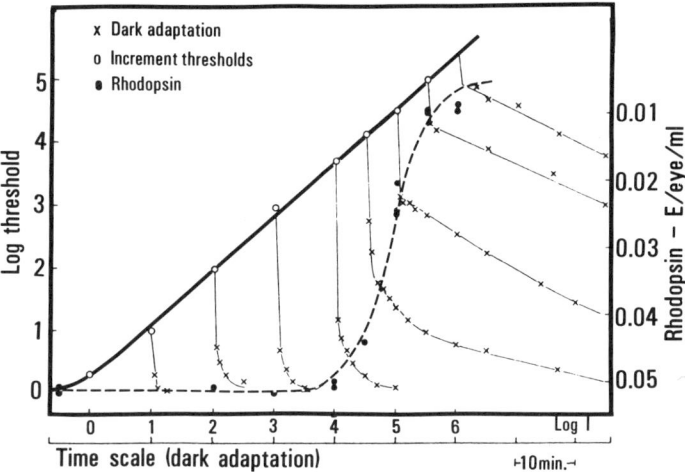

Figure 2-22 In a rat retina, the effect of five minutes of light adaptation at various luminances on the rhodopsin content (black dots along broken line), on increment thresholds of the ERG (outline dots along solid line), and on dark-adaptation ERG thresholds (crosses on the thin line). The left ordinate is the log increment threshold (expressed as log multiple of the absolute increment threshold; in other words, log threshold = 2 means that at this value, the increment threshold was 100 absolute threshold). The right ordinate is the rhodopsin concentration. The abscissa is the log-adapting illuminance, relative to increment threshold (upper) and relative time scale (each division = 10 min).

The log increment threshold rises linearly with the log-adapting intensity once Log I (abscissa) is above 0.5. The rhodopsin concentration, however, does not significantly fall until an adapting intensity of 4 log units is reached. Similarly, the time course of dark adaptation is rapid up to this point, the retina returning to a dark-adapted status within 10 minutes. Once photochemical bleaching of the rhodopsin occurs, readaptation takes much longer. Thus, dark and light adaptation are seen to consist of two processes: a neural process occurring with low background luminance from which recovery is rapid; and a photochemical process occurring only at higher background intensities from which recovery is relatively slow. (With permission from Dowling.[24])

receptor, it apparently generates a potential that is "shared" or "pooled" with nearby receptors. Although Rushton thought that the signal generated in a single rod is shared throughout the entire retina, the phenomenon is actually much more localized. Signal pooling causes the electrical response recorded in a given receptor to be much greater than would otherwise be expected from the number of photons falling on the retina and thereby increases sensitivity in the dark-adapted state. With slightly higher illumination, this effect may tend to push the rod slightly further along its operating curve toward saturation and thus to decrease the response per increment illumination. At still higher levels, the effect may become insignificant compared with photopigment bleaching. Potential sharing has been demonstrated to occur via interreceptor gap junctions in some fish and amphibia. How and whether it occurs in other species is in doubt. Enhanced retinal sensitivity is also accomplished by spatial summation, where multiple receptors feed one bipolar cell, which in turn joins with other bipolars to converge on one ganglion cell. Indeed, both mechanisms—potential sharing and spatial summation—may well be at play in the human retina, since cones exclusively exhibit gap junctions, while lateral summation is more prominent with the rods. Finally, horizontal cell activity causes a shift of the bipolar operating curve so that electrical response varies according to input from the receptors. A similar shifting occurs in the operating curve of the ganglion cells. Although the majority of the sensitivity control is undoubtedly due to changes in the photoreceptors themselves, these "downstream" adjustments can account for several log units of change in the threshold.

Regardless of the cause, a knowledge of dark-adaptation curves from a purely descriptive basis is of use to the perimetrist in the performance of the visual field test. The dark-adaptation curve of a normal subject shows two limbs, as is illustrated in Figure 2-23. The upper curve, labeled "cones," is due largely to adaptation of the cones and is relatively short, on the order of 10 minutes. The break in the curve corresponds to equal sensitivity of rods and cones, or mesopic conditions, whereas farther down the curve the rods are much more sensitive than the cones, and these are considered to be scotopic conditions. Since there are no rods in the fovea, one would expect there to be a relative central scotoma under scotopic conditions, and these may be seen in Aulhorn's curves, illustrated in Figure 1-7. When the perimetrist uses photopic backgrounds, dark-adaptation times are short, namely, on the order of 10 minutes. With scotopic tests, much longer times are required, namely, on the order of 30 minutes at a minimum and up to several hours in high levels of luminance, such as at the beach.[10] Changing of the dark-adaptation status during the test is disastrous; spiraling fields or huge amounts of scatter result. This problem can be avoided only by scrupulously dark-adapting every patient or by choosing photopic perimetry. We prefer the latter course.

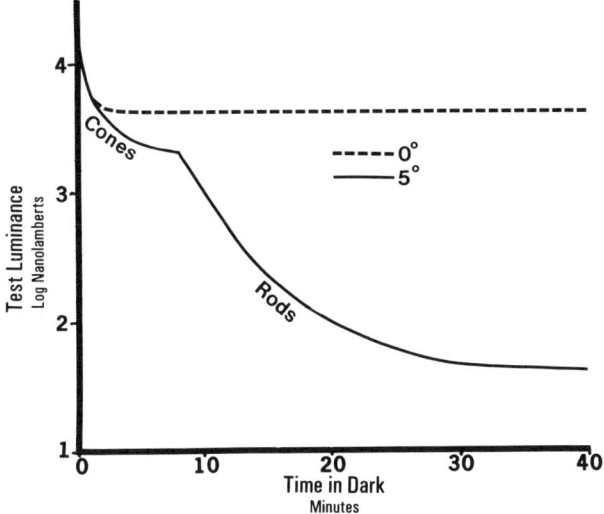

Figure 2-23 Dark-adaptation curves for the human at 0° and 5° eccentricity. Note that centrally, adaptation is virtually complete within 3–5 minutes, whereas at 5° the process continues for over 30 minutes. The discontinuity in the 5° curve is known as the rod-cone break. The timing and intensity at which this break occurs vary with retinal location.

The Organization of the Higher Centers

Further integration of the visual signals coming from the retina occurs at the lateral geniculate body[13,19,52,55] and the visual cortex.[19,53,54] The receptive fields of the lateral geniculate body have an organization reminiscent of the retina. Four cell types are present in the lateral geniculate body: an "on" cell, an "off" cell, an "on-off" cell, and a cell that decreases the frequency of its discharge during illumination. The receptive fields show concentric "center-surround" organization just as in the retina. Little binocular interaction is noted at the level of the lateral geniculate. Input from nonvisual sources is present at the lateral geniculate and may conceivably modify the visual response. Lateral geniculate cells respond well to diffuse retinal illumination and in some ways seem less specific to direction and motion than the retinal cells themselves. Hubel feels that the main function of the lateral geniculate body is in responding to spatial differences of retinal illumination and thereby increasing the contrast between small spots of light and the background.[52,55]

Cortical organization is far more complex than that seen at lower levels. We owe much of our knowledge of cortical activity to the studies by Hubel[52,53] who meticulously mapped out the receptive fields of cortical cells to stationary and moving lights. These receptive fields differ from those of the retina and lateral geniculate body in that they have a large variety of shapes and are not simply concentric circles. Furthermore, binocular interaction is seen for the first time as an almost constant feature.

The conditions of the stimulus are more important in determining the type of response in the cortex than in any of the lower visual centers. Diffuse illumination of the retina does not seem to have much effect on the cortex, but diffuse illumination does affect the retina and therefore must alter the input to the cortex. An appropriately placed point source of illumination produces a response in most cortical cells, and movement of this spot of light is especially effective in producing widespread cortical activity. The cortical cells respond selectively to direction of movement or, in the case of a moving edge of light, even to the orientation of the edge with respect to the direction of movement.

It is not unusual to find one cortical cell which is influenced by a retinal area of five millimeters diameter, whereas the retinal receptive field in that zone is found to measure only two millimeters. This differential seems to imply that the cortex does not truly represent the retina in a point-to-point manner but that specific cortical cells are involved in processing various types of information arising from relatively limited but not minuscule areas of the retina.

Organization of the cortical receptive fields, like the retina, can be divided into two types: simple and complex. The simple fields in the cortex detect the orientation of stationary bars or edges of light on the retina. These receptive fields can be thought of as rectangles with a stripe down the center, the center stripe being analogous to either "on" or "off" centers and the surrounding area being antagonistic to the center reponse. Thus, if a visible bar is oriented so its cortical representation is along "on" center, the cell will fire. If the bar is then rotated 90° such that more of the "off" surround is exposed to the bar than the "on" center, nothing will happen. If the cell lies obliquely such that slightly more center area is stimulated than surround, a weak response may be obtained. Complex cortical fields also respond to edges and their orientation, but they do not discriminate with regard to position. Like the complex receptive fields of the retina, these respond to motion. Hubel has suggested that the "simple" cortical cells receive input directly from the lateral geniculate body whereas the complex cortical cells receive input from numerous simple cortical cells and represent a higher level of integration. Thus, a complex cortical cell that responds to movement of a bar with a given orientation receives its input from a huge number of simple cortical cells, all of which have receptive fields with a similar orientation. This implies that a staggering amount of interconnection and integration occurs at the cortex, and one would expect that the cortical cells must have a very precise arrangement in order to make this possible. Hubel has found that functionally the cortex is divided into a multitude of columns of cells that extend from the surface down to the white matter with the cells in each column having the same receptive field orientations. There are numerous interconnections between the cells vertically so that the net result is that each of these columns forms an integrative center in which simple cells receive input directly from the lateral geniculate body and in turn provide output to the complex cell. Thus, the organization at the cortical level is such that differences in brightness are the most important visual stimuli.

Physiological and Psychophysical Correlations

The foregoing physiological studies provide an important background for the understanding of clinical perimetry. In fact, one can predict many of the dictums that have been discovered through the years.

One example of this concerns the behavior of the eye at different states of dark-light adaptation to small spots of light. In Figure 2-10 one sees that the curve of threshold increment stimulus versus background brightness at different states of dark adaptation is nonlinear until one reaches the photopic level. Once the background luminance rises above about -1 log Asb, the curve flattens. At this stage, the cones begin to function, colors are appreciated, and visual acuity improves. From about $+1$ log Asb, the curve is linear throughout the remaining visual range. This is explained by the fact that at scotopic levels the rods are the predominating receptor, and as we have seen, their response curve is nonlinear. In the mesopic range the rods have begun to saturate and the cones have begun to function. In the photopic range the rods are saturated and they contribute very little to the operating curve of the retina. The cones, which behave linearly over their operating range, therefore produce a linear plot. This part of the plot may be said to obey Weber's Law,* since the Weber fraction ($\triangle B/B$) is constant over the photopic range. This constancy is of great practical importance for the perimetrist. Visual field tests done in the photopic range with equipment that permits both the background and the test object to receive their illumination from the same light are practically immune to small variations in the light output due to bulb aging, line voltage fluctuation, and so forth. Because the ratio of a given test's stimulus to background luminance remains constant, the thresholds at different absolute values still lie on the same curve, leaving isopter lines unchanged. If the perimetrist chooses to work in the mesopic or scotopic ranges, this disregard for absolute values will not be valid since $\triangle B/B$ is not constant in either of these brightness ranges. It is for these reasons that the

---

*Weber's Law states that a just noticeable change in stimulus divided by the stimulus is a constant. This is usually written as

$$\frac{\triangle B}{B} = K$$

Goldmann Perimeter is designed so that the projected test and the background light are provided by the same bulb.

Kinetic Versus Static Perimetry

The foregoing physiological data provides us with a far deeper insight than merely to aid in the choice of which light range we choose to perform our perimetry. The anatomical and electrophysiological findings would seem to indicate there are basic differences in the physiological functions tested by kinetic and static perimetry, and that the two sets of test results are not completely interconvertible. For clinical purposes it is far simpler to think of kinetic perimetry as the measuring of a visual island by the moving of a test spot in the "horizontal" direction, whereas profile or static perimetry is the measuring of a visual island in the "vertical" direction. There are, however, some subtle differences between the two techniques.

Perhaps the first studies to differentiate the perception of movement from the perception of form were those by George Riddoch, a British physician, who published in 1917 a series of cases of patients who had suffered occipital injuries.[77] His patients had large areas of the visual field in which stationary stimuli could not be seen, but movement was readily recognized. Figure 2-24 shows an example of the visual fields of one of Dr. Riddoch's patients. Later Zappia et al [107] published a series of cases that show the Riddoch phenomenon is associated with lesions other than those in the occipital lobe, notably with lesions in the optic tract.

McColgin carried out perimetry on normal subjects in which the perception of motion was the end point.[68] He found that an individual's movement sensitivity decreases linearly from the fovea to the retinal periphery. The isograms obtained for either rotary or linear motion are elliptical in shape with the horizontal axis approximately twice as long as the vertical axis. He also noted that the sensitivity to rotary movement is less for a uniocular field than for binocular fields. Finally, Fankhauser and Schmidt[36] showed in a beautiful set of curves (Fig. 2-25) that static thresholds are generally slightly higher than kinetic thresholds at the periphery of the visual field, whereas the reverse is true centrally. This means that a subthreshold peripheral stationary spot of light can be made to appear by moving it slowly, whereas near to fovea a stationary spot of light that is just visible can be made to disappear by moving it. This result correlates with the smaller receptive fields that are generally found near the fovea. These smaller receptive fields theoretically decrease the opportunity for lateral interaction.

These data put to rest the idea that kinetic and static fields are exactly identical, although the differences are subtle ones and for practical clinical purposes they may be considered as equivalent. Nevertheless, the fact that

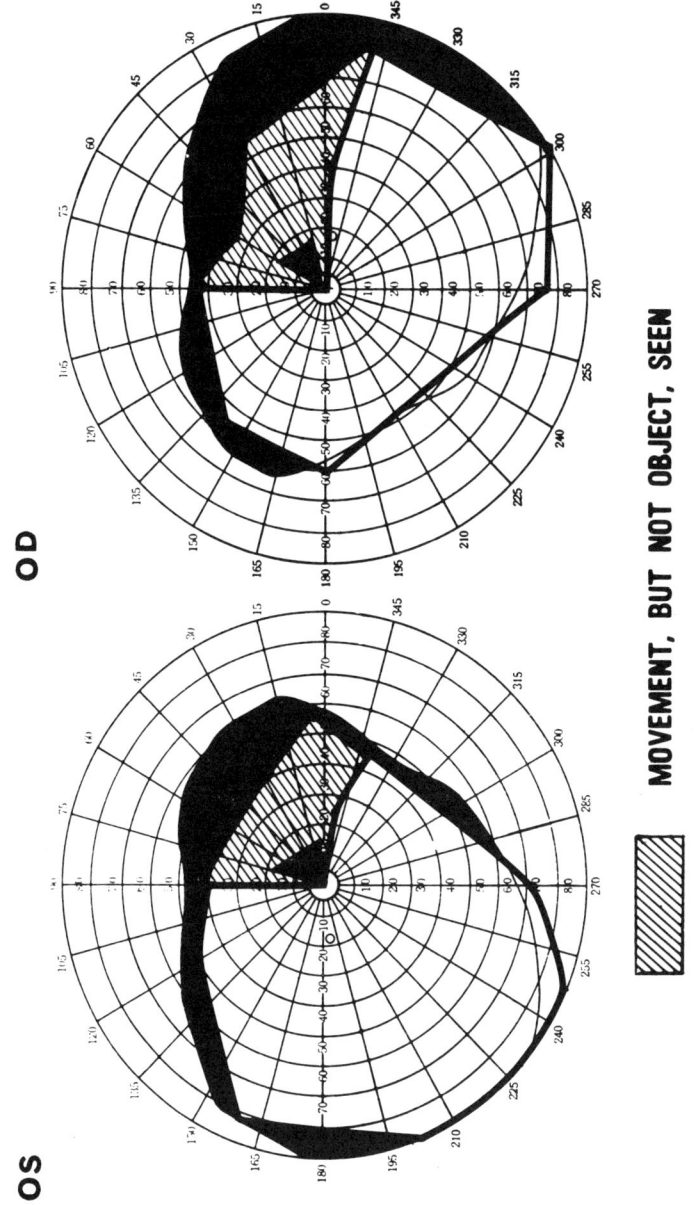

Figure 2-24 Fields demonstrating the Riddoch phenomena. The black area shows an area of field in which neither movement nor a stationary object can be seen. The diagonally shaded area corresponds to area in which movement but no stationary objects, however large, can be seen. (Redrawn from Riddoch.[77])

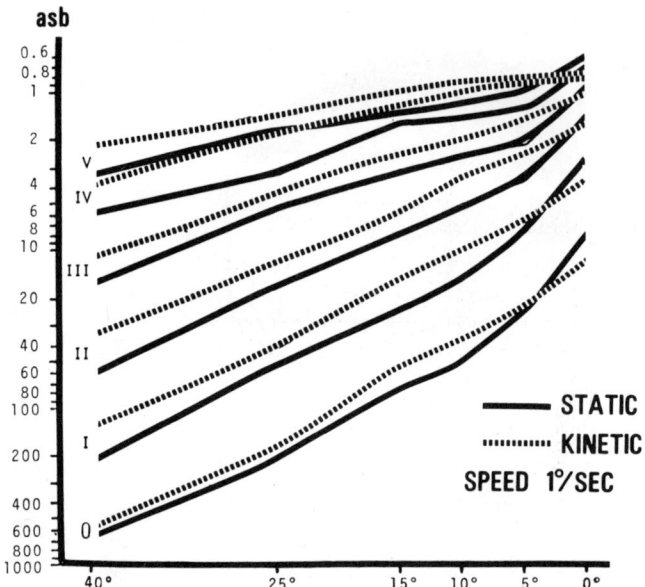

Figure 2-25 The difference in threshold value found in normal subjects with static (solid line) and kinetic (dotted line) perimetry. The ordinate is the test luminance in asb. The abscissa is the eccentricity in degrees. The roman numeral (0 through V) to the left of each pair of lines gives the corresponding size of the test object on the Goldmann Perimeter. Note that kinetic thresholds are lower (thus, a higher line) in the periphery than static thresholds, where the reverse is true centrally. (Redrawn from Fankhauser and Schmidt.[36])

movement itself is a stimulus to the retina means that the kinetic perimetrist must be careful to standardize the test velocity.

Goldmann has suggested five degrees per second peripherally,[39] whereas Fankhauser feels that two degrees per second is a bit better[33] because it allows slightly more precise resolution of scotomas when the combined reaction time of the patient and the doctor is taken into account. Although there may be sound reasons for varying the object speed from test to test because of patient reaction time, distraction, or other reasons, one should be aware that variable velocities cause variable thresholds. It should also be emphasized that resolution of small scotomas is a function of target speed, and one cannot find tiny areas of defect utilizing a high velocity.

Temporal and Spatial Summation

Large, long-lasting spots are empirically more effective as visual stimuli than spots of a small size and short duration. Spatial and temporal summation (or integration) operate quantitatively within limits that are small and brief. Temporal integration means that there are transmission delays along the visual pathway and that additional photons, in striking a given receptor, cause an increase in that receptor's potential if they arrive before the effects of the preceding photons have worn off completely. Spatial summation means that impulses from many adjacent receptor cells converge potentially on a single ganglion cell; hence, the more receptor cells are stimulated by increasing the area of the stimulus, the more the combined outputs these receptor cells are likely to reach the threshold of their ganglion cell. Both of these summation mechanisms are progressively active in eccentric retinal positions.

Temporal integration is described by Bloch's law (B·T = constant). This applies only to very small targets for short exposures since the light difference sensitivity fails to increase once the exposure passes a certain length of time (Bloch's time). Aulhorn and Harms have investigated this phenomenon[5] and find that with exposure times longer than 0.5 second, no further decrease in the light difference threshold is noted (Fig. 2-26). This has been substantiated by Alexandres[1] who notes that the time to saturation for the temporal summation effect also varies somewhat as a function of retinal location as well as the light–dark adaptation status of the eye. Therefore, if exposure times during static perimetry are kept as long as one second, the effect of temporal integration is effectively neutralized. This solution is less than ideal, for with long

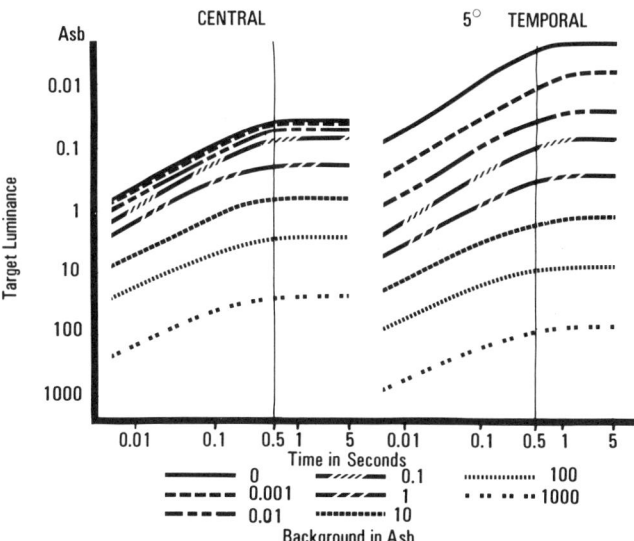

Figure 2-26 Temporal summation: the effect of different exposure times on light difference thresholds in normal subjects under differing degrees of adaptation. The ordinate is the increment threshold, Asb. The abscissa is the exposure time in seconds. The parameter on each curve is the background luminance. (Redrawn from Aulhorn and Harms.[5])

stimulus times, fixation often wanders. Greve[43] observes that the interindividual variance in temporal summation is small and feels that electric shutters with short stimulus presentations provide a more suitable solution to the problem of temporal summation in clinical patients who fixate irregularly. With kinetic perimetry, the temporal summation effect cannot be neutralized, and the degree to which it influences the threshold is uncertain, largely because reaction time variance often exceeds the summation effect. The combined effects of temporal and spatial summation may make the shape of the test object just as important to the kinetic perimetrist as the area. A small rectangle with its short axis parallel to the direction of movement is a less efficient stimulus under some conditions than with its long axis parallel to the direction of movement, since the opportunity for temporal summation is decreased in the former case.

Spatial summation is a different question and is of great pertinence to perimetry, for spatial summation is the mechanism by which the stimulus value increases with increasing size of test objects in devices that employ test objects of various sizes such as the Goldmann Perimeter or the tangent screen. The basic concept of spatial summation is that an increase in area may be substituted for an increase in the brightness of a test stimulus. When summation is complete, one expects that the sum of the logarithm of the luminance of the test object and the logarithm of its area will be equal to a constant, that is, $\log B + \log A = C$. In practice, summation is usually incomplete so this equation is modified to read $\log B + K \log A = C$ where the constant K is called the summation coefficient or the summation exponent (since this equation may also be written $BA^K = C$). When $K = 1$, we say Ricco's law holds. Piper's law is said to hold when $K = 0.5$, and Pieron's law corresponds to $K = 0.33$. This plethora of laws describing the same fundamental process indicates that the summation constant is a function of retinal position and the adaptational status of the retina.[3] This would be expected, of course, from the receptive field data discussed previously. During his initial studies,[39,40] Goldmann was well aware that there is a small variation in K over the retina, but concluded that a summation coefficient of about 0.8 is a useful approximation for the purposes of clinical perimetry. Thus, the areas of the standard test objects on the Goldmann Perimeter differ from the next larger spot by 0.6 log units (i.e., they increase by a factor of 4) whereas the luminances of the standard test objects differ from the next brighter spot by 0.5 log units, (i.e., they increase by a factor of 3.16). Sloan has examined this question in great detail and finds that the summation coefficient in reality varies from 0.55 at the fovea to 0.9 at 45° nasally (Fig. 2-27).[80,81]
These values were all obtained under photopic conditions, and Fankhauser and Schmidt[36] point out that the summation ability of the retina increases as the retina becomes more dark adapted. They agree that the summation coefficient is not constant across the entire retina. Aulhorn and Luddeke (personal communication) have also examined the problem and find that K also varies to some

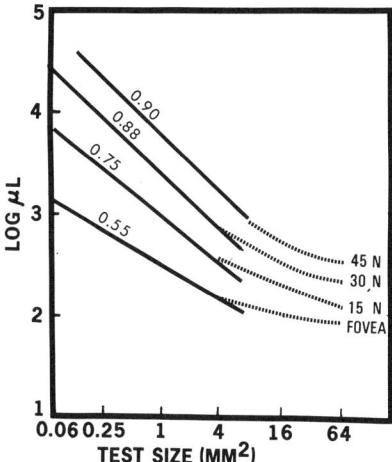

Figure 2-27 The relationship of retinal location to summation coefficient, K. The ordinate is the target luminance in log micro-Lamberts. The abscissa is the target area in square millimeters. The parameters above each curve are the summation coefficients, while the parameters to the right of each curve give retinal position in degrees from fixation (here, all nasal). Although the principle of a K that varies with retinal location is undoubtedly true, other investigators have found different values for K, and that K also depends on target size (as did Sloan, et al, for areas over 4mm^2) and differing adaptation conditions. (Redrawn from Sloan and Brown.[81])

extent with the size of the test object. One must thus be very careful in assuming that the size and brightness steps on the Goldmann Perimeter are as interchangeable as one might assume. Although they are approximately equal under normal conditions, they are not sufficiently close to permit the interchanging of, for example, an I-4-e isopter with a IV-1-e isopter and the drawing of valid conclusions about any change present between the two visual fields. In clinical practice, then, the procedure seems clear: one should adopt the standard series of sizes and luminances with the Goldmann Perimeter and stick to it unless other factors dictate a change in technique.

The topics of temporal and spatial summation along with the "frequency of seeing" curve are closely related to the phenomenon of scatter seen with kinetic perimetry. These phenomena serve to underscore the difference between the static and kinetic techniques. A "frequency of seeing" curve for a given area in the visual field may be plotted by repeatedly presenting a test spot of a given size at each of a graded series of luminances and by recording the subjective response to each presentation. The results of such an effort do reveal a range of luminances over which the spot is *never* seen (probability of seeing = 0), a range over which the spot is *always* seen (probability of seeing = 100%), and a range of luminances over which the spot is seen some of the time (Fig. 2-28). This "uncertain range" spans approximately 0.3 log units in *trained* observers.

110   Principles of Quantitative Perimetry

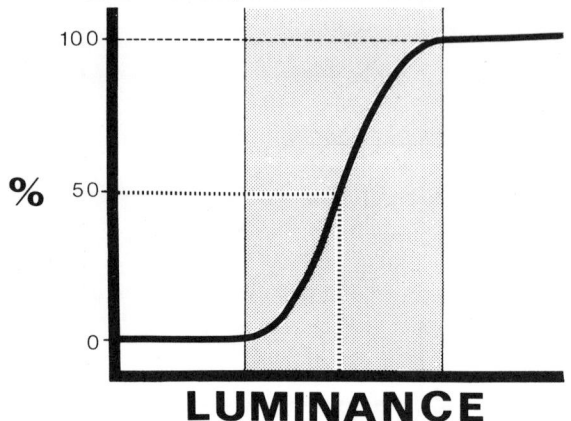

Figure 2-28   Example of a frequency of seeing curve. The grey "partial response zone" represents the luminance range over which the subject changes from never responding to a test object (0%) to always responding to a test object (100%). The ordinate is the percent of tests seen at a given brightness. The abscissa is the luminance.

Since in any current form of clinical perimetry the stimulus is gradually brought closer and closer to threshold until it is seen once and the position marked, a certain percentage of the responses will be seen "early" (toward the low end of the frequency of seeing zone) where others will penetrate more deeply before being seen. The width of this zone of uncertainty varies with the sensitivity gradient, or slope of that portion of the field under investigation (Fig. 2-29).

This difficulty is compounded by the two types of summation; the opportunity for temporal summation to influence threshold occurs only within a certain brightness range, whereas spatial summation is a topographic phenomenon. If the slope of the field is shallow enough, these two phenomena will act over a considerable expanse of retina, whereas with a steep slope, their ability to influence the threshold is limited (Fig. 2-29). This is compounded by the existence of the "uncertain zone" and in areas with a flat slope, one may find closely spaced isopters (e.g., those that differ by 0.1 to 0.3 log units) may scatter into one another. In fact, it may not even be possible to plot an isopter reproducibly through such areas. The scatter phenomenon varies with velocity of movement (which affects the temporal summation mechanism, cells that are responsive to motion, and also scatter because of variances in reaction time) and with spot size (which always affects spatial summation and, since the target is moving, temporal summation as well). These interactions are nonquantitative and poorly understood, but their existence should be noted by anyone undertaking a study of kinetic perimetry. It has been suggested[43] that the cotangent of the slope of the visual field (which is higher as the slope is flatter) gives a rough measure of the likelihood of scatter related to these interactions in a kinetic examination. A

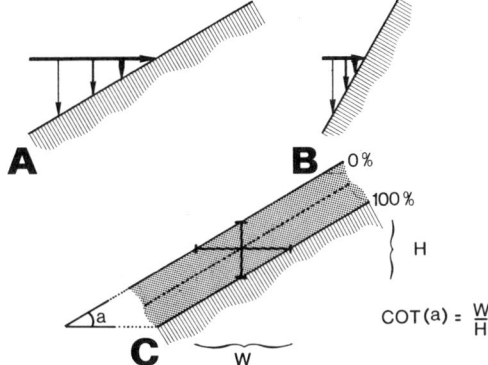

Figure 2-29 Diagrammatic representation of how spatial summation and the "frequency of seeing curve" affect scatter in kinetic thresholds. A and B show that with a flat slope, spatial summation may occur over a wider range than with a steep slope, and that the closer one comes to the "surface" (i.e., 100% response, hatched area), the stronger the summation is. C attempts to show the quantitative aspects of the problem. The distance H is a function of the underlying receptor and is thus more or less independent of slope. W is the length of the path that a kinetic stimulus must traverse through the "partial response zone" to get to the 100% response surface; thus, the length of W is somewhat proportional to the chance for scatter. Since the slope can be measured from the field, whereas the length of W cannot, the cotangent of the slope a provides us with a convenient measure of scatter. Since W is dependent on slope and H is not, one would also expect that a flat slope would be far more damaging to a kinetic field than a steep slope would be to a static field.

similar phenomenon occurs in static perimetry along very *steep* slopes, but here it is possible to neutralize temporal and spatial summation to a greater extent than possible with kinetic perimetry. Since steeply sloped areas can only cover a limited portion of any visual field, the potential confusion arising from scatter along such areas is minimal.

Finally, it should be noted that the steepest any slope can be is when it is approached perpendicular to the isopter. The more obliquely the slope is approached, the flatter it appears, and if the isopter is paralleled, the slope is perfectly flat. Although this phenomenon does not get out of hand so long as the line of aproach is within 30° of perpendicular to the isopter, every effort should be made to keep the line of approach as close to perpendicular as possible if scatter is to be held to an absolute minimum in kinetic testing.

One other related topic that deserves comment is the subject of photometric disharmony. Dubois-Poulsen[28] has long been an advocate of photometric disharmony as an indicator of retinal or optic nerve pathology. The basic assumption is that when equivalent Goldmann isopters do not overlap exactly, then photometric disharmony is present and pathology should be suspected. Dubois-Poulsen originally called the phenomenon *maladie de summation* ("difficulty with summation"), a misnomer since large, dim test objects are usually seen better.

Although the phenomenon of photometric disharmony does exist,[81] it can be measured in a particular subject only by determining carefully the summation coefficient at each retinal location and comparing these findings to normal values for each location. Merely noting a disparity in two isopters is not sufficient, since isopters tend to be "egg shaped" and thus tend to lie at different eccentricities in different parts of the field rather than to circle the fovea at constant radius. The summation coefficient will vary along the isopter; hence "photometric disharmony" of the sort that can be observed by plotting two supposedly equivalent Goldmann isopters will exist, to some extent, in almost every field. Dubois-Poulsen counters this criticism by stating that differences in symmetry, as opposed to differences in position, are more important in determining the presence or absence of pathology. Nevertheless, photometric disharmony remains a relatively unimportant part of the perimetrist's armamentarium.

Fixation

Although reasonably stable fixation is required for the accurate performance of a visual field examination, completely stable fixation does not exist under the usual clinical conditions. Greve[43] has reviewed the findings of numerous workers and concludes that at least three types of physiological fixation nystagmus have been demonstrated in alert, cooperative research subjects.

The first type of fixation nystagmus is a tremor of small amplitude, with both linear (from 5 to 30 seconds of arc) and torsional (about 45 seconds of arc) components. This tremor is of irregular high frequency that ranges from 70 to 90 Hz. The second type of fixation nystagmus consists of slow drifts. These occur with a frequency of about 2 Hz and have an amplitude that ranges from 0.8 to 6.0 minutes of arc with a velocity of about 6 minutes of arc/sec. Both of these types of fixation nystagmus are probably related to oculomotor instability, although the drifts may function to prevent fading of the target. The third type of eye movement during attempted fixation is rapid microsaccades that occur irregularly and have a range of amplitude from 2.0 minutes to 50 minutes of arc. These seem to correct fixation errors resulting from drifts.

From the foregoing, it appears that stable fixation to within 1° is possible if not easy to attain. Although the effect of torsional movements has not been well studied, Greve notes that horizontal movements can be controlled within 0.5° of arc (30 minutes), but the combination of torsional and vertical movements range over 4.0° of arc in trained subjects. Results are even worse in persons with poor visual acuity.

Border Contrast

If the background screen of a perimeter is divided by a sharp edge into a light and a dark field, one would expect some sort of phenomenon to occur at the border between the different brightnesses. One might reason that the receptive field organization of the retina is such that those cells right along the border will have only half of their surround illuminated while the other half will be in darkness. Also, the conditions of center illumination will differ from those across the border; thus, the operating characteristics of those cells lying on one side of the border will change from those of their fellows on the other side of the border. Since the eye is never perfectly still, even with the best voluntary fixation available, there is slight movement, and near the border, an edge will move back and forth over the receptive fields of cells and may cause some additional effects as a result of this movement. Since cortical cells respond exquisitely well to moving edges, some modification of the response at this level is likely.

Such border phenomena have long been known to psychophysiological investigators in the form of Mach bands. These occur as subjective sensations upon viewing a moving edge, namely, just adjacent to the border there is a narrow whiter band present on the white side and a similar darker band present on the dark side. Harms and Aulhorn[46] have studied this phenomenon from a perimetric point of view. Their findings are given in Figure 2-30 and may be summed up basically by saying that there is a depression of the sensitivity of the retina for light objects at such borders. Since the subjective sensation is one of a darkening at the dark border, and a lightening on the light side of the border, one would expect this curve to be biphasic, yet no such increase in sensitivity is observed empirically. Aulhorn also reported (personal communication) that this depression occurs even when the border is presented essentially at the same time as the test, or when the border contrast is so low that it disappears as a result of local adaptation. From a practical standpoint, the perimetrist must maintain a uniform background, since changes in the retinal sensitivity above and beyond those produced by the adaptive state are caused by the presence of borders in the visual field.

The Effect of Blur on Perimetric Thresholds

If a spot of light is sharply focused on a surface and then progressively blurred by defocusing, two things may be observed to happen simultaneously. The first is that the spot becomes dimmer; the second is that it becomes larger in diameter. How this affects its stimulus value will depend upon what part of the retina is being stimulated by the light. Area is a more efficient stimulus for vision in the periphery than near the fovea. The original size of the focused spot is also of some interest since defocusing a large spot produces less diminution of brightness and relatively less enlargement for a given amount of blur than does a small spot. The effect of this phenomenon on perimetric thresholds has been investigated by numerous workers.[34,80,81] Fankhauser and Enoch[34] demonstrated that the increment thresholds over the central 30° are markedly affected by blur (Fig. 2-31). Sloan has also investigated this phenomenon and notes that there is indeed a change in thresholds for test object size I and II on the

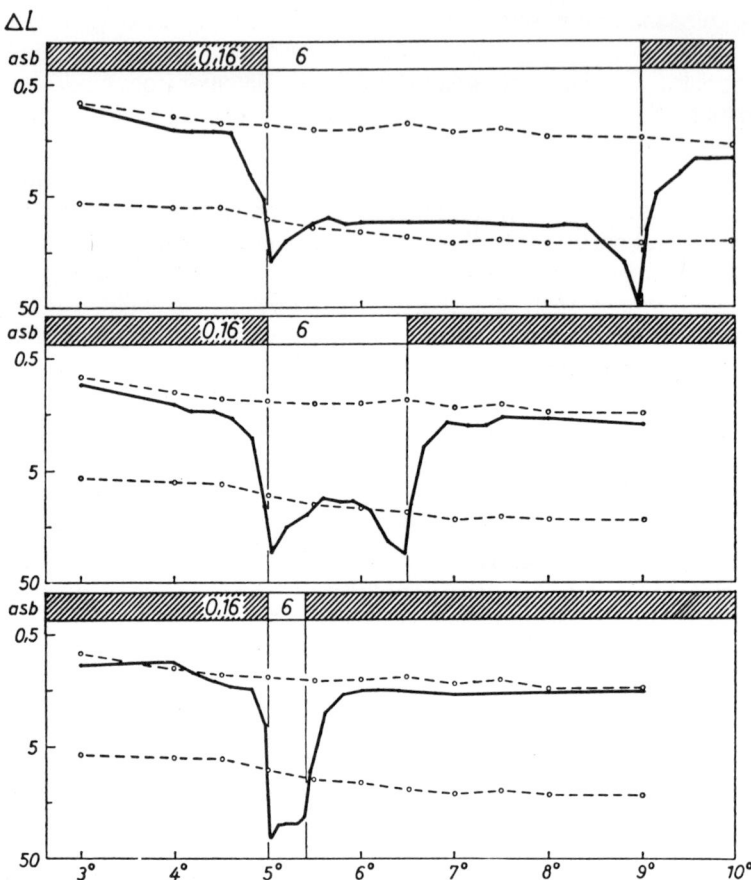

Figure 2-30 The effect of border contrast on increment threshold. The background contains areas of differing luminances, thus producing areas of different retinal light adaptation. Contrast across the area of demarcation is 1:37. Width of brighter portion varies from 4° in the top figure to 2° in the middle figure to 25' in the bottom figure. Luminance of the darker background is 0.16 Asb; luminance of the brighter is 6 Asb. The ordinate is the increment threshold, Asb. The abscissa is the eccentricity from fixation in degrees. The dotted lines show the threshold found in the same area across a uniform light (bottom line) or dark background (top line, each figure). The solid line is the increment threshold. Note the depression on both the dark and light sides of the border. (With permission from Aulhorn and Harms.[5])

Goldmann Perimeter but that with the larger spot sizes (III, IV, and V) this effect is not seen. According to present data, the effect of blur on perimetric thresholds is minimal beyond about 35° to 40° with any size object. This may be due to the fact that when the fundus periphery is compared with the center it tends to be more hypermetropic, has more off-axis aberrations, and has better spatial summation than the central area.

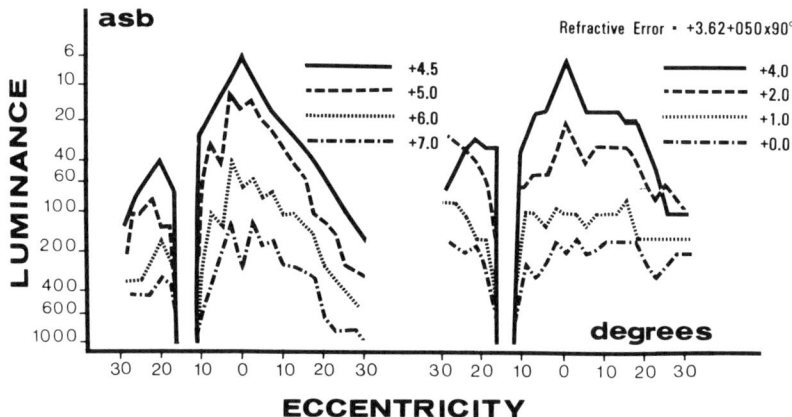

Figure 2-31 The effect of changing refraction on increment threshold. A patient with a refractive error at 30 cm of +3.62 +0.50 ×90° underwent perimetry with various degress of overplus (left) and overminus (right). The overplus corresponded from +0.62 (top line left, refraction +4.50) to +4.12 (bottom line left, refraction +7.00). The overminus ranged from +0.12 (actually a slight overplus, essentially emmetropic) (top line right, refraction +4.00) to -3.87 (bottom line right, refraction plano). Note that a refractive error of only one diopter can change the threshold by about half a log unit. A greater error, such as 4 diopters, depresses the threshold by about 1½ log units. This effect is more marked centrally than peripherally. The ordinate is the increment threshold in asb. The abscissa is the eccentricity from fixation in degrees. (Redrawn from Fankhauser and Enoch.[34])

Certain fundus pathology that induces blur can certainly have a profound effect on perimetric thresholds. Several authors[33,39,40,79] have called attention to the fact that refractive scotomas may appear, but none shows more graphically than that of Figure 2-32 which is from the work of Theodore Schmidt.[79] This field is from a patient having fundus ectasia, essentially a herniation or staphyloma of the posterior part of the eye. The superior temporal field in the upper part of Figure 2-32 shows a large scotoma to the I-3 isopter. With a −2.0 diopter refraction, however, the lower part of that same area is the only zone sensitive enough to see an I-2 isopter. Thus, the alert perimetrist will always consider the possibility of refractive scotomas and will attempt to see how altering the patient's refraction changes the threshold of the area in question.

The Response of the Eye to Flicker

The response of the eye to a flickering visual stimulus is an extremely complex matter. A thorough explanation of how the eye works in this regard can take one deep into the mathematical swamp of Fourier analysis and linear filter theory. Even though we set out on this journey with the intention of being fearless explorers, an exhaustive discussion of the physiology involved in flicker would be an effort far out of proportion to its clinical usefulness. A nice explana-

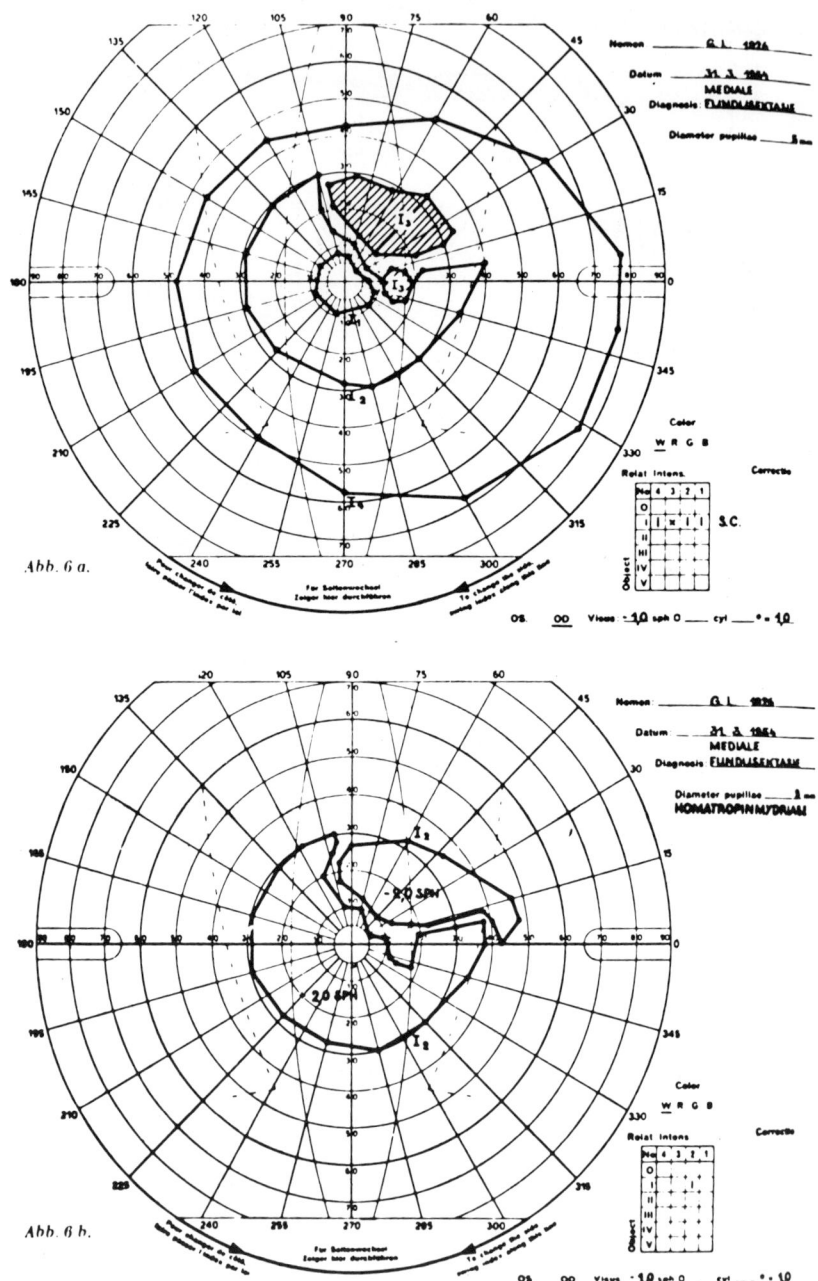

Abb. 6 a.

Abb. 6 b.

tion by Gerard Shickman may be found in Chapter 20 of Adler's *Physiology of the Eye*.[2] However, the really dedicated explorer will insist upon reading the papers by Delang,[21-23] Kelley,[58-60] Sperling,[82] and Luddeke[67] in order to round out his understanding of the topic. Clinical studies on flicker have been done by numerous authors.[56, 64, 66, 69-71]

One of the basic laws to the study of the flicker-fusion phenomenon is Talbot's law. Simply stated, this law says that the subjectively fused flickering light and an objectively constant light with equal subjective brightness have the same average luminous energy per unit of time. This is a precisely valid law. In many studies of flicker, it is custom to talk about "Talbot brightness," which is the equivalent steady brightness predicted by Talbot's law for a flashing light.

Another law of great interest is the so-called Ferry-Porter law. The Ferry-Porter law states essentially that the critical flicker frequency is linearly proportional to the retinal illumination. This law holds for a range of retinal illuminance that extends for about four log units and varies from the linear curve only at high illuminances. The law is described for the fovea that deals with only one type of cell, the cones. When eccentric spots are studied, a hump is seen (as in Fig. 2-33) in the curve at low illuminance because of the action of the rods. Particularly under dark-adapted conditions, the wavelength of the light itself is of some importance and influences the critical fusion frequency (Fig. 2-33). It will be noted from the figure that the longer wavelengths, such as red, deviate least from the Ferry-Porter predictions even at low illuminances, whereas the hump is most marked for the short wavelengths in the blues and violets.

The critical flicker frequency is a function of many things other than retinal illumination and spectral composition. The size of the test object; the wave form of the test light; the duty cycle (i.e., the relative proportion of light time to dark time), the shape of the test object; the luminance of the background; the adaptive state of the observer; the age of the observer, his general physiological state, and his personality; and any brain damage away from the visual tract have all been demonstrated to influence the critical flicker frequency. The result of all these variables has been that almost no investigator's work has been comparable to other studies. Ernst Wolf and his co-workers have done a great deal to standardize the conditions of the clinical test, and anyone desiring to use

---

Figure 2-32 A classic example of the effect that a change in refraction can have on the form of a visual field. The patient was a 28-year-old man with a minimal myopia (-1.00 for the right eye as shown) with vision correctable to 20/20. Ophthalmoscopic exam revealed a myopic fundus with a fundus ectasia inferonasal to the disk. Visual field on the Goldmann Perimeter (above) reveals a superiortemporal scotoma to the I-3-e and I-2-e isopters. Similar findings (not illustrated) could have suggested a pituitary lesion. Exam with -2.00 sphere correction (below, top isopter), however changed matters such that the previous area of scotoma is now the only area clearly seen. The I-2-e isopter with a $+2.00$ lens (below, bottom isopter) once again shows the defect. (With permission from Schmidt.[79])

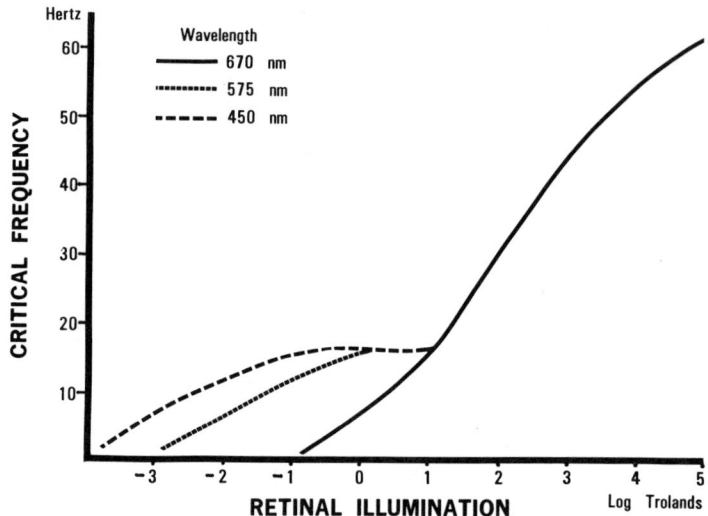

Figure 2-33 The influence of wavelength and retinal illumination, the Ferry-Porter law. In the photopic region (above 1 log Troland) all wavelengths follow the solid curve, and the CFF is linearly proportional to retinal illumination. With dark adaptation, however, linearity holds only for red light, with the shorter wavelengths departing from this law and forming a "scotopic hump" on the curve. The shorter the wavelength, the more marked the deviation is. The ordinate is the CFF in Hz (cycles per second). The abscissa is the retinal illumination in log Trolands. (Redrawn after Hecht, as quoted in Adler.[2])

flicker clinically would be well advised to become familiar with their work.[101-105]

One common problem that arises with the clinical determination of critical flicker frequency is that of duty cycle. There are two major ways of presenting flicker stimulus to the observer. One involves the use of a sector disc (i.e., an episcotister), which rotates at variable speeds and thereby has a constant duty cycle for increasing frequency. The other is by the use of a stroboscope, which has a flash of short duration, and as the frequency of flashes increases, the duty cycle increases, since the flash duration remains constant while the dark time decreases. Wolf feels that the optimum duty cycle is 50% and should be kept constant if possible with increase in frequency. This one factor alone accounts for much variance in clinical flicker perimetry from one investigator to another.

The subject of background luminance also deserves comment. In general, the highest critical flicker frequency is obtained if one uses a background luminance that is equal to the Talbot brightness of the test area. If one is using a stroboscope, the Talbot brightness of the test object will increase as the frequency of the presentation is increased. If the duty cycle is held constant, then the background brightness may be matched to the Talbot brightness of the flickering object for all frequencies of flicker.

Object size is a third important variable. Flicker studies have been carried out with objects varying in size from 0.5° to 10° or more. Wolf and others who have studied this parameter recommend an object size of about one to two degrees. The same size object should be used for all flicker studies. The Granit-Harper law states that the critical flicker frequency increases linearly with the logarithm of the stimulus area, and therefore different-sized flicker targets will give different values for critical flicker frequency.

Another variable is in the method of performing the test. The most widely accepted method is to start with the frequency higher than fusion frequency and gradually to decrease it until the subject perceives flicker. Therefore, many authors refer to this frequency as the critical *flicker* frequency whereas the measurement obtained in the opposite direction, that is, with the light flickering and its frequency gradually increased until fusion is reached, is the critical *fusion* frequency. Although these frequencies are close, more scatter is seen in the critical fusion frequency determinations than in critical flicker frequency determinations.

From a practical standpoint, one must question if the determination of critical flicker frequency provides any useful clinical information. Although the critical flicker frequency doubtlessly has many factors brought to bear on it throughout the entire visual and even the nonvisual portions of the nervous system, it probably adds very little information to that obtainable by standard perimetric techniques. Best[12] has examined the critical flicker frequency in normals under scotopic conditions and finds that if the stimulus intensity is a constant multiple of the threshold stimulus at that point, the critical flicker frequency, with scatter taken into account, is constant over the retina. Harms and Aulhorn[47] have examined critical flicker frequency and compared it with static perimetric results in patients in both health and disease. They find that the results are qualitatively similar in each case, although the flicker studies show a great deal more scatter than standard static perimetry. Luddeke, working in Aulhorn's laboratory, has examined the subject of flicker in all of its parameters.[67] He feels (personal communication) that flicker studies in which the frequency is held constant and the illumination is increased until flicker appears may be of some clinical value. Nevertheless, at the present time, it seems that in patients with opacities in the optical media, such as cataracts, flicker perimetry may be easier to carry out than standard light sense perimetry, but beyond this, it seems to offer little that is of diagnostic value.

Local Adaptation

When an illuminated test spot is presented at various eccentricities from fixation to a perfectly fixating observer, the spot disappears after a few seconds. This phenomenon was first described by Troxler in 1802 and is therefore called

120   Principles of Quantitative Perimetry

the Troxler effect. It has been studied in detail by Cibis.[17,18] It occurs most rapidly at greater eccentricities from fixation and least rapidly near the fovea, with center of fovea apparently never adapting at all. Curves of this phenomenon may be seen in Figure 2-34. It is seen that for virtually the entire retina, the local adaptation phenomenon is complete within two minutes and that for the retina outside approximately five degrees, the local adaptation phenomenon is complete within 20 seconds. The phenomenon occurs during stimulation with white or colored stimuli, and will occur even if the colored stimulus has the same brightness as the background. Thus, it occurs not only with differences in brightness, but with differences in hue. Exactly what this phenomenon represents is not known, although it apparently does not involve the same mechanisms as adaptation of the retina by photochemical means. It has been suggested by Aulhorn and Harms[5,45] that local adaptation times measured by static perimetric techniques may give some deeper insight into retinal disease processes. It is certain, however, that such a technique would require an im-

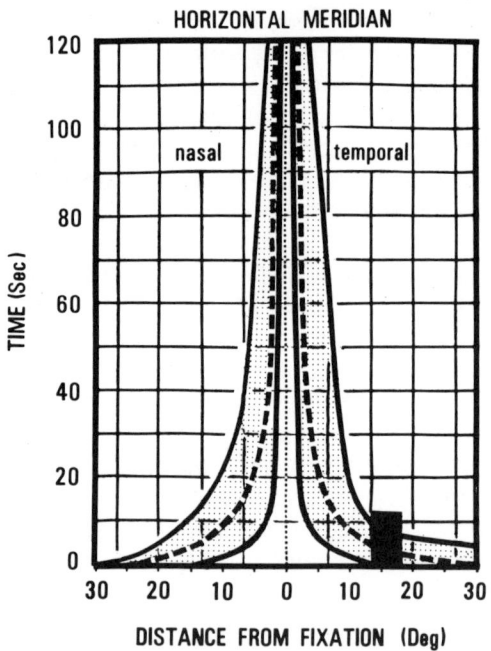

Figure 2-34   Local adaptation times as a function of retinal eccentricity. The ordinate represents the time in seconds for the test spot to disappear with as perfect free fixation as possible. The Abscissa is the distance in degrees from fixation along the horizontal meridian. The dotted line is the mean value. The shaded area represents deviations, and the black area temporally corresponds to the normal blind spot. (Redrawn from Cibis.[17])

practical amount of time if anything resembling a thorough testing of the retina is to be performed.

The phenomenon was also investigated by Yarbus[106] who used projectors fixed to contact lenses to provide absolutely stable retinal images. Yarbus reported that the entire field disappeared within three seconds, and that the center was *not* spared as reported by Cibis. Thus, it seems plausible that Cibis's results may be explained by the fact that peripherally, the receptive fields are large enough to keep the spot within them during the small movements that occur with even the best free fixation, whereas foveally this is not true.

From the standpoint of the perimetrist, the phenomenon of local adaptation is responsible for an increase in the threshold found in experimental static perimetry when a point is gradually brightened as opposed to presenting multiple, interrupted stimuli of increasing brightnesses. The difference in the thresholds obtained by these two techniques varies depending on a number of factors, but is on the order of 0.3 log unit.

Psychophysical and Psychological Phenomena

The previous sections have dealt mainly with the physiology of the isolated retina or the psychophysics of the visual system as a whole in research subjects. The clinical perimetrist does not have the luxury of dealing only with such isolated entities for invariably there is a patient attached, and certain features of his or her psyche may modify the results obtained perimetrically. Obviously the patient intent on malingering, or one who is hysterical, can profoundly influence the results that the perimetrist obtains, even if the visual apparatus is totally normal. A perfectly cooperative patient with full intention to provide the perimetrist with the best, most reliable results possible may still have his performance altered, however, by psychological influences. Psychological phenomena may make reliable testing of some patients with definite pathology impossible with certain varieties of tests.

One pitfall of a specific type of visual-field study technique is the so-called completion phenomenon. It has been pointed out by several authors[35,40] that patients with damage to their posterior visual pathway may not be adequately tested for progression of their lesion by devices such as the Amsler grid.* These patients tend to complete repeating patterns or objects of a familiar shape in the blind field. Goldmann[40] cites the case of a young railroad worker who had a skull

---

*An Amsler grid is any one of a set of cards bearing a grid pattern of varying designs first described by the Swiss ophthalmologist, Marc Amsler. The standard grid is 10 cm square and is marked off in 5 mm squares. It subtends a visual angle of about 10°, and is used primarily in the evaluation of macular disease.

fracture with damage to the left parietal lobe which caused aphasia and alexia. When the patient was followed with an Amsler grid to test for his hemianopsia, the defect was noted to recede. When standard Goldmann perimetry was performed, however, a full dense hemianopsia was found to persist. Despite the patient's awareness of the results of the visual field test and despite good fixation, the entire Amsler grid continued to be perceived. When the patient looked at the nose of the examining physician, he thought he saw the entire face. If the half of the Amsler grid corresponding to his hemianopsia was covered with a sheet of paper, however, the paper reached the midline before it was initially seen by the patient.

The tendency of the human eye to complete figures has been examined by Fankhauser and Geiger,[35] who find that most normals tend to organize random arrays of points into figures. Other workers have found that the presence of multiple spots can influence the apparent brightness of each individual spot and even change the flicker frequency.[41, 90] Binocular presentation of stimuli may vary their threshold as well as their critical flicker frequency. Nevertheless, multiple-stimulus devices may be clinically useful as rapid screeners.[38, 43, 48]

Patients with parieto-occipital lesions may show the so-called "extinction phenomenon" when examined by a simultaneous double stimulation technique. Bender[11] has investigated the extinction phenomenon in many sensory systems, including the tactile, auditory, and visual. He found that extinction is normally a part of tactile sensation but is made more prominent by cortical disease. He has reported several patients whose visual fields were "normal" when tested by routine perimetric techniques showed a hemianopic defect when investigated with double simultaneous stimulation. He did not thoroughly investigate the extinction phenomenon perimetrically but rather concentrated on the other sensory systems.

Lynn and Aulhorn (unpublished data) investigated the visual fields of normal individuals and glaucoma patients by double simultaneous stimulation and were unable to detect extinction in this group of subjects. Greve[43] likewise carried out multiple-stimulus perimetry in a similar group of subjects and found no threshold shift with up to eight simultaneous stimuli. Thus, it would appear that extinction with regards to the monocular visual field is likely to occur only in persons with disease of the higher centers.

The use of simultaneous multiple-stimulus screeners in disease processes affecting the anterior visual pathway is therefore regarded as visually equivalent to sequential stimuli in the same locations. The proper use of multiple stimuli may not only facilite the detection of pathology by its increased speed but also direct further perimetric studies. An even greater bonus of this technique is to screen out disease; for correct answers as to the number of spots that are seen eliminate the time that must be used to learn which tests were not seen. In disease of the higher centers, multiple stimuli may offer a unique advantage in the detection of pathology, so long as one avoids patterns containing easily completed figures, such as grids, crosses, or other geometric shapes.

Training is another factor that influences the perimetric threshold of a subject. Aulhorn and Harms[5] have studied the influence of training on perimetric threshold and find that there may be nearly an entire log unit shift in threshold with practice. This effect is greatest in the early trial sessions, and tends to be maintained in subsequent test sessions (Fig. 2-35). The amount of feedback given a patient can speed his learning and improve his performance significantly. It has been shown that when the patient is forced to make a choice as to the direction in which he sees the test object, and is then told immediately whether his choice was right or wrong, he will attain lower thresholds (i.e., greater sensitivity) with less scatter sooner than by other methods.[14] These results underscore the importance of immediately telling the patient when his performance is not adequate during the test and how he can correct it to obtain optimal reproducible results.

The foregoing variables all relate to and influence a phenomenon known as the *criterion effect*. Simply stated, this is a temporal variation in response to a stimulus as the subject's criterion for making a response changes. A common example with an untrained subject is waiting until the spot is clearly visible before making a response. As the subject learns to "see the spot" further eccentrically, the isopter enlarges. Nothing has changed physiologically; the

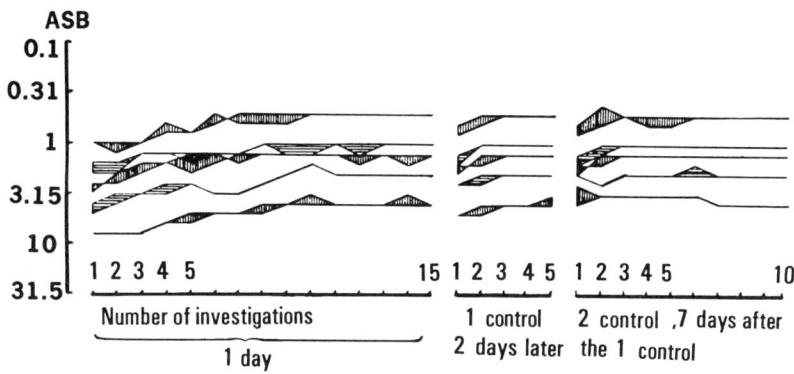

Figure 2-35 The effect of training on static thresholds initially, then two and nine days later. All five lines are from the same observer, taken at 0°, 2.5°, 5°, 10°, and 18° eccentricity from top to bottom. Two thresholds were consecutively determined for each location. Once each eccentricity had been tested, the cycle was repeated for 15 cycles (total of 30 tests at each eccentricity) on the first day, five cycles two days later, and 10 cycles one week following the second session. The difference between the two consecutive thresholds for a given time is represented by the shaded area. A single line indicates that the two determinations were identical. Note that threshold improves a few tenths of a log unit with practice and the scatter likewise decreases. Moreover, the effect of practice seems to persist. (Redrawn after Aulhorn and Harms.[4])

subject's criterion for reporting a seen stimulus has changed. The opposite effect may occur as a trained, alert subject tires, becomes indifferent to the spots, and requires a more intense stimulus. Improvements of the field that result only from a change in the response criterion may occur when the patient is extraordinarily motivated (e.g., "If this field is worse, Mrs. Jones, we will have to operate"). Such variations are best managed by training the patient carefully and trying to avoid field examinations when the patient is under extraordinary emotional stress of one sort or another.

Simply stated, the stimulus strength that a subject is willing to report as "seen" is influenced by psychological factors that affect his perception of how important it is to be *sure* he sees the test spot versus the importance of not missing a spot, even though he produces some "false alarms." This process of changing one's response criteria lends itself to a mathematical description through the language of signal detection theory.[42,72,84] Baumgartner provides a criticism of the signal detection approach to perimetry.[10] Although a detailed discussion of statistical decision theory and signal detection theory are beyond the scope of this chapter (see Appendix A), suffice it to say that it is the opinion of many workers in this area that a subject's responses are colored by his psychological state, a fact certainly borne out by clinical experience.

Obviously, these factors only scratch the surface of psychological variables. Fatigue, anxiety, preoccupation, hunger, thirst, drugs, and many other factors can influence the patient's performance during a visual field test. Some of these may be recognized and neutralized and some cannot. Thus, when the perimetrist notes a degradation in performance from previous studies, she or he should inquire about extraneous factors that may be influencing the patient's performance. If the presence of such distractions is confirmed, or even strongly suspected, the patient should be rescheduled for repeat perimetry on a different day before any important therapeutic decisions, such as surgical intervention, are made.

SUMMARY

In this chapter, we have tried to give the reader a deeper insight into those principles that form the basis of perimetry. The main point of this chapter, however, is simply to say that there are good reasons for performing tests of visual fields in the recommended manner. There are many pertinent points that have been discussed in this section: The use of photopic, evenly illuminated backgrounds; the use of standard size test objects; the importance of uniform movement in performing kinetic perimetry; the extreme importance of refraction when testing the central field; and the importance of controlling the patient's psychological variables to the maximum extent possible. Methods of achieving these goals will be examined in greater detail in subsequent chapters.

REFERENCES

1. Alexandridis E: Spatial and temporal summation of pupillomotor contraction upon light stimulation in man. Albrecht von Graefes Arch Klin Ophthalmol 180:12, 1970
2. Adler F: Adler's Physiology of the Eye, RA Moses (rev), St. Louis, C V Mosby, 1970
3. Aulhorn E: Psychophysische Gesetzmässigkeiten des normalen Sehens. Ber Dtsche Ophthalmol Ges 66:144, 1964
4. Aulhorn E, Harms H: Early visual field defects in glaucoma. Glaucoma Symp, Tutzing Castle, 1966. Basel, Karger, 1967
5. Aulhorn E, Harms H: Visual perimetry, in Jameson D, Hurvich LM (eds): Handbook of Sensory Physiology. Berlin, Springer-Verlag, 1972, vol 7(pt 4)
6. Bair HL: Some fundamental physiologic principles in study of the visual field. Arch Ophthalmol 24:10, 1940
7. Barlow HB, Hill RM, Levick WR: Retinal ganglion cells responding selectively to direction and speed of image motion in the rabbit. J Physiol (Lond) 173:377, 1964
8. Barlow HB, Levick WR: The mechanism of directionally selective units in rabbit's retina. J Physiol (Lond) 178:477, 1965
9. Bartoli F, Liuzzi L: Laser Perimetry: Diagnostic application in six cases of pituitary chromophobe adenoma. Acta Ophthalmol (kfh) 51:841, 1973
10. Baumgartner E: Threshold quantal problems, in Jameson D, Hurvich LM (eds): Handbook of Sensory Physiology. Berlin, Springer-Verlag, 1972, vol 7 (pt 4)
11. Bender MB: Disorders in Perception. Springfield, Illinois, Charles C Thomas, 1952
12. Best W: Die Abhangigkeit der Flimmerfrequenz von der Reizflachengrösse und dem Ort der gereizten Netzhautstelle unter besonderer Berucksichtigung der Schwellenreizlichtstärke. Albrecht von Graefes Arch Klin Ophthalmol 152:99, 1951
13. Bishop PO, Kozak W, Levick WR, Vakkur GJ: The determination of the projection of the visual field onto the lateral geniculate nucleus in the cat. J Physiol (Lond) 163:503, 1962
14. Blackwell HR: Studies of psychophysical methods for measuring visual thresholds. J Opt Soc Am 42:606, 1952
15. Burkhardt DA: Sensitization and Center-Surround Antagonism in Necturus Retina. J. Physiol (Lond.) 236:593, 1974
16. Campbell FW, Grubisch RW: Optical quality of the human eye. J Physiol (Lond) 186:558, 1966
17. Cibis P: Zur Pathologie der Lokaladaptation. I. Mitteilung. Albrecht von Graefes Arch Klin Ophthalmol 148:1, 1947
18. Cibis P: Zur Pathologie der Lokaladaptation. II. Mitteilung. Albrecht von Graefes Arch Klin Ophthalmol 148:216, 1948
19. Clark WEL: The visual centres of the brain and their connexions. Physiol Rev 22:205, 1942
20. Dawson WW, Perez JM: Unusual retinal cells in the dolphin eye. Science 181:747, 1973

21. De Lange Dzn H: Relationship between critical flicker-frequency and a set of low-frequency characteristics of the eye. J Opt Soc Am 44:380, 1954
22. De Lange Dzn H: Research into the dynamic nature of the human fovea-cortex systems with intermittent and modulated Light. I. Attenuation characteristics with white and colored light. J Opt Soc Am 48:777, 1958
23. De Lange Dzn H: Research into the dynamic nature of the human fovea-cortex systems with intermittent and modulated light. II. Phase shift in brightness and delay in color perception. J Opt Soc Am 48:784, 1958
24. Dowling JE: Neural and photochemical mechanisms of visual adaptation in the rat. J Gen Physiol 46:1287, 1963
25. Dowling JE: Organization of vertebrate retinas. Invest Ophthalmol 9:655, 1970
26. Dowling JE, Boycott BB: Organization of the primate retina: electron microscopy. Proc R Soc Lond [Biol] 166:80, 1966
27. Dowling JE, Ehinger B: Synaptic organization of the amine-containing interplexiform cells of the goldfish and Cebus monkey retinas. Science 188:270, 1975
28. Dubois-Poulsen A: Etude critique des techniques d'examen de la vision peripherique. Can J Ophthalmol 1:24, 1966
29. Egan JP: Signal Detection Theory and ROC Analysis. New York, Academic Press; 1975
30. Enoch JM, Sunga RN, Bachmann E: Static perimetric technique believed to test receptive field properties. I. Extension of Westheimer's experiments on spatial interaction. Am J Ophthalmol 70:113, 1970
31. Enoch JM, Sunga RN, Bachmann E: Static perimetric technique believed to test receptive field properties. II. Adaption of the method to the quantitative perimeter. Am J Ophthalmol 70:126, 1970
32. Fain GL: Quantum sensitivity of rods in the toad retina. Science 187:838, 1975
33. Frankhauser F: Kinetische Perimetrie. Ophthalmologica 158:406, 1969
34. Fankhauser F, Enoch JM: The effects of blur upon perimetric thresholds. Arch Ophthalmol 68:240, 1962
35. Fankhauser F, Giger H: Die Perzeptorische Organisation von Punktfeldern. Vision Res 8:1349, 1968
36. Fankhauser F, Schmidt TH: Die optimalen Bedingungen für die Untersuchung der räumlichen Summation mit stehender Reizmarke nach der Methode der quantitativen Lichtsinnperimetrie. Ophthalmologica 139:409, 1960
37. Francois J, Verriest G, Israel A: Perimetrie statique colorée effectuée à l'aide de l'appariel de Goldmann. Resultats obtenus en pathologie oculaire. Ann Oculist 199:113, 1966
38. Friedmann AI: Serial analysis of changes in visual field defects, employing a new instrument, to determine the activity of diseases involving the visual pathways. Ophthalmologica 152:1, 1966
39. Goldmann H: Grundlagen exakter Perimetrie. Ophthalmologica 109:57, 1945
40. Goldmann H: Lichtsinn mit besonderer Berücksichtigung der Perimetrie. Ophthalmologica 158:362, 1969
41. Granit R, Harper P: Comparative studies on the peripheral and central retina. Am J Physiol 95:211, 1930
42. Green DM: Signal Detection Theory and Psychophysics. New York, John Wiley and Sons, 1966

43. Greve EL: Single and multiple stimulus static perimetry in glaucoma: the two phases of perimetry. Doc Ophthalmol 36: 1973
44. Greve EL, Verduin WM, Ledeboer M: Two-colour threshold in static perimetry. Mod Probl Ophthalmol 13:113, 1974
45. Harms H: Die technik der statischen Perimetrie. Ophthalmologica 158:387, 1969
46. Harms H, Aulhorn E: Studien über den Grenzkontrast. I. Mitteilung. Ein neues Grenzphänomen. Albrecht von Graefes Arch Klin Ophthalmol 157:3, 1955
47. Harms H, Aulhorn E: Vergleichende Untersuchungen über den Wert der Quantitativen Perimetrie, Skiaskotometrie und Verschmelzungsfrequenz für die Erkennung beginnender Gesichtsfeldstorungen beim Glaukom. Doc Ophthalmologica 13:303, 1959
48. Harrington DO, Flocks M: The multiple pattern method of visual field examination. Trans Am Acad Ophthalmol Otolaryngol 59:126, 1955
49. Hartline HK: Inhibitory interaction in the retina, in Straatsma et al (eds): The Retina. Berkeley, University of California Press, 1969, p 297
50. Hartline HK: The receptive fields of optic nerve fibers. Am J Physiol 130:690, 1940
51. Hogan MJ, Alvarado JA, Wendell JE: Histology of the Human Eye. Philadelphia, WB Sanders, 1971, p 687
52. Hubel DH: Single unit activity in lateral geniculate body and optic tract of unrestrained cats. J Physiol (Lond) 150:91, 1960
53. Hubel DH: Single unit activity in striate cortex of unrestrained cats. J Physiol (Lond) 147:226, 1959
54. Hubel DH: The visual cortex of the brain. Sci Am 209:54, 1963
55. Hubel DH, Wiesel TN: Integrative action in the cat's lateral geniculate body. J Physiol (Lond) 155:385, 1961
56. Hylkema BS: Flicker fusion frequency in a few eye disturbances. Ophthalmologica 132:202, 1956
57. Jay BS: The effective pupillary area at varying perimetric angles. Vision Res 1:418, 1961
58. Kelly DH: Sine waves and flicker fusion. Doc Ophthalmologica 18:16, 1964
59. Kelly DH: Visual responses to time-dependent stimuli. I. Amplitude sensitivity measurements. J Opt Soc Am 51:422, 1961
60. Kelly DH: Visual responses to time-dependent stimuli. IV. Effects of chromatic adaptation. J Opt Soc Am 52:940, 1961
61. Kuffler SW: Discharge patterns and functional organization of mammalian retina. J Neurophysiol 16:37, 1953
62. Laties AM: Specific neurohistology comes of age: A look back and a look forward. Invest Ophthalmol 11:555, 1972
63. LeGrand Y: Light, Colour and Vision. London, Chapman and Hall, 1957
64. Levinson JZ: Flicker fusion phenomena. Science 160:21, 1968
65. Liebman PA: Handbook of Sensory Physiology, HJA Dartnall (ed), Berlin, Springer-Verlag, 1972. vol 7 (pt 1), p 481
66. Lovekin LG, Chandler MR: The range of normal for visual fields by flicker fusion. Arch Ophthalmol 62:588, 1959
67. Luddeke H: CFF and Visual Field Threshold. Annee Ther Clin Ophthalmol 25:236, 1974

68. McColgin FH: Movement thresholds in peripheral vision. J Opt Soc Am 50:774, 1960
69. Miles PW: Flicker fusion fields. I. The effect of age and pupil size. Am J Ophthalmol 33:769, 1950
70. Miles PW: Flicker fusion fields. II. Technique and interpretation. Am J Ophthalmol 33:1060, 1950
71. Miles PW: Flicker fusion fields. III. Findings in early glaucoma. Arch Ophthalmol 43:661, 1950
72. Nachmias J: Signal Detection Theory and its Application to Problems in Vision, in Jameson D, Hurvich LM (eds): Handbook of Sensory Physiology. Berlin, Springer-Verlag, 1972, pp 56–77
73. Normann RA, Werblin FS: Control of retinal sensitivity. I. Light and dark adaptation of vertebrate rods and cones. J Gen Physiol 63:37, 1974
74. Norton AL, Spekreijse H, Wagner HG, Wolbarsht ML: Responses to directional stimuli in retinal preganglionic units. J Physiol (Lond) 206:93, 1970
75. Pirenne MH: Vision and the Eye. London, Chapman & Hall Ltd., 1967
76. Purkinje JE: Beobachtungen und Versuche zur Physiologie der Sinne. Prague, 1819–23. As quoted by Duke-Elder.
77. Riddoch G: Dissociation of visual perceptions due to occipital injuries, with especial reference to appreciation of movement. Brain 40:15, 1917
78. Rushton WAH: Visual adaptation. Proc R Soc Lond [Biol] 162:20, 1965
79. Schmidt T: Perimetrie relativer skotome. Ophthalmol 129:303, 1955
80. Sloan LL: Area and luminance of test object as variables in examination of the visual field by projection perimetry. Vision Res 1:121, 1961
81. Sloan LL, Brown DJ: Area and luminance of test object as variables in projection perimetry. Vision Res 2:527, 1962
82. Sperling G: Linear theory and the psychophysics of flicker. Doc Ophthalmol 18:3, 1969
83. Spring KH, Stiles WS: Apparent shape and size of the pupil viewed obliquely. Br J Ophthalmol 32:347, 1948
84. Swets JA, Tanner WP, Birdsall TC: Decision processes in perception. Psychol Rev 68:301, 1961
85. Teller DY: Sensitization by annular surrounds: temporal (masking) properties. Vision Res 11:1325, 1971
86. Teller DY: Visual sensitization by annular surrounds. J Opt Soc Am 59:509, 1969
87. Teller DY, Gestrin PJ: Sensitization by annular surrounds: sensitization and dark adaptation. Vision Res 9:1481, 1969
88. Teller DY, Lindsey B: Sensitization by annular surrounds: individual differences. Vision Res 10:1045, 1970
89. Teller DY, Matter CF, Phillips WD: Sensitization by annular surrounds: spatial summation properties. Vision Res 10:549, 1970
90. Thomas JP: Brightness-contrast effects among several points of light. J Opt Soc Am 55:323, 1965
91. Verriest G, Israel A: Application du perimètre statique de Goldmann au relief topographique des seuils differentiels de luminance pour de petits objects colorés projetés sur un fond blanc. Vision Res 5:151, 1965

92. Verriest G, Padmos P, Greve EL: Calibration of the Tüebingen perimeter for colour perimetry. Mod Probl Ophthalmol 13:109, 1974
93. Werblin FS: Control of retinal sensitivity. II. Lateral interactions at the outer plexiform layer. J Gen Physiol 63:62, 1974
94. Werblin FS: Response of retinal cells to moving spots: Intracellular recording in nectrus maculosus. J Neurophysiol 33:342, 1970
95. Werblin FS, Copenhagen DR: Control of retinal sensitivity. III. Lateral interactions at the inner plexiform layer. J Gen Physiol 63:88, 1974
96. Westheimer G: Spatial interaction in the human retina during scotopic vision. J Physiol (Lond) 181:881, 1965
97. Westheimer G: Spatial interaction in human cone vision. J Physiol (Lond) 190:139, 1967
98. Westheimer G: Bleached rhodopsin and retinal interaction. J Physiol (Lond) 195:97, 1968
99. Wiesel TN: Receptive fields of ganglion cells in the cat's retina. J Physiol (Lond) 153:583, 1960
100. Witkovsky P, Shakib M, Ripps H: Interreceptoral junctions in the teleost retina. Invest Ophthalmol 13:996, 1974
101. Wolf, E: Flicker perimetry: Methods and interpretation of flicker fields. Postgraduate Course in Ophthalmology, Harvard Medical School, 1972
102. Wolf E, Gaeta AM, Geer SE: Critical flicker frequencies in flicker perimetry. Arch Ophthalmol 80:347, 1968
103. Wolf E, McGowan BK: The effect of light-time: Dark-time ratio and luminance on peripheral sensitivity to flicker. Arch Ophthalmol 69:241, 1963
104. Wolf E, Schraffa AM: Relationship between critical flicker frequency and age in flicker perimetry. Arch Ophthalmol 72:832, 1964
105. Wolf E, Vincent RJ: Effect of target size on critical flicker frequency in flicker perimetry. Vision Res 3:523, 1963
106. Yarbus AL: Eye Movements and Vision. B Haigh and LA Riggs (trans), New York, Plenum Press. 1967
107. Zappia RJ, Enoch JM, Stamper R, Winkelman JZ, Gay AJ: The Riddoch phenomenon revealed in non-occipital lobe lesions. Br J Ophthalmol 55:416, 1971

3
Available Visual Field Devices and Their Limitations

There is no single visual field device available that will suit the needs of every practitioner, nor is there ever likely to be one. A neuro-ophthalmologist will frequently opt for a tangent screen and colored test objects, since his interest is mainly in rapid, diagnostic fields. A person whose practice is skewed heavily toward glaucoma will require quantitative, reproducible fields and hence should choose a perimeter capable of producing them. A person whose main concern is occupational medicine may find that a screener of some variety answers his needs. The real secret of reaping bountiful rather than barren results from visual field testing is to choose a device and a technique that are compatible with one's needs.

FULL-FIELD DEVICES

The Goldmann Perimeter

The Goldmann Perimeter is, in the authors' opinion, the device best suited to the average ophthalmologist's practice. It is simple to set up and to use; and it is capable of high quality, quantitative fields to truly delight all but the research-oriented perimetrist. Very adequate central field exams and static perimetry are possible with this device, although it is inadequate for use with color perimetry. Exotic tests, such as flicker-fusion studies, are not available with the device. As compared with a tangent screen, the eye to screen distance is small (30 cm), and special care must be given to the patient's refraction. Finally, the telescope used to monitor fixation serves also as the fixation spot and thus makes it impossible to test the central 2° without using a special device (1-dot–4-dot projector) to shift the fixation point to the side. The versatility of the Goldmann equipment more than compensates for these minor shortcomings. In over seventeen years, Lynn has not once encountered a patient with a visual field defect that could be mapped in any instrument and not be analyzed adequately with the Goldmann Perimeter.

Physically, the Goldmann Perimeter is a bowl perimeter, which makes full-field studies possible (Fig. 3–1). The same light source provides background and test spot illumination so that calibration problems are simplified. On the Goldmann produced by Haag-Streit, this is accomplished by a variant of "grease-spot" photometer, although some other manufacturers utilize a photoelectric meter, an extremely unfortunate choice since the eye is far more sensitive in calibrating test spots than any but the most sensitive of meters. The spot size may be varied from an area of 1/16 mm^2 to 64 mm^2, and the brightness varied by neutral gray filters, ranging from a transmission of 0.0125 (0.0001 on model 940-ST) to 1.00 in twenty steps (sixty steps on model 940-ST). Thus, the brightness can span a range of two log units in increments of 0.1 log unit on the

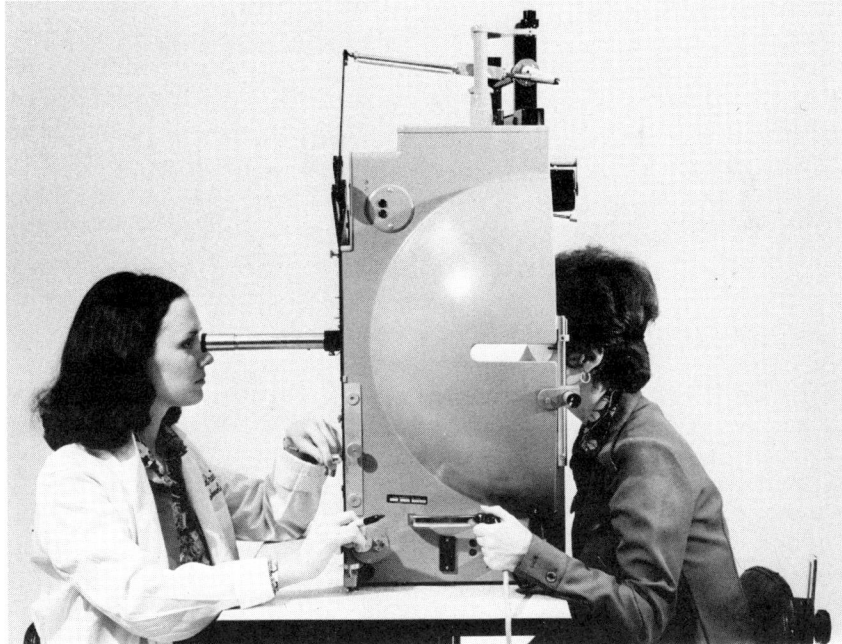

Figure 3–1 The Goldmann Perimeter, seen from the side. The operator controls the pantograph arm with her left hand, the shutter with her right; and she monitors fixation through the telescope.

standard model and six log units on the model 940-ST. The device utilizes preprinted charts that are back-illuminated. These charts provide landmarks for the perimetrist as well as a convenient permanent record. (The Goldmann Perimeter is described in greater detail in Chapter 5.)

The Tübinger Perimeter (Oculus)

The Tübinger Perimeter is without a doubt one of the most versatile, accurate perimeters available today (Fig. 3–2). It lends itself to kinetic studies and is the perimeter par excellance for static perimetry. It easily handles extra tasks such as examination of central and peripheral visual acuity, examination of flicker-fusion fields, examination with multiple-colored spots and/or backgrounds, dark adaptation, adaptoperimetry, and is useful in other kinds of testing besides. There is a variable control linkage between the registration mechanisms and the target projector, which thereby enables the central field to be magnified on the chart and thus be plotted with greater accuracy. In our opinion, the Tübinger Perimeter is the finest piece of equipment on the market today for the testing of visual fields, be they of a clinical or a research nature. Unfortunately, the device is relatively expensive and the very flexibility that makes it such a useful re-

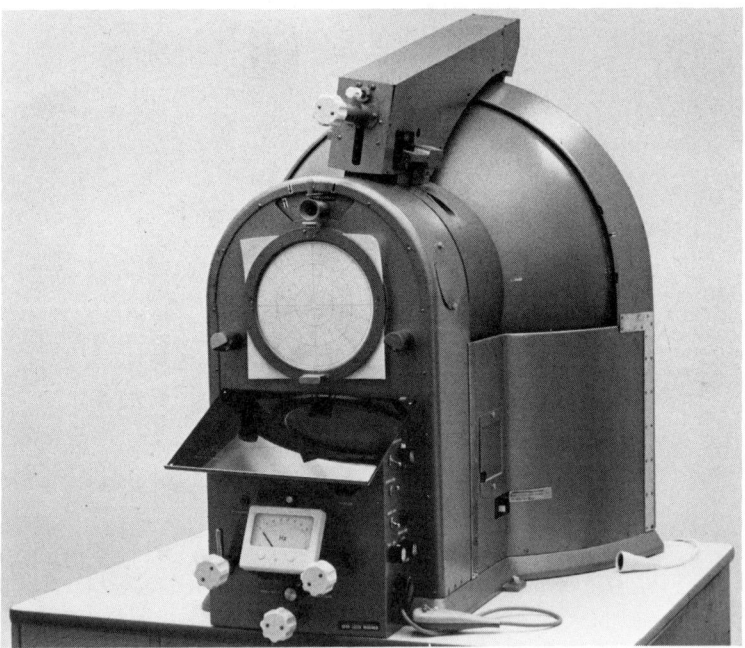

Figure 3-2   The Tübinger Perimeter of Harms and Aulhorn as seen from the operator console.

search tool can make it a bit cumbersome for the physician or technician who has no need for its special capabilities. These factors tend to limit the availability of the machine to those centers that have a research interest in either visual fields or glaucoma, and it is not, therefore, so widely available as the Goldmann. This detracts slightly from its usefulness, since it is not so easy to obtain comparable fields from one geographic area to another. Nevertheless, a physician who demands the finest quality device available, one that will give him the utmost flexibility, can do no better than the Tübinger Perimeter.

Other Bowl Perimeters

There are a number of other bowl perimeters on the market, which range from a tiny five-inch opalescent bowl (the "Eye Cup" perimeter, suitable only for screening bedside fields) to a huge two-meter diameter fully quantitative perimeter constructed by Donaldson at the Howe Laboratories at the Massachusetts Eye and Ear Infirmary in Boston, Massachusetts (Fig. 3-3). Two

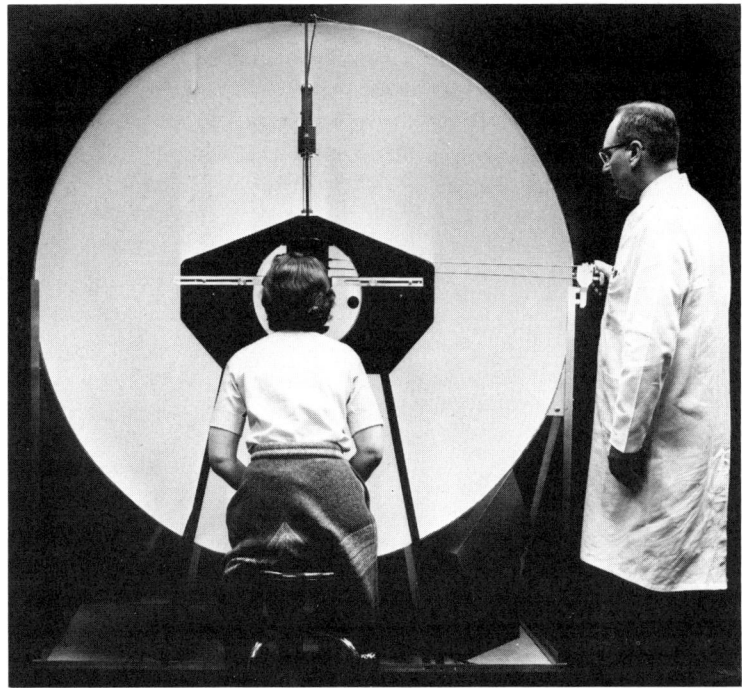

Figure 3-3 The Donaldson Perimeter. This machine, with its two meter diameter bowl, is a candidate for the title of largest perimeter ever constructed. (Photo courtesy of Dr. Donaldson.)

134   *Principles of Quantitative Perimetry*

other bowl perimeters that are commercially available and suitable for quantitative studies are the Gambs and the Rodenstock Perimeters.

The Gambs is a translucent bowl with a handheld projector that is applied to the outside of the bowl (Fig. 3–4). The device has several pitfalls that should be avoided. The manufacturer suggests marking on the bowl itself, a technique that increases the likelihood of nonreproducible fields. All the same, this device can be calibrated and can give good results if used with care.

The Rodenstock Perimeter is a large projection perimeter similar in quality and capability to the Goldmann. It is an excellent machine but suffers from an awkward appearance and is slightly less convenient in operation than the Goldmann.

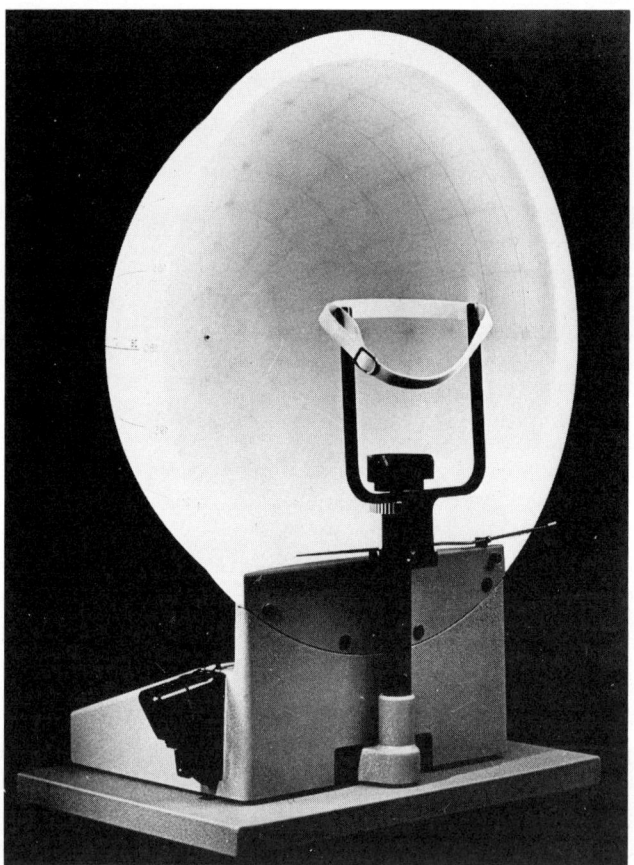

Figure 3-4   The Gambs Perimeter is unique among the full size bowl perimeters in that the bowl is translucent and the stimulus is projected through, rather than onto, the bowl. (Photo courtesy of House of Vision.)

DEVICES FOR TESTING THE CENTRAL FIELD: CAMPIMETERS

The Tangent Screen

The tangent screen is undoubtedly *the* classic visual field device. It has been used by such great practitioners in the art as Bjerrum, Rönne, and Traquair with good results, and it is familiar to virtually every student of ophthalmology. The tangent screen stands as silent proof of the truth of Traquair's famous quote, "Perimetry is not done by the perimeter but by the perimetrist." One would be hard pressed to design a more austere device or visual field test with more potential pitfalls for the perimetrist than the tangent screen. In its classic form, the screen consists of a 40-inch square plane of black wool felt that has black stitching to outline its various meridia and eccentricities. Most tangent screens also have outlines with the blind spot stitched onto them. Better ones have a solid background to prevent wrinkling, stretching, or variations in shape. This background may be made of cork to permit small black pins with a matte finish to be inserted or of metal to permit small black magnets with a similar finish to adhere on the tangent screen to mark the limits of the isopter being tested. The tangent screen has been modified by a number of workers so that the test can either be done with projection techniques or recorded automatically by photography. Nevertheless, all of these devices share some of the same problems.

If the tangent screen is used in the classical fashion, using wand-mounted targets, then basically three choices of test objects are available. These are spherical beads (Fig. 3–5), flat discs, or self-luminous targets, such as the Jenkel-Davidson Lumiwand (Fig. 3–6). Each has its own pitfalls. For example, spherical targets of a given diameter may vary greatly in size from one bead to the next. Requests to the supplier for beads of research quality do not secure more uniform targets. Thus, if one wishes to use beads, one should measure his set. Care must be taken to insure that the beads stay clean, and that new beads are purchased when the present set becomes unalterably soiled.

One way around this problem is to use circular disc targets. These are of two sorts. One is supplied similarly to the beads with the size and the color determined by the manufacturer (e.g., "Traquair Targets"). Although these too have the disadvantage of becoming dirty, they do have the advantage of usually being somewhat more uniform in size than beads. The disadvantage of the flat discs is that they are not strictly comparable to a spherical target in stimulus value, although under practical conditions this difference is probably not significant (See Chapter 1). The other type of flat disc consists of utilizing a paper punch and clean white or other colored paper. This has the advantage that the discs are always of a uniform size, and that they are always as clean as possible. However, they do represent a bit more trouble for the perimetrist. Any flat

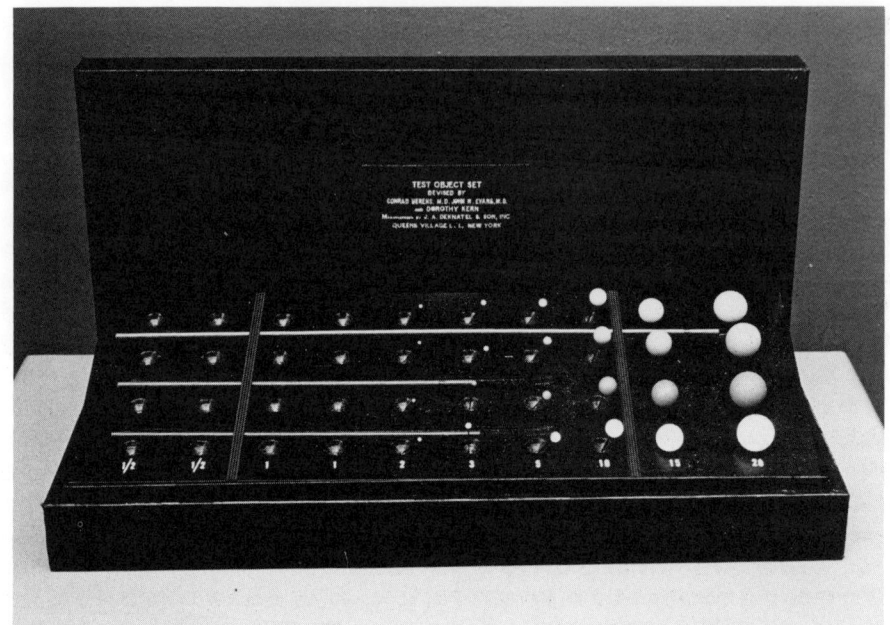

Figure 3-5 The Berens Test Targets for use with the tangent screen. Such sets are available with beads of graded sizes and in several colors. Other sets with disciform targets are also available. (Photo courtesy of House of Vision.)

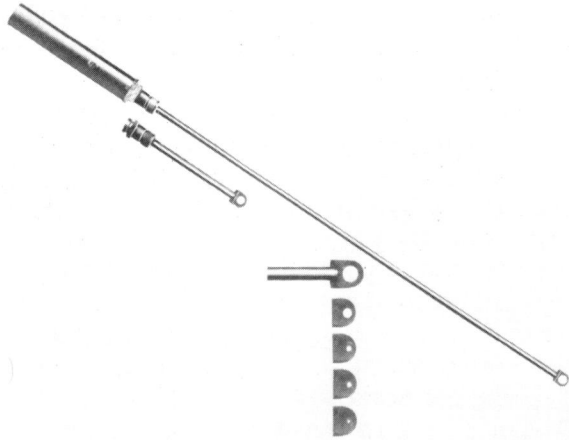

Figure 3-6 The Jenkel-Davidson Lumiwand. This is a self-illuminated wand for tangent screen fields under mesopic or scotopic conditions. A series of caps with graded apertures (center, below) slip over the luminous element to control object size. (Photo courtesy of House of Vision.)

target suffers from variations in its stimulus value if that target is rotated slightly from the plane of the tangent screen.

The final set of devices are self-illuminated wands, such as the Lumiwand. These are battery powered devices, and are more or less the same stimulus strength from one use to the next. The size of the stimulus area is constant but can be changed by variable-sized apertures that slip over the luminous element. The major disadvantage is that the field should be done under scotopic or mesopic conditions for the wand to be of optimal usefulness. This makes the recording of the field somewhat difficult and also requires a longer period for dark adaptation of the patient, otherwise spiraling fields will expand as the patient adapts to the dark during the performance of the field.

The second area of difficulty for the perimetrist is with the screen itself. Care must be taken to make sure that the screen is illuminated uniformly and reproducibly from test to test. The background must be kept scrupulously clean in order to obtain anything resembling reproducible fields. The practice of marking the position of the isopters on the background felt with chalk is therefore strongly condemned. Also, as the screen collects dust, it will become grayer and must be frequently cleaned or replaced. Those screens on rollers that are rolled up and down invariably develop wrinkles on their surface and thus make it difficult to maintain a uniformly illuminated background or to determine the exact eccentricity of the test object.

Finally, the perimetrist must provide for the disappearance of the test target. White beads sitting nakedly on the end of a probe are a totally unsuitable test target for two reasons. The first is that it is impossible to introduce the bead in an unseen fashion from an area of seeing into an area of scotoma, such as the normal blind spot. It is likewise impossible to make sure that the subject is reacting to the presence of the bead and not to the wand itself. The best wands are those that are covered with black felt, like the screen, and are therefore nonreflecting. The pins forming the test objects can be fixed to the side (not the tip) of the wand by inserting them through the black felt, and the wand may be rotated about its long axis to allow the spot to be either presented or not. Those wands that carry disc-shaped targets should have a black matte surface on one side of the disc and the target carried on the other. The Lumiwand is turned on and off simply by pushing a button to supply current to the illuminated test object. The use of tip-mounted, half-blackened beads is to be avoided because of the possibility of minor rotations changing the stimulus value of the bead.

The refraction of the patient is not so critical as with the Goldmann because the working distance (one meter or more) with the tangent screen is greater. One should make sure that the patient has their best correction, however, since the entire test is done within the central field. Although it is not characteristically done by those employing tangent screens, it is best in those patients who are more than 55 years old to add one diopter to the distance prescription for use with the one meter tangent screen. Of course, if the patient has single-vision glasses, these are often suitable, but if the patient has graduated into bifocals or trifocals these may not be suitable for use during the examination if the segment is so high that it encroaches upon the central field. In this case, one should use a trial frame containing the proper prescription.

Fixation may be a bit of a problem for the perimetrist who prefers the tangent screen since he is forced to observe the patient's eye obliquely. With skill and experience this difficulty can be minimized. The orientation of the patient and the performance of the test are similar to those carried out on the Goldmann.

Once the visual field has been performed, the problem of recording the results remains. Classically, the position of the isopters is marked on the screen itself by use of pins or magnets and later transcribed onto a field chart. Some workers keep the chart handy and transcribe the results as the test progresses without the intermediate steps of marking the screen. A number of devices also exist that make the task of recording the field easier. One of the most imaginative is the use of a Polaroid camera and strobe light which the patient trips everytime they see the object. Most of these have their drawbacks, however, (such as playing havoc with the light-adapted state of the patient in the previous example) and the simple paper chart remains about the best means available.

The isopters in a tangent screen exam are coded as a common fraction with the numerator representing the diameter of the test object in millimeters and the denominator the distance in millimeters at which the test is performed. Thus, an isopter performed with a three millimeter object at a distance of two meters would be coded as a 3/2000 isopter. This ratio represents the visual angle subtended by the test object expressed in radians. Isopters coded with equivalent fractions (e.g., 1/1000 and 2/2000) should be seen at the same eccentricity.

Certain types of field testing are better done on the tangent screen than with a bowl perimeter such as the Goldmann or the Tübinger. A particular case is the hysterical patient. If one plots an isopter with the patient one meter from the screen and then again with the patient two meters from the screen, but with the same size test object, one would expect the angular eccentricity of the isopter to fall. Alternatively, doubling both the distance and the test object should cause the angular eccentricity to remain constant. This frequently does not happen with the hysterical or the malingering patient, and many of these patients plot the same physical size of isopter regardless of the combination of distance and test object used. This is diagnostic of these conditions. Other ploys suitable for use with the bowl perimeters exist and will be discussed later in the book (Chapter 8).

It has been said that perimetry with the tangent screen has many shortcomings. Yet, in spite of them, the tangent screen is probably the most widely used visual field device in ophthalmology today. The virtues of providing quick, flexible visual fields—to say nothing of being available at low cost—permit this

Available Visual Field Devices and Their Limitations

piece of equipment to be present in the examining room of every busy practitioner. In addition, its accuracy in establishing diagnostic fields more than outweighs its shortcomings in the judgment of many. To be aware of its limitations is to know how to deal with them. Such knowledge also makes it easier to plot fields that are comparable and reasonably reproducible within a given laboratory. There is no way, however, that tangent screen fields will be exactly comparable from one laboratory to another because of the number of variables that must be controlled.

The Autoplot (Bausch & Lomb)

The Autoplot is essentially a tangent screen (Fig. 3-7). It adds refinement, speed, and mechanical convenience; and it makes for a more accurate and repeatable tangent field examination than the classical felt screen. It is also more expensive. It has a device that moves the target and also at the same time marks a chart, a feature that eases the task of transcribing the data from the tangent screen to a permanent record. The Autoplot is a projection device, which means that the test objects are clean and uniform in size. The results

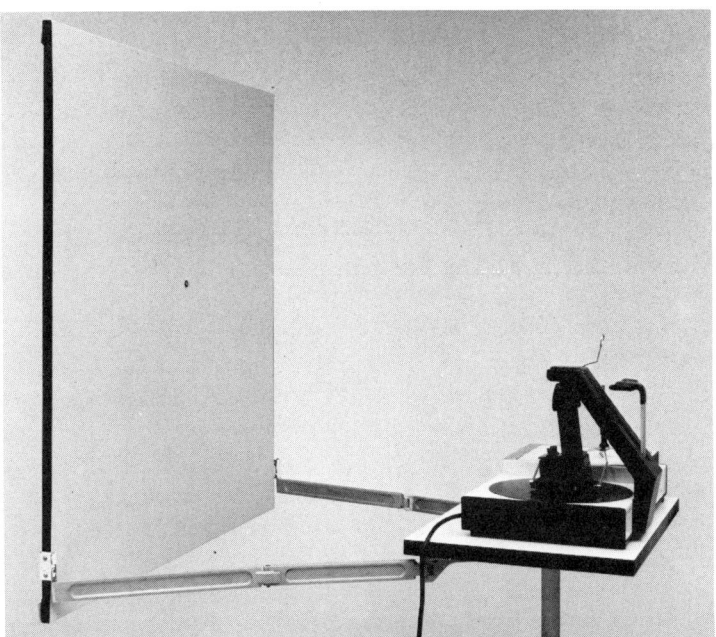

Figure 3-7 The Bausch & Lomb Autoplot, shown with its grey vinyl screen. This device is one of the most convenient of the tangent screen devices available today.

140 *Principles of Quantitative Perimetry*

obtained with any projection campimeter will not be quite compatible, however, with those obtained on a standard tangent screen, since the size of the spots will be slightly larger in the periphery than in the center. The Autoplot is used with a gray vinyl plastic screen that allows uniformity of target brightness over its entire surface area and enhances target contrast under photopic conditions. One may select test stimuli of sizes ranging from 0.5 mm to 15 mm in diameter; and the color of the test may be one of four: white, red, green, or blue. In addition, the device has a switch in its lower left-hand corner which permits the examiner to extinguish the test stimulus and to make a blind presentation of the test to the patient. It is certainly simple to operate, having only an on/off switch, an extinguish switch, and two knobs on the projector to control stimulus size and color.

In use, the patient is positioned on the device with his glasses correction in place and the pointer is placed over fixation on the chart. The device is turned on and the examiner makes sure that the projected spot corresponds to the fixation mark on the screen. If it does not, an adjustment is made either in the fixation mark (if a magnetic fixation mark is used) or by moving the device slightly. The scheme of testing with the device is very similar to that with the Goldmann. The Autoplot is probably the best tangent screen device on the market today, insofar as reproducibility from field to field is concerned. Nevertheless, since this device has no provision for controlling background illumination, the fields may vary from time to time, a factor that must be taken into consideration by the examiner.

The Juler Scotometer

The Juler Scotometer is a handheld device that permits projection campimetry (Fig. 3–8). The size of the object can be changed from a 0.5 mm to 30 mm in diameter, depending on lens-to-screen distance, and the test object may either be red, white, or green in color. Additionally, it has on its handle a switch for extinguishing the spot. It is designed for use with a one-meter tangent

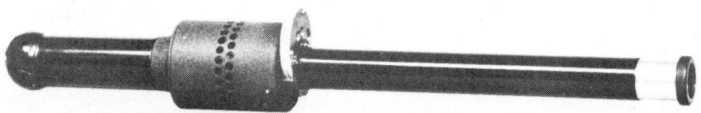

Figure 3-8   The Juler Scotometer is a handheld device that permits rapid projection campimetry suitable for diagnostic fields. The circular wheel on the lamp housing permits the selection of spots of various sizes and colors. (Photo courtesy of House of Vision.)

screen, which is preferably gray. The Juler Scotometer however, has several drawbacks that must be recognized by anyone choosing to use this device. If the examiner sits very eccentrically, the test objects will be larger on one side of the screen than the other. Varying the distance to and from the screen varies the size and stimulus value of the spot. Nevertheless, the device is rapid, easy to use, and capable of supplying adequate diagnostic visual fields. It is totally unsuitable for quantitative fields.

Arc Perimeters

All arc perimeters share in common the same two major defects: they are useful only for testing the peripheral fields; and they provide little, if any, surprise since the subject soon learns the test stimulus will be coming somewhere along the meridian in which the arc is positioned. The arc itself subtends little area, so it should be placed in front of a uniform background with approximately the same or slightly less luminance as the arc if uniform test conditions are to be maintained. Nevertheless, the examiner who chooses to utilize one of the tangent screen devices (which are only capable of testing the central field) must utilize either an arc or a bowl perimeter if the periphery of the field is to be tested. The practice of going back and forth between an arc perimeter and a tangent screen has its problems. Since the test is done under two sets of circumstances, it is extremely difficult to make sure the peripheral isopters are comparable to the central isopters in any meaningful way. Nevertheless, arc perimeters are capable of providing adequate results when used properly.

Aimark Projection Perimeter

The AIMARK is the original projection arc perimeter. It is silent in operation and has automatic recording (Fig. 3-9). Since it is a projection device, the perimetrist faces no problems with test objects of varying size and degrees of cleanliness. He must, however, keep the background of the arc itself scrupulously clean. The size of the test objects are controlled by three milled wheels, one of which allows the selection of test object size from 1 mm to 10 mm in diameter, another provides colors (white, red, green, and blue), and the third modulates the intensity of the spot by transposing neutral density filters in the projection path. The device also has an on/off switch that permits the test spot to be presented or extinguished silently. Fixation is by viewing illuminated cross hairs or, as an alternative for those patients with central scotoma, an illuminated white ring. An automatic recording is made by a pin that perforates the chart at a position corresponding to the meridian and eccentricity of the patient's response. This or very similar devices are manufactured by several companies.

142 *Principles of Quantitative Perimetry*

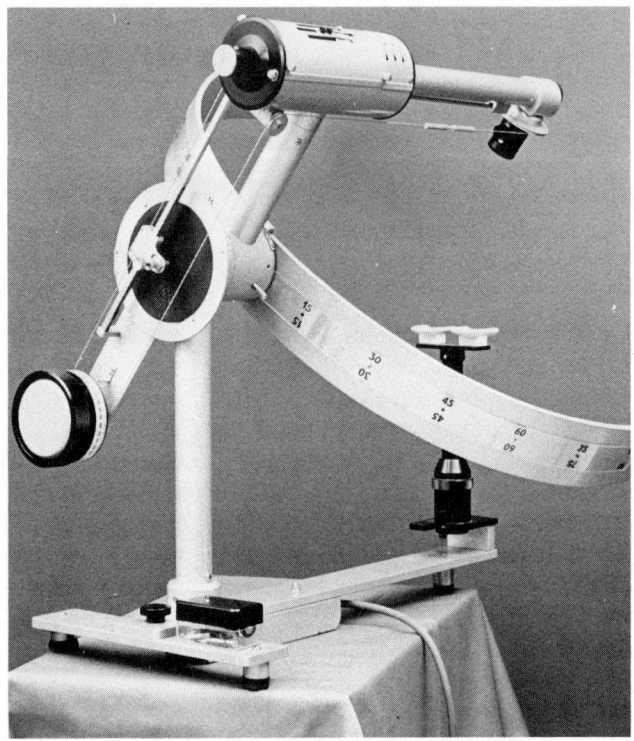

Figure 3-9 The AIMARK Projection Perimeter. The projector assembly is toward the upper right of the picture. The white centered knob at the lower left controls the position of the test spot along the arc. A chart can be mounted on the circular wheel in the center. (Photo courtesy of House of Vision.)

Schweigger Hand Perimeter

The Schweigger is a simple, portable hand perimeter. It finds its main use in screening, in providing diagnostic peripheral fields, and in permitting the neuro-ophthalmologist to take a slightly more quantitative approach in screening of the bedside patient. It consists of an arc of about a foot radius which is marked off in degrees. The central fixation device is rather clever since it consists of a small mirror at which the average person finds it nearly irresistible to stare, for in it he sees the reflection of his own eye. It is used with a separate set of test objects. Alternatively, it may be a useful instrument in the practice of strabismology when squints, angle kappa, and other factors must be measured.

Screening Devices

The clinician who undertakes the use of screening devices should understand several things about them. First of all, one may use a very adequate perimeter as a screening device. Armaly, among others, has proposed several screening patterns for use with the Goldmann Perimeter which can be done quickly by even the most unskilled of office help, and can provide just as much or more information as any of the other screeners on the market. Secondly, the use of a screener *alone* is never adequate if the results suggest a visual field defect or if one is strongly suspected on clinical grounds. It is possible for a defect that is found by the screener to decrease in size, increase in size, or change in depth without any change being shown by the screener. A positive screener test thus calls for a full, carefully done, visual field exam. In addition, many practitioners may wish to include a screener examination as part of routine eye examinations on patients who are not otherwise suspect. If a patient has a disease condition that is commonly associated with a visual field defect, or is suspected of having such a condition, one should be wary in using a screener because it is possible under such circumstances to fail to detect the pertinent defects. A complete set of indications and contraindications for screening examinations is discussed elsewhere.

The Harrington-Flocks Screener

The Harrington-Flocks Screener is a multiple-pattern screening test. It consists of a tablet of a variety of patterns that are printed in fluorescent ink and that are quite invisible by normal light. Each sheet of the tablet also contains a fixation cross, which may be seen either by black light or by white light. In the performance of the test, the subject is asked to fixate the cross and the examiner presses a button that flashes the ultraviolet tube for a short period of time and renders the various test patterns visible. The patient is then asked how many test spots he sees. Should he give an incorrect number, he is asked the locations of the spots. The defects are noted by the examiner on an accompanying chart.

The Freedman Analyzer

This device consists of a covered flash tube that evenly illuminates a face plate containing a number of holes through which the light can pass. This arrangement allows for a variable number and geometry of stimuli to be presented to the patient. Various filters of different densities may be placed in the light beam, making it possible to detect relative scotomas. The device thus utilizes some of the better principles of multiple stimulus static perimetry. It is one of the sounder devices for screening on the market.

Illuminated Screeners

In this group are a number of bowl or tangent screen devices that work by flashing a light of a given brightness at various positions in the visual field and by recording whether or not the patient sees them. Devices of this nature are made by Ocutron, Biotronics, Biometrics, and others. Although some have a photoelectric fixation control, this is generally a weak point of these devices. These generally work either by perforating or by otherwise marking a chart at the location where a light stimulus was presented. The Biometrics unit utilized a shift in eye position to mark a chart.

Amsler Grids

Although not strictly a visual field test, the Amsler charts make it possible to pick up disturbances of visual function that may accompany maculopathies or similar lesions. The Amsler chart is particularly useful in following chorioretinitis patients with defects near fixation. In these patients it is recommended that each patient be given a standard Amsler Grid (white background with black lines) and instructed to look at the grid daily. Any change in the appearance of the grid may signal a reactivation of his uveitis and should alert the patient to report to his physician immediately.

Automatic Perimetry Devices

Two automatic perimetry devices are currently available, with two additional devices forthcoming. These devices, in contrast to the screeners, are threshold-seeking devices capable of doing either kinetic or static testing and "thinking" their way out of complex perimetric situations, much as a human perimetrist would. This is made possible by utilizing a small computer to control a more or less standard perimeter.

Automatic perimetry, however, must be done in a more sophisticated fashion if it is to succeed. The computer lacks the eyes and ears of the human, and if the designers have neglected to provide it with the appropriate sensors, automatic perimetry can rapidly degenerate into a horrifying experience for the subject and a profitless exercise for the physician. It is thus important that anyone contemplating the purchase of such a device be well acquainted with the special problems of automatic testing so he can evaluate the device in an intelligent manner. For this reason, we have decided to devote a special chapter to this subject alone. We will attempt to discuss the basic problems as well as evaluate the devices—including one developed by the authors—as objectively as possible.

4
Indications for Perimetry and the Perimetrist

The most fundamental dilemmas facing the physician who wishes to utilize visual fields in his practice are when to test, how thoroughly to test, and who (or what) should perform the test. Too frequent performance of field studies is wasteful of valuable health care resources and unnecessarily expensive to the patient, while failing to perform them in a timely and adequate fashion can lead to disaster. Steering an unfailing course between the Scylla of waste and the Charybdis of unsuspected progression of a disease requires careful analysis of the patient's problem, an awareness of exactly what sort of information is necessary for its correct management, and a knowledge of what field techniques, if any, are appropriate means of acquiring this knowledge.

We find it useful to think of the indications for perimetry by stages. Some patients deserve only a screening examination or a confrontation field, whereas with others it becomes mandatory to perform multiple isopter, reproducible fields. Thus Stage I is a screening visual field examination, which can be done by confrontation, fingercounting, face description, Amsler Grid, or one of the other devices such as the classic Harrington-Flocks Screener, the Friedman Analyzer, or one of the newer screeners currently available. In addition, any quantitative instrument such as the Goldmann can be used as a screener.

Stage II is the plotting of one isopter. Equipment suitable for this stage is limited to devices capable of plotting an isopter such as a tangent screen, an autoplot, or one of the more quantitative instruments such as the Goldmann or the Tübinger. Stage III consists of plotting several, but not necessarily reproducible, isopters, while Stage IV is a full, multiple isopter quantitatively reproducible field. Reproducible isopters can be done with most of this same equipment, but they are more easily performed with devices such as the Goldmann Perimeter. Those variables that must be controlled for diagnostic isopters as well as those additional variables that must be controlled to produce reproducible isopters over a period of time are listed in Chapter 5.

146   Principles of Quantitative Perimetry

The indications for doing at least a screening field include a wide variety of complaints from the general medical, the neurological, or ophthalmic histories and several findings from the ophthalmological examination (Table 4-1). In many of these findings (e.g., papilledema), a visual field is obviously not sufficient workup, and these patients may need x-ray studies, examinations by other specialists, such as neurologists, or other laboratory examinations. However, we will not dwell on management of these problems other than to insist on the need for perimetry.

Screening visual fields are also useful for screening normal populations. A surprising incidence of unexpected pathology can be uncovered (Table 4-2). Visual field screening can be done by unskilled persons and provides a good compromise for the performance of fields on supposedly normal patients. In certain areas of occupational medicine where full fields are important, such as in aerospace medicine, screeners may very well provide a suitable means of testing the intactness of the visual system.

Although screening is recommended in a wide variety of conditions in Table 4-1, one should not merely screen a patient if one strongly suspects intracranial pathology damaging the visual system. For here we move to Stage II, which is the mapping of one isopter only. Here the goal is to obtain a diagnostic pattern or to define completely the extent of a visual field. The indications for a Stage II examination include those cases in which no screening was done. This level is also appropriate when the information about the patient strongly suggests a diagnosis that is not expected to be progressive and that requires only an abnormal pattern for confirmation. Examples are chorioretinal scars, old optic atrophy, and so forth. It should be commented, however, that chorioretinitis which may be recurrently active should probably be examined by Stage IV techniques, at least over portions of the field, since this provides us with an objective record of activity in the lesion. If the screening examination gives results that are not normal but not diagnostic of a disease, one should plot at least one isopter. This may occur when screening suggests a fiber bundle defect or some sort of hemianopsia such as the bitemporal or homonymous in particular. Isopters are necessary because screening will neither provide information about the degree of congruity present nor permit localization of a lesion to the anterior or posterior chiasm in bitemporal defects. In addition, patients who are applying for vocational rehabilitation or for aid to the blind are at present required by law in many states to have the extent of the visual field determined by one (and only one) isopter. Finally, if a patient is stable, but has a visual disability, one isopter may provide enough information to counsel the patient about his limitations. Should he drive his car? Can he improve his reading ability by turning the page? Can he improve his visual efficiency by scanning? These are all questions that require at least an isopter to answer adequately.

One progresses to multiple isopters—Stage III—whenever the questions that

I. History	II. Examination

A. General medical problems
  1. cardiovascular disease
  2. diabetes
  3. demyelinating disease
  4. syphilis
B. Neurological problems
  1. headache, particularly if associated with vomiting or if varies with posture
  2. paraesthesias, numbness
  3. transient weakness of limbs
  4. head injury
C. Ophthalmological problems
  1. diplopia, particularly associated with cranial nerve palsy
  2. poor vision on one side of body
    a. bumping into objects on one side
    b. difficulty reading (inability to find or keep on line)
  3. visual hallucinations, formed or unformed
	A. Ophthalmologic
	  1. pallor of the disc
	  2. cupping of the disc, particularly if C/D > 0.5 or asymmetric
	  3. papilledema of *any* degree
	  4. proptosis, particularly if unilateral
	  5. retinal or choroidal disease
	  6. elevated intraocular pressure
	  7. abnormalities of pupils or motility
	B. Roentgenologic
	  1. displacement of calcified pineal gland to one side
	  2. destruction or hyperostosis of bone, particularly around the sella
	  3. enlarged (or small) optic foramina
	  4. calcification, which may point to tumor or aneurysm

Table 4-1 Indications for perimetry. (Adapted from Reed and Drance.[2])

Researcher	Number of cases	Selection	Positive[a] (%)	False positive[b] (%)	Positive minus false positive (%)
Robertson	5630	factory	3.8	50	1.9
Roberts	1500	eye clinic	9	33	6
Hilton	607	(eye?) clinic	3.1	15.8	2.6
Cassidy	1536	eye clinic	13	19	10.5
McGough	4968	?	2[c]	9?	?
Graham	1339	population over 40 years	13	24	7
Linfield	1078	factory	1.85	40	?
Greve	1834	routine x-ray unit	1.95	5.5	1.84

Table 4-2 Results of mass visual field investigations. [a] Percentage of total number screened. [b] Percentage of positive results. [c] After reexamination in quiet room. Presumably, this value actually represents the number of positives minus false positives. (Adapted from Greve.[1])

one asks of a Stage II examination are not answered by a single isopter, and the possibility exists that unexplored space might provide these answers. Multiple isopters should be done whenever the first isopter is not consistent with clinical findings. Another indication for a Stage III examination is the need to gain some idea about the activity of a lesion, and thus the prognosis for return of function after treatment. In order to do this, some information about the slope of the field defect is required. This mandates at least two and often more isopters in the defective area. If a patient is suspected of hysteria or malingering, multiple isopters and tests done at different distances may be required.

Stage IV perimetry is the most exacting, for it demands multiple isopters that are reproducible. In these fields, the isopters should be close (about every 10°), and care should be taken to ensure uniformity of conditions from one time to the next. Stage IV fields are required whenever studies for following a patient are needed. A family history of glaucoma, suspected glaucoma for any reason, abiotrophies such as retinitis pigmentosa or taptoretinal degenerations where one wishes to follow their progression, and patients receiving potentially retinotoxic medication such as chloroquin are all prime candidates for Stage IV fields. Diseases that are capable of progression or regression are also important indications for quantitative perimetry. Follow-up changes must be easily detectible if the visual fields are to be valuable in the patient's management. Such diseases include pituitary adenoma, glaucoma, and, in some instances, chorioretinitis or papillitis as well as a host of other pathological processes.

The decision to perform a field of a given stage by no means ends the physician's problems but rather serves to unlock a new Pandora's box of questions that rise up shrieking demands for answers. The choice of equipment is often specified by either the stage field required or by the equipment available. The question of who should perform the field is a thorny problem and the subject of some controversy even among experts.

The dilemma is simply this: Must the physician spend his valuable time performing the field test himself, or can he rely on a technician or trust an automatic perimeter for this task? Many esteemed ophthalmologists of old have counseled the physician not to delegate the task, and many excellent men still hew to this line. Undoubtedly, there are rare instances when the physician can do a superior job, but in general we feel that the physician need not perform visual field studies himself. It is perfectly feasible to hire persons of average intelligence and dedication and to have them perform visual fields of high quality and good reproducibility in a reasonable period of time. Most of the major centers in the world employ perimetric technicians to perform the vast bulk of visual fields that are either for clinical use or for research study. The harried ophthalmologist would do well to benefit from this experience rather than try to rush through fields himself, or worse, to neglect them entirely.

In the past year, the exciting possibility that a computer can be harnessed to a perimeter to perform visual fields of a quality that rivals (and potentially exceeds) the best manual fields available, has become a reality, and several such machines are either in the marketplace or soon will be. These machines offer the advantages of being free from the problems of boredom, bias, mood variations, and fatigueability of the technician. In addition, they are unlikely to terminate their employment capriciously. Admittedly, they are unable to perform other tasks about the office or even exchange pleasantries over a cup of coffee during a lull in the day's business. Nonetheless, they offer a viable alternative to those who wish to rely more on efficiency than on human warmth. The factors peculiar to the use of automatic devices are discussed at length in Chapter 9.

The physician planning to employ a technician should be aware of several things. The first is that it requires about six months of on-the-job training for most technicians to become fully competent and confident in making visual fields that are reproducible from one sitting to the next. During this period of time, they will need frequent counselling by their supervisors. They should have their failures (such as forgetting to plot a blind spot, for example) pointed out to them promptly but kindly and be told how to correct them. Constructive suggestions rather than mere chastising of the technician are the key. It is important to realize that the technician is not a physician, should not be expected to be a physician, and therefore should not be expected either to make diagnoses or to decide just how extensive a field should be outside of specific guidelines. Without any information to the contrary, the technician should assume a Stage IV test. If the physician requests a less extensive examination, the technician will eventually learn that when a Stage II or III test reveals certain defects, additional isopters must be plotted, but this knowledge should not be expected immediately.

It should also be realized that the technician is a professional and should be treated as such. Stage IV visual field testing takes a long time and should be scheduled by appointment. The perimetrist should not be required to stay in the perimetry room all day doing nothing but one visual field after the other, since this is a very short road to insanity. It is wise to allow the perimetrist to have other duties during the day to break the monotony. Approximately four to five bilateral Stage IV fields a day borders on being above and beyond the call of duty. The physician who desires extensive static testing should expect an even lower output. The perimetry technician, like any other human, will tend to take short cuts when given the chance and when tired and bored will push even harder for short cuts. Therefore, injecting some variety into the routine and evaluating performance frequently is necessary if top quality competence is to be acquired by the technician.

Real advantages are associated with the use of either a technician or a fully automated service. Perhaps one of the most important is that it frees the doctor's time for tasks that he or she alone is capable of doing. Since neither the technician nor the machine knows the suspected diagnosis or the exact pathology in each case, the technician can be much more objective. A brief orientation is all right for Stage IV fields, but more orientation is necessary if the technician is to do a good job with a Stage II or III examination. When only a few isopters are employed, the defect may be missed unless the choice of isopter is fortuitous or one has a fair amount of knowledge concerning the nature of the expected defect. Similarly, the use of a computerized perimeter in this type of testing requires less examination time if the area of interest is specified.

Thus, the value of technicians is as great or as little as their supervisors will allow. When forced to use inadequate equipment, harried by too little time and too much work, when relatively unsupervised and untrained, the output of technicians will doubtlessly be utter garbage. If given good perimetric equipment, sufficient time to perform the examinations, sufficient training, and adequate supervision, perimetric technicians are probably one of the most valuable additions possible to the offices of ophthalmologists.

REFERENCES

1. Greve EL, Verduin WM: Mass visual field investigation in 1834 persons with supposedly normal eyes. Albrecht von Graefes Arch Klin Ophthalmol 183:286, 1972
2. Reed H, Drance SM: The Essentials of Perimetry, 2nd ed. London, Oxford University Press, 1972

5

Testing the Visual Field with the Goldmann Perimeter: A Sequential Guide

This chapter is a guide to the use of the Goldmann Perimeter. The first section outlines the method of setting up and calibrating the instrument. The second section gives the technique for performing the test. Although the second section also uses the Goldmann as an example, the methods advocated are equally valid for other devices as well.

As a teaching aid, both sections are given in the form of flow charts (Fig. 5-1 and Fig. 5-9). In addition, the location of the controls of the Goldmann are shown in Figures 5-2 and 5-3, while the field chart is explained in Figure 5-4. Repeated reference to these figures (or to an actual perimeter) while reading the text should benefit the inexperienced Goldmann user.

PREPARING TO TEST

1. Check the patient's best corrected visual acuity in each eye and enter the value obtained on the visual field chart. If visual acuity is less than 20/20, ask the patient if he or she has undergone a recent refraction, and, if not, re-refract prior to perimetric testing. (See Figure 5-1 for actual logic of Steps 1 and 2.)

2. Ask for the patient's distance-corrected glasses and read them out on the lensometer. Use spherical equivalent of any cylinder having 0.75 diopter or less power. (A recently performed refraction already recorded is preferable to this readout, but Step 1 should be repeated with trial frames containing the new prescription if visual acuity is found to be reduced in Step 1.)

3. Seat the patient before the perimeter, with the instrument lights on, room lights off. Tell the patient you want his eyes to grow accustomed to this level of light. If one plans a standard photopic field, five to ten minutes will suffice.

4. Look up the appropriate addition to the patient's refraction for the patient's age:

Range of Age (yrs)	Addition (Diopters)
under 30	none
30-39	+0.50
40-44	+1.00
45-49	+1.50
50-54	+2.25
55-59	+3.00
60 or more	+3.50

5. Check to see if the signs of the sphere and the cylinder are different after adding the values obtained in Steps 2 and 4 above. If so, check to see if the absolute value of the sphere is more than 1/2 that of the cylinder. If both conditions are met, the prescription for use in the perimeter should be transposed by:

a. adding algebraically old sphere and old cylinder to obtain the value and sign of new sphere
b. changing the old cylinder's sign (+ to − or − to +) to obtain the sign of the new cylinder
c. keeping the old cylinder's power the same in the new Rx
d. changing the old cylinder's axis by 90° to obtain the new axis (adding 90° to axes of 90° or less, subtracting 90° from axes of 91° to 180°)

This step allows the use of lenses of the minimum power to correct the vision, and consequently, reduces the chance of distortion by the trial lenses. A good rule to follow is to use negative cylinders for myopes; positive cylinders for hyperopes.

6. Insert the perimeter prescription for the better eye into the instrument's lens holder (see Fig. 5-5); using *thin-rimmed,* large-size trial lenses, have the patient place his or her chin on the headrest, forehead against the headstrap, and adjust the screw to bring the lens into contact either with the brow or just short of the lashes, whichever occurs first. Do this after patching the nontested eye with the translucent occluder provided by the manufacturer and shifting the headrest all the way over toward the patched eye. *Do not* use an opaque occluder of any sort, since it will change the state of light adaptation of the patched eye.

7. Ask the patient to look at the small light inside the black circle in the center of the perimeter bowl and to tell you whether it is more clearly seen when:

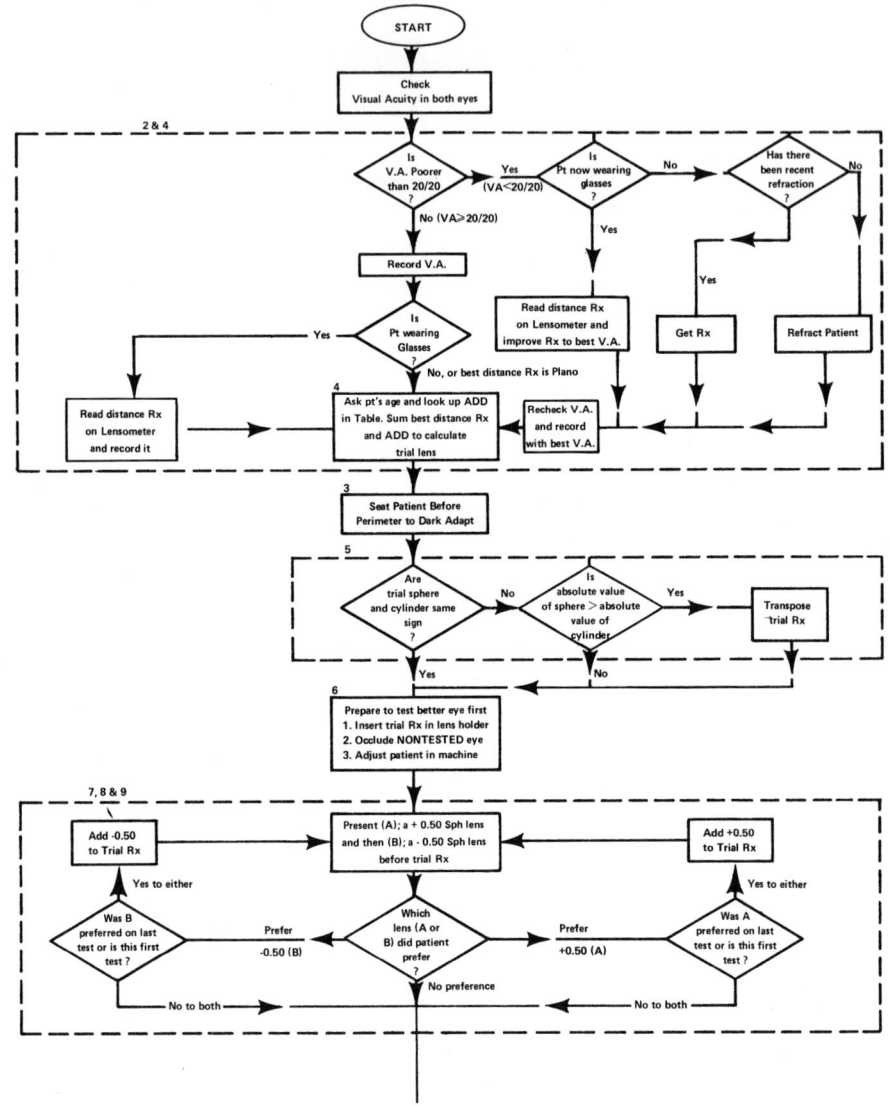

Figure 5-1 Flow chart that shows how to begin to test with a Goldmann Perimeter (see text). Block numbers correspond to step numbers in the text. In the block immediately following Step 6 (Step 7), *a* is defined as the trial prescription in the holder.

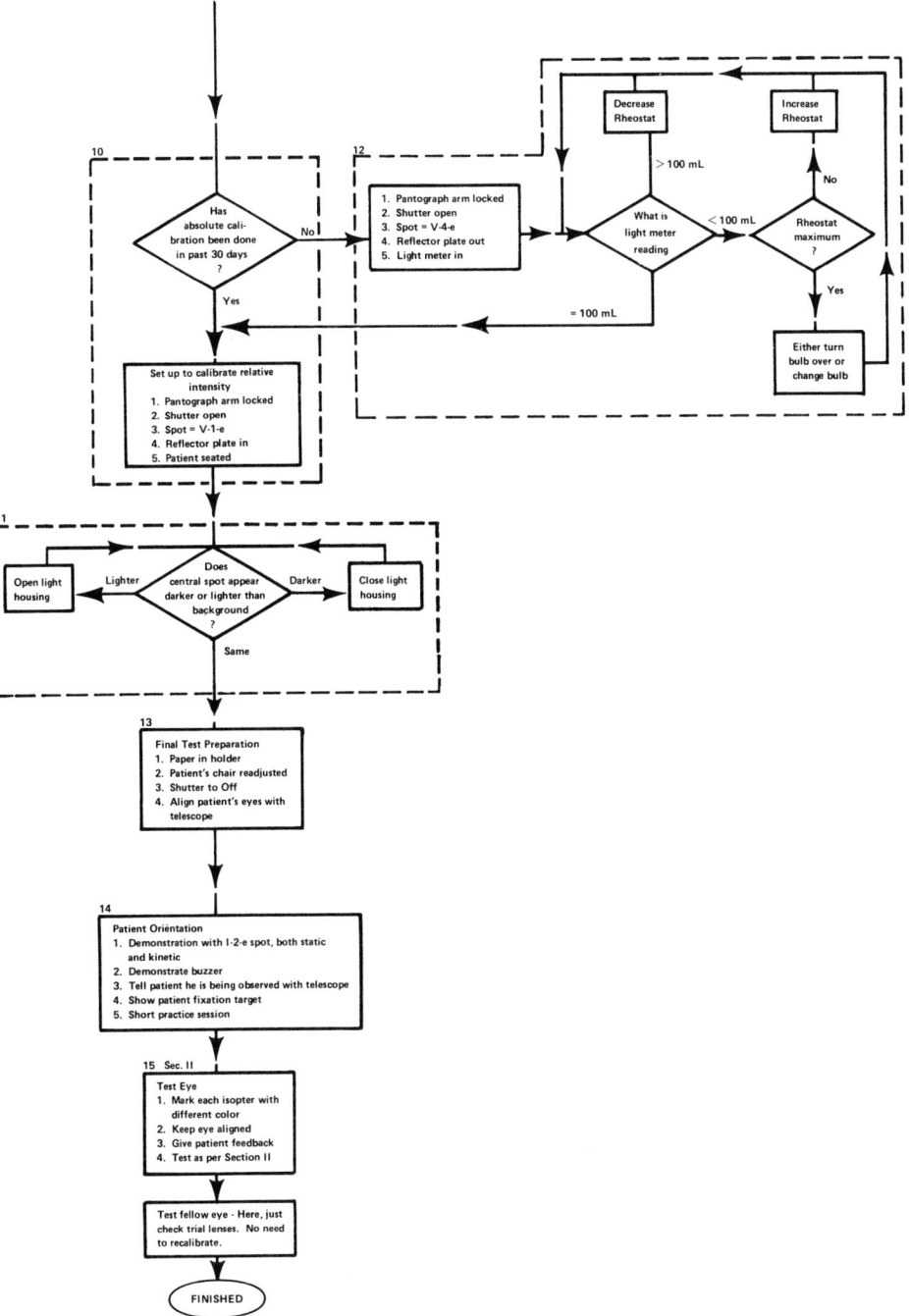

156 *Principles of Quantitative Perimetry*

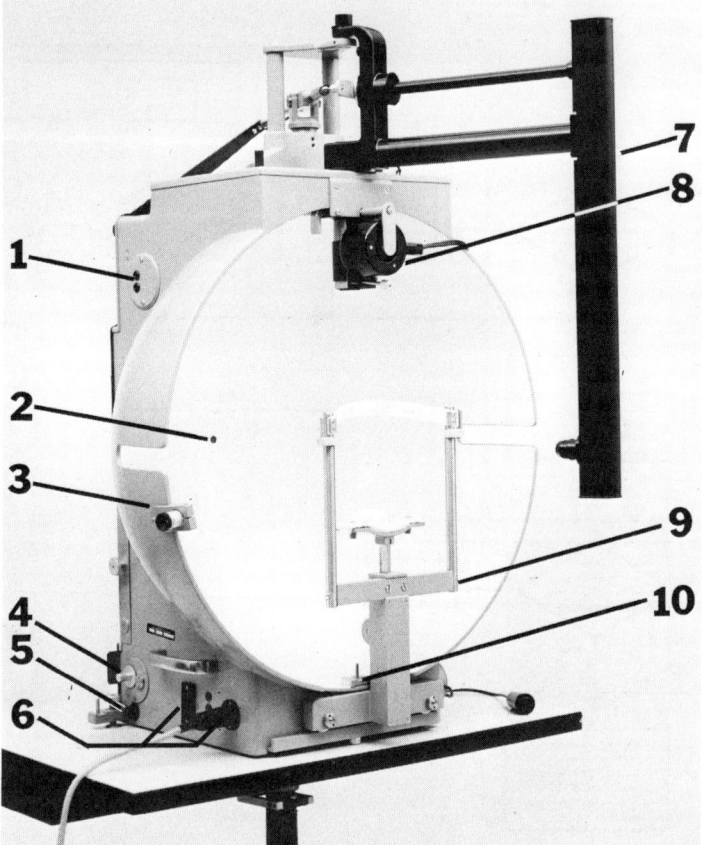

Figure 5-2 The Goldmann Perimeter from the patient's side: (1) accessory socket; (2) patient's view of telescope which serves as fixation target; (3) calibration telescopic magnifier; (4) shutter; (5) fuse; (6) power switch and cord; (7) projector arm; (8) lamp house; (9) headrest; (10) pin to center lens holder.

    a.   a clean handheld +0.50 sphere is held in front of the instrument-supported lenses, or
    b.   a clean handheld −0.50 sphere is held in front of the instrument-supported lenses. (Do not give the patient the option of comparing the "a" and "b" views with the view having neither lens in front of the original perimeter Rx.).

    8.   If the patient says neither lens is preferable, no change is indicated. If, by choosing 7a, the patient shows that more plus is desired, a slightly stronger plus sphere (or weaker minus sphere) would be substituted for the sphere calculated in Step 5 above. If by choosing 7b, the patient prefers minus, a weaker plus or stronger minus sphere should then be used.

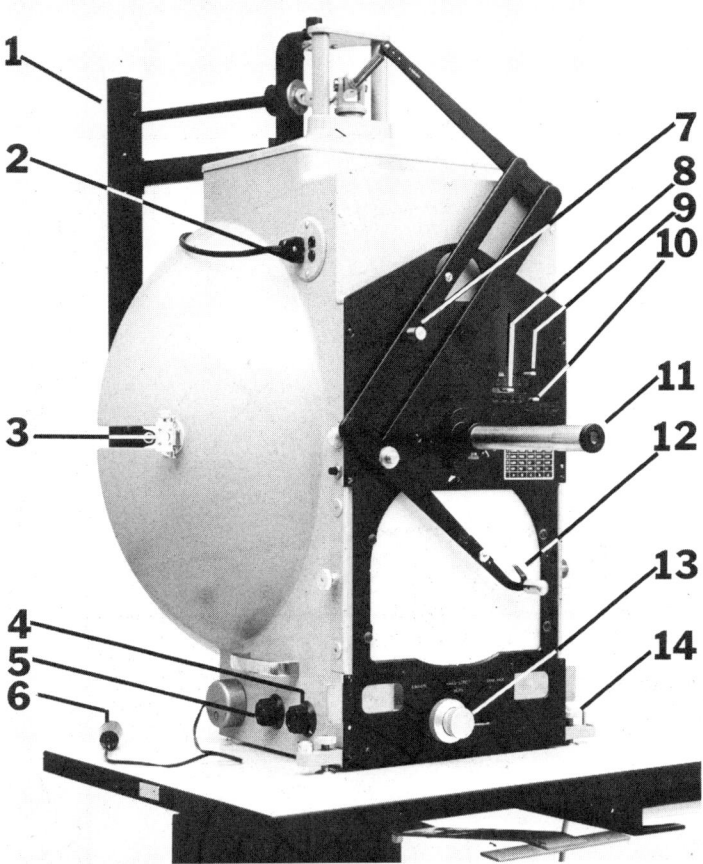

Figure 5-3 The Goldmann Perimeter from the operator's side: (1) projector; (2) socket with cable for main bulb and accessory socket; (3) light-meter bracket and calibration screen; (4) control for chart illumination; (5) control for main bulb brightness; (6) push button for buzzer; (7) pantograph arm lock for calibration; (8) neutral density filter, 0.5 l.u.; (9) neutral density filter, 0.1 l.u.; (10) spot size control; (11) telescope to monitor fixation; (12) handle of pantograph; (13) knobs to adjust headrest; (14) leveling knob.

9. Steps 7 and 8 should be repeated until the patient fluctuates from preferring plus each time to preferring minus and vice versa, or the patient reaches a Rx that gives him no preference. (The *final* perimeter prescription might still be altered by repeating Steps 7 and 8 if the patient seems to tire because of long accommodation during testing or if he pays too little attention to his answer during Step 7.) The examiner knows to retest Step 7 if the patient says the center is fading in and out or if the examiner himself notes that the central field has too much scatter or variability of test results compared with earlier or more peripheral isopters.

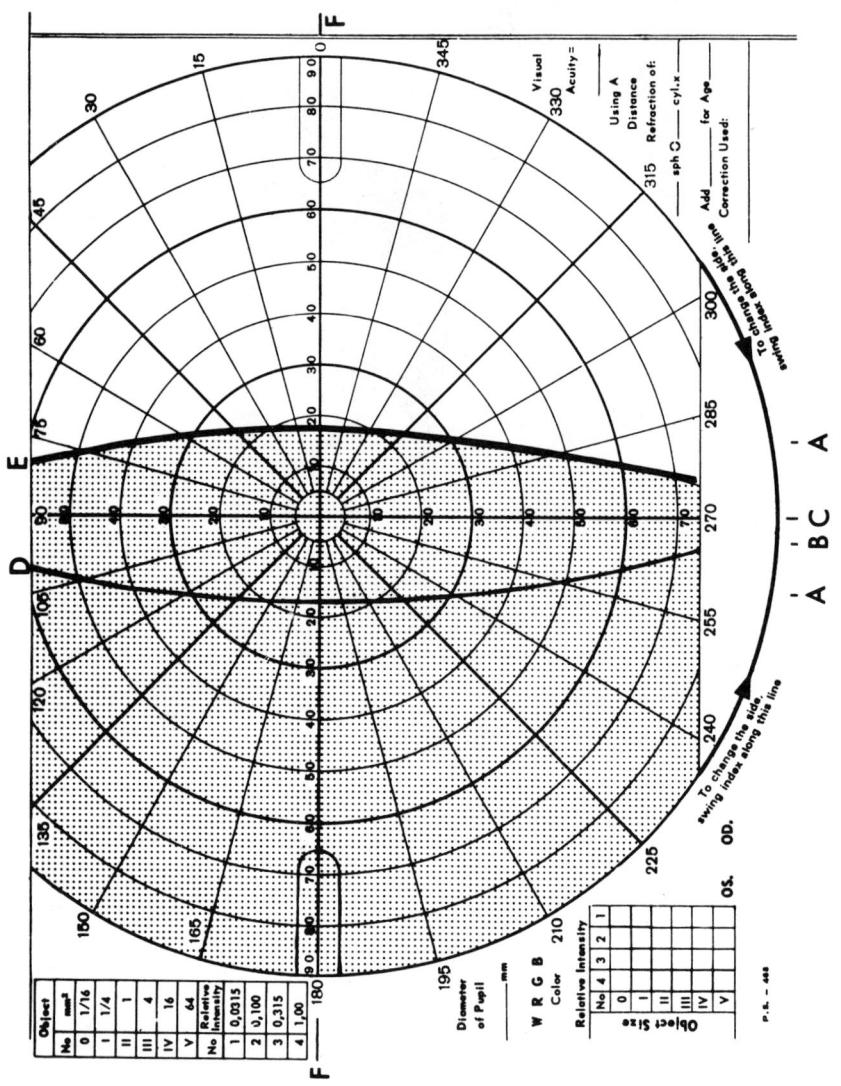

Testing the Visual Field with the Goldmann Perimeter 159

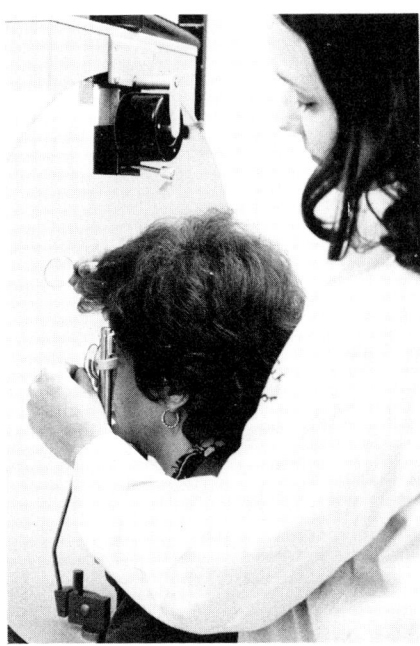

Figure 5-5 The patient's refraction, with additional diopters for age, is placed in lens holder and refined with plus and minus half-diopter spheres (see Fig. 5-1, blocks 7,8, and 9).

10. At this point the machine must be calibrated. If absolute calibration has not been accomplished within the preceeding 30 days, it should be done first (see Step 12 and Fig. 5-6). Otherwise, the contrast is calibrated by setting the test spot projector to V-1-e (a spot of 64 sq mm that adds 3.15 millilamberts of light to the background luminance) and by placing the shutter in the constantly "on" position (see Figs. 5-2 and 5-3). The pantograph arm is fixed by a special lock to point toward the reflector plate located 70° out on the right horizontal meridian. Notice the curved lines to each side of the vertical meridian on the chart paper. (Fig. 5-4). If the pantograph pointer is to the right, as it is for calibrations, it will move easily to any point on the right side of the paper (corresponding to the patient's right side inside the hemisphere) and will move to the left of the center only as far as the curved line. The pantograph pointer may be changed from side to side by swinging it evenly below along the arc marked on the standard Goldmann chart.

Figure 5-4 Chart for Goldmann Perimeter. The shaded area shows that area which can be tested with the pantograph arm to the left. Lines D and E mark the limits of test for the right and left pantograph positions. Lines F and C mark the center of the chart for normal use. B marks the horizontal displacement necessary when the 1-dot–4-dot device is used, and lines A mark the position for the central scotoma device (see Chapter 6).

160   Principles of Quantitative Perimetry

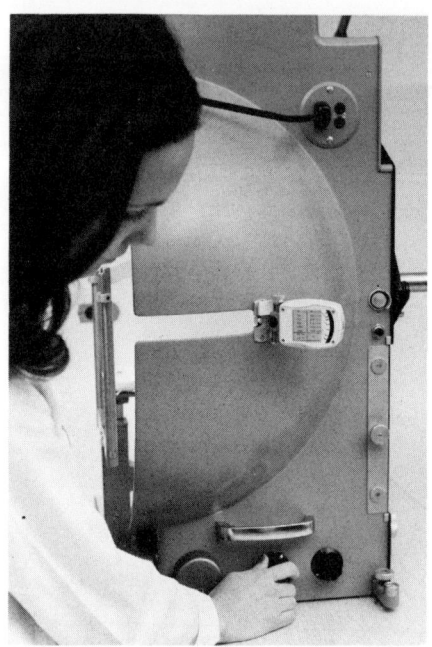

Figure 5-6   Calibration of bulb brightness on Goldmann. The projector arm is clamped into position; the machine set to V-4-e; a light meter is affixed to the bowl; and the rheostat is adjusted until the meter reads 100 ml (1000 asb). (See Fig. 5-1, block 12)

   11.   With patient still seated before the perimeter, the cover over the light at the top of the hemisphere (see Fig. 5-7) is adjusted up and down while the examiner observes the reflector plate to the patient's right from the observer telescope or hole in the hemisphere rim to the patient's left. When the light from the reflector plate so evenly matches the light from the hemisphere's inner surface that they fade together and have the same luminance or brightness, the light cover is left in that position, and the instrument is calibrated relatively for that patient.
   12.   Absolute calibration consists of Step 10, but changing the projector setting to V-4-e (100 millilamberts) and pushing the reflector plate out of the way so that all the light passes through a hole in the rear part of the reflector plate. A light meter, shielded from room light exposures to keep it accurate, is clipped on the back of the reflector plate (see Fig. 5-6), and a plate to the left side of the examiner's pantograph is swung open to illuminate the light meter. The meter's reading is adjusted to read 1000 ASB (100 millilamberts) by turning the rheostat knob on the side of the perimeter below the light meter. (Relative calibration should be done every time a different patient is to be tested. Absolute calibrations need only be done about once each month or so.)

Testing the Visual Field with the Goldmann Perimeter

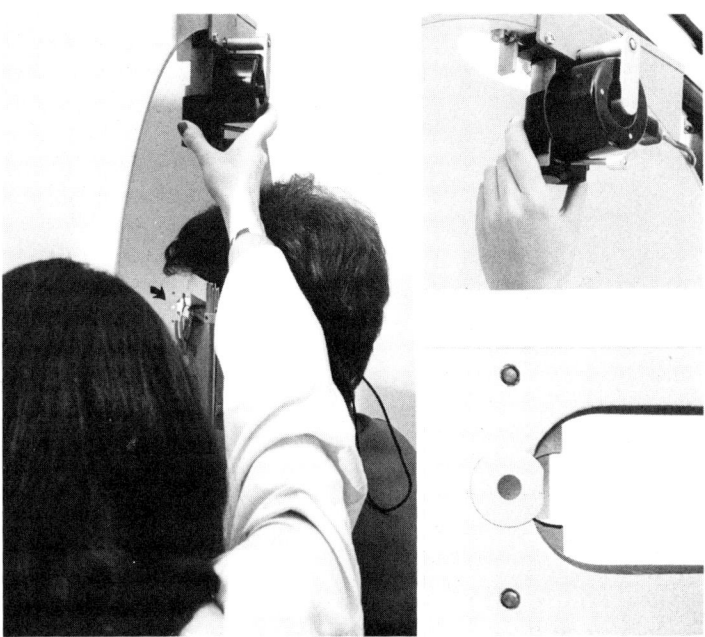

Figure 5-7 Calibration of background on the Goldmann Perimeter. After the patient is seated at the perimeter, the filters are set to V-1-e, the pantograph arm locked, and the shutter opened. The operator (left) peers through the small telescope on side of bowl (Figure 5-2, #3) at the "grease spot" photometer (arrow) across the bowl. The shutter on the lamp housing (upper right) is adjusted until the center spot is the same brightness as the bowl. In the picture on the left, this spot is too light. In the picture at lower right, it is too dark. (See Fig. 5-1, blocks 10 and 11.)

13. The patient should be told how to adjust the height of the machine relative to his chair by turning the wheel below the perimeter and be encouraged to keep himself comfortable. While he does this the examiner should insert paper in the pantograph so that printed lines (lines F and C on Figure 5-4) go into the notches at right, left, and bottom (see Fig. 5-4). Rotate the shutter switch so that when it is released, the spot is "off."

14. The patient should be told:

The idea of this test is to check your side vision. To do that, you must help by signaling *(place the patient's hand on the buzzer and press for him)* when you see a spot like this one which is moving around before you *(present I-2-e)*, whether it is moving in from the edges, moving out, or standing still *(describe and demonstrate simultaneously)*. The most important thing you have to do, however, is look steadily at the little light in the middle of the black spot, which is a telescope opening so I can look at your eye. *(Flash the extra mirror to the operator's right at the base of the telescope.)* Now, please, don't look at this spot *(move the test spot)*. Just press the buzzer *(press)* whenever you think you see it, and it will disappear *(close the shutter)*. Remember to keep looking here *(mirror*

162   *Principles of Quantitative Perimetry*

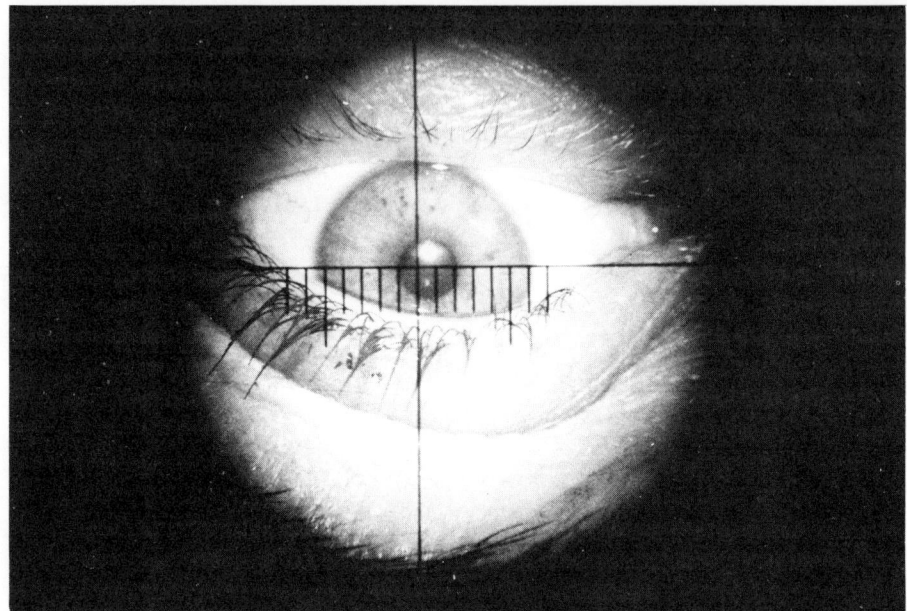

Figure 5-8   View of the patient through the fixation telescope. Note that the eye appears inverted. The pupil diameter may be measured by use of the graticule; the diameter of this one is 3 mm.

flash), not at this one *(test spot "on" near middle).* When you see this one, press immediately and make it go away *(close the shutter).* Remember, keep your forehead against the strap, chin against its rest, your eye on the middle, and press when you see this light *(I-2-e "on" near middle).* Now, you are ready, here it comes. The first 3 or 4 don't count, so you can practice with the button.

15.   Position the levers to I-2-e, choose the color of pen or pencil you will generally use to record this standard test (we use red), and mark the "e" box with this color where roman I crosses arabic 2. Look at the patient's eye through the telescope to be sure it is centered on the cross hairs (Fig. 5-8). Make any corrective adjustments necessary by turning the large concentric knobs below the pantograph (see Fig. 5-3, 13).

At this point, we are ready to begin the test.

DOING THE TEST

The principles here, though illustrated on the Goldmann perimeter, are valid for any device.

1.   With an I-2-e setting, start the pantographic pointer 40° out, just to the right or left of the upper vertical meridian, and move it downward at the rate of 4°

or 5°/sec until the patient presses the buzzer. Never purposely oscillate any test spot. Do not plan to mark the first 3 or 4 presentations, but look intently through the telescope at the patient's eye, waiting for any sign of shifting fixation. If the patient's eye does not move during this period, yet the buzzer is sounded at roughly appropriate times (or at least reproducibly in the event of a severe visual field defect), the patient should be encouraged verbally by a comment that he or she is doing a good job of holding fixation. The patient should be encouraged to blink, if necessary, right *after* pushing the buzzer.

If the patient has not been tested on several previous occasions he is very likely to move his eye about, trying to find the spot and thus ignoring earlier instructions. If so, this should be recognized the first time it occurs, and the examiner should say, firmly but gently:

> No, no, Mr. (Ms.) Smith! Remember that you must not look away from this center spot *(flash the mirror on the telescope)*. I am watching your eye through this telescope and know you didn't understand how important it is to keep looking steadily at the light in the center of the black spot. Push the buzzer only when you first notice this other spot *(turn on the test spot and move it around the center)* out of the corner of your eye. Don't look at it to be sure you are right; I'll keep track of that. You must hold the middle and let me know with the buzzer just as soon as you think you see the test spot. I'll let you know if you are signalling when you are not really seeing it, but don't you look around to try to find it. Now hold the middle and tell me. Are you ready? Here it comes.

Do not wait until late in the test—when results are irregular—to check up and find the patient has never fixated. Try to catch him moving early in the test, and make the above or similar speech. Giving the patient immediate feedback, both positive and negative, as to his behavior with regards to fixation and signalling is very important, particularly on the first few visual fields. This aids the patient in learning how to take the examination.

2. The first 4 or 5 spots should move at the same rate as subsequent ones, come in from the periphery, and move relentlessly and steadily toward the center until the buzzer sounds. Within the limits of the examiner's capability, these passes should come from random directions. Randomness and unchanging speed of movement are fairly easy until the examiner becomes interested in working out the details of a suspected defect. Despite the temptation, the presentations should remain random, starting 10°-15° outside the expected isopter and moving steadily to intersect this line at a right angle (see Fig. 5-10).

3. The time between presentations of test spots should be brief to prevent anxiety and boredom, but they should not be so brief the patient cannot be prepared to respond. If the time between presentations is too regular, the patient may learn the rhythm and merely keep pushing the buzzer whether he sees the spot or not. Purposely randomizing the time intervals between spots is strongly recommended.

4. As the sixth and subsequent test spot presentations are made, the examiner should make a short line on the test chart at the location where the spot

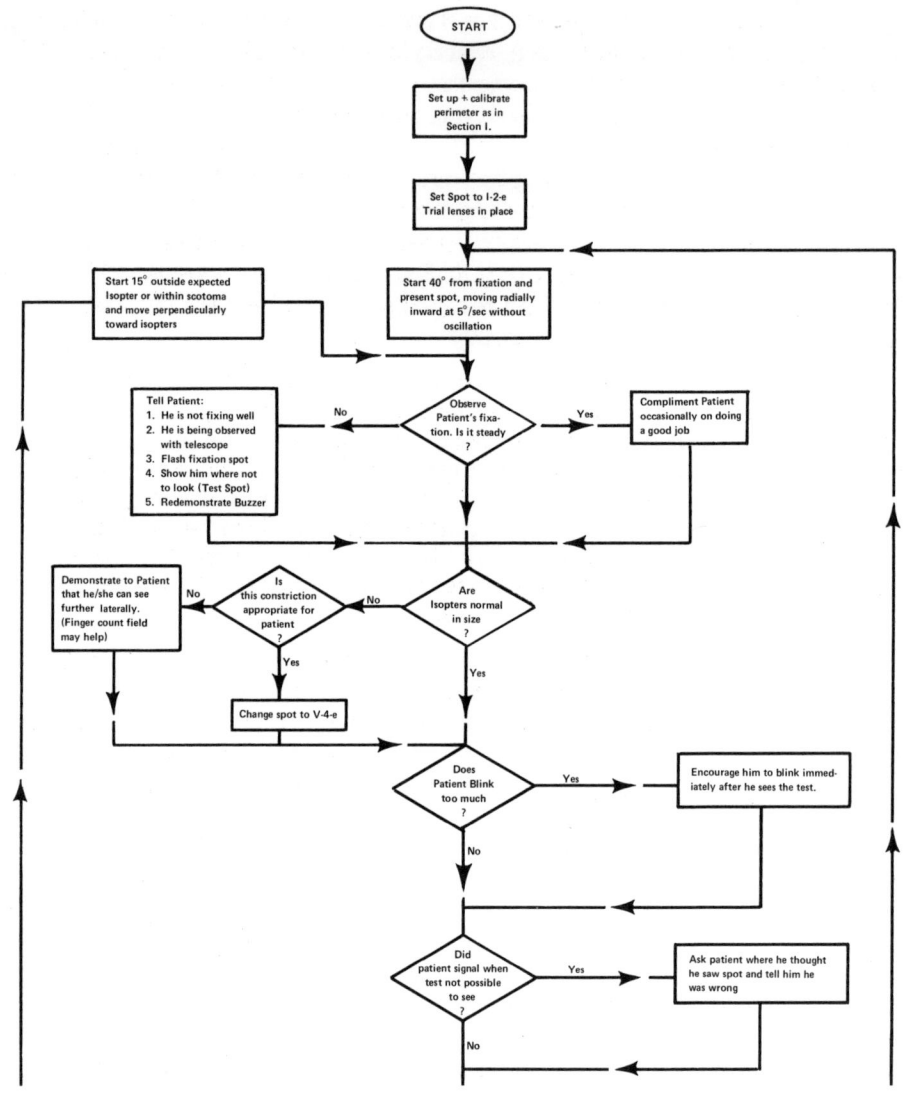

Figure 5-9   Flow chart that shows how to do the test.

was presented. Direction of movement can be indicated in most instances by making a dash (–) perpendicular to the direction of test object movement. Where events are confused through irregular borders, etc, the response location may be marked by a "T" shaped mark, with the cross bar of the "T" serving as the usual dash (–) and the stem indicating the direction from which the test object moved to the dash or cross bar.

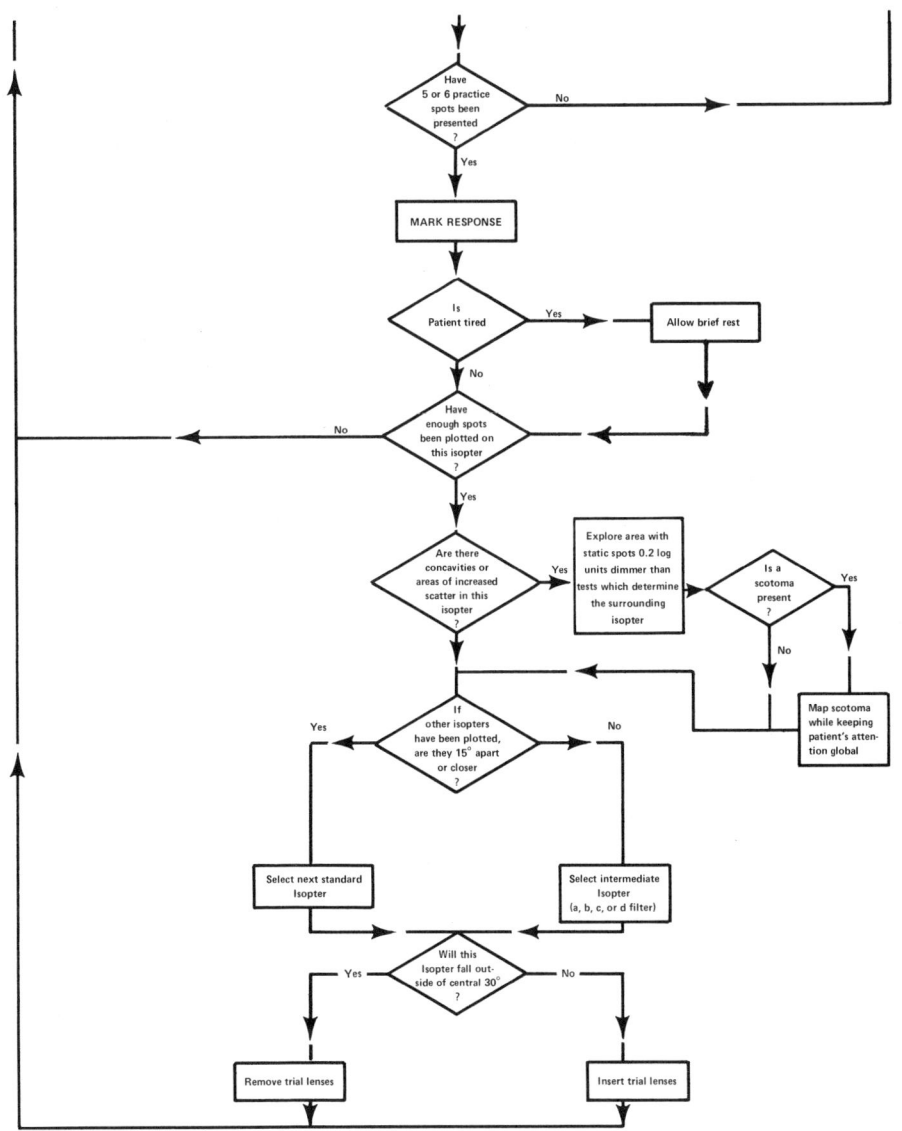

This procedure applies to other perimeters in addition to Goldmann.

5. Enough testing should be done with the I-2-e spot to enable the examiner to predict with accuracy where the same test spot will be seen. Any spots that penetrate the expected isopter or occur outside it should be recorded unless the eye was closed or deviated from fixation. Deep penetrations often occur when a scotoma lies within a given isopter. Also, in most cases scatter is expected to some extent and a record of it helps interpretation.

166   *Principles of Quantitative Perimetry*

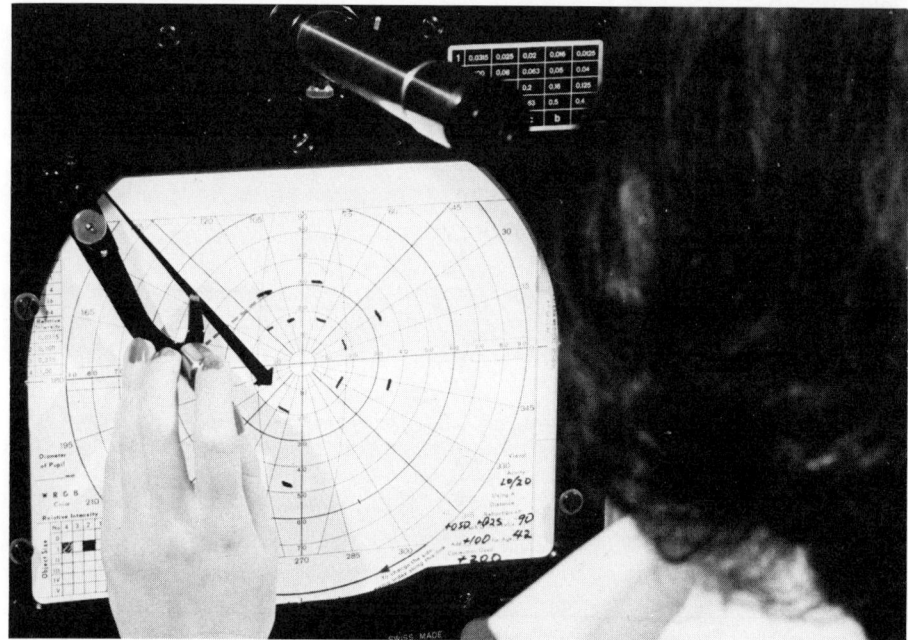

Figure 5-10   Illustration of the method of tracking inward toward the expected isopter boundary. The operator mentally constructs a straight line between points (dotted line) and tracks inward along this line's perpendicular bisector (arrow), *not* toward fixation.

6. When the patient grows tired, his responses grow more irregular and slow. Avoid this fatigue by frequent, short periods of rest; and utilize any time when testing must be interrupted to reset the instrument or to record data. Simply say: "Now, sit back and close your eyes for just a moment. *(pause)* Okay, I'm ready to go again, are you? Just put your head back against the head rest, chin down, and let me be sure you are centered." Light conversation during the pause may serve to put an anxious patient at ease, or answer any questions that he or she may have concerning the testing procedure.

7. If the patient has good visual acuity, he or she must have good light sense at least centrally. If the patient's visual acuity is poor, the central light sense must be down, but the peripheral light sense may be good. Use of I-2-e should be followed by I-3-e, also through the lenses if I-2-e was mostly inside 20°. If I-2-e was at 30° or so, I-3-e must be tested later, after the lenses are removed. An isopter using the I-1-e setting should be recorded routinely as a standard isopter and can always be seen if the vision is decent; it can often be seen in the paramacular area when the visual acuity is down. If this or any larger or brighter standard test cannot be seen, a letter "T" (for "tested and not seen anywhere") should be entered in the color code table at the appropriate

intersection of size and brightness to indicate the greatest standard stimulus value that was presented but not seen anywhere at all. Standard stimuli are: 0-1-e, I-1-e, I-2-e, I-3-e, I-4-e, II-4-e, III-4-e, IV-4-e, and V-4-e. Adding the roman and arabic numbers together gives a combined "stimulus value" for these of 1,2,3,4,5,6,7,8, and 9. The second through fifth test spots differ in projected intensity by 1/2 log unit from their adjacent listing; the last five differ from one another by an equivalent fourfold change in area. (For further discussion of this topic, see Chapter 1.)

8. Relative defects in the visual field may show up as complete cuts, as scotomas, or as normal seeing areas, depending upon the size and intensity of the spot used to test them. Too small a stimulus value may fail to elicit any response at all in the questionable area of field. Too large a stimulus may be seen in an area shown clearly to be defective with a smaller spot. We use the smaller standard isopters until the lens edge is reached (25° for aphakes; 45° for patients with high myopia). Then a maximum isopter is performed with the lens and its holder removed, and intermediate isopters (standard, if possible) are added until no distance greater than 10° exists between isopters.

9. Where irregularities in a given part of an isopter occur, where penetrations have been noted well inside an isopter yet the eye was open, and where larger expanses of untested space exist (more than 10°-15° between isopters), we suggest an intermediate isopter, using the filters a,b,c, or d with the major setting of the surrounding (i.e., larger) isopter. The defect might be picked up by scotoma testing that uses the test size and brightness of the isopter just surrounding the zone of the suspected defect. (For examples of irregularities that arouse the suspicion of a scotoma, see Figs. 5-9, 5-11.)

10. Scotoma testing, as exemplified by mapping of the normal blind spot, is accomplished by presenting a stationary test object inside that part of the field surroundable by the test object's isopter. If it is seen within 1.5 to 2 seconds, it is probably not a scotoma, for the patient may be primarily ready to report moving spots. If it is not seen in two seconds, the spot should be moved in a straight line until it is seen and an appropriate dash or "T" mark is recorded to indicate that location. We strongly urge mixing the isopter determination randomly with the normal blind spot check to accustom the patient to paying global attention, not focal. Where brief scotoma checking has been tried between isopters, we indicate this by making "x" marks in the test areas where the spot was seen, using the color coding of the isopter corresponding to the same size and brightness as the test spot.

The importance of the two-second wait must be emphasized. If the spot is moved as soon as it is presented, the movement during the patient's reaction time will permit a scotoma to be plotted—even where none exists!

11. When no test is seen for a prolonged period during early testing, a large defect is the usual explanation. Use of a very large test object will outline the

168   *Principles of Quantitative Perimetry*

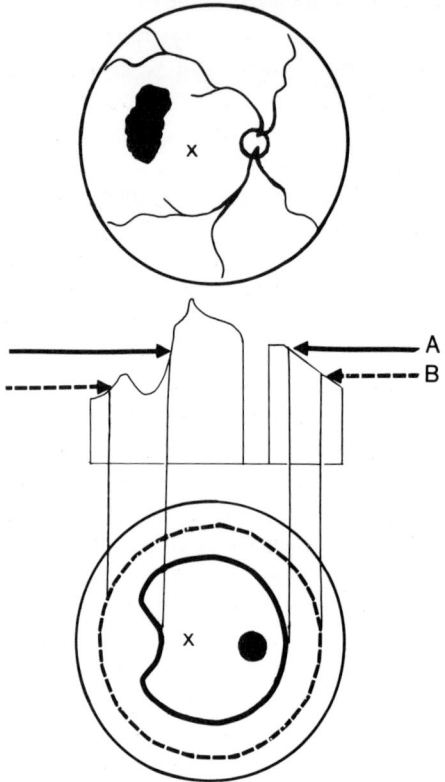

Figure 5-11   Illustration showing how to suspect the location of scotomas. Fundus view with lesion, above kinetic field, causes a field defect (static cut, middle below). If the kinetic target is too dim to explore rim of scotoma, it will pass across top and strike the "wall" of remaining vision, thus appearing as a concavity. A slightly dimmer test, which just grazed across the top of the rim of normal field, would show up as an area of scatter.

maximum limits of the field for smaller stimuli. In patients with poor vision, particularly of a refractive nature (i.e., corneal defects), the use of larger test objects with approximately the same stimulus value may be an aid (e.g., the IV-1-e and the I-4-e have about the same stimulus value, but differ in size; see Chapters 1 and 2).

12.   Record the pupillary diameter, date, and patient's name as well as the refraction finally utilized and any comments regarding the patient's cooperation or reliability. Be sure visual acuity was noted earlier. These data will prove invaluable in later attempts at interpretation or comparison with other fields.

13.   Change the eye patch, headrest location, patient's chair position, paper in the pantograph, and lenses, being sure to check the lens value (see prepar-

ing to Test, Steps 7 and 8). The second eye should be tested, even if the only vision recorded is light perception. If perception is poor, the test will be brief. If light projection is present, a *very* valuable field may result from what is usually regarded as a "blind" eye (see Fig. 1-33). Assuming the fellow eye sees, fixation may be greatly facilitated by use of the central scotoma device (see Chapter 6).

The principles given above are illustrated in Figure 5-12, A through L, which reconstruct the testing of an actual visual field.

TROUBLESHOOTING

On rare occasions (initially, perhaps, as frequently as every third test), one will encounter a visual field that is difficult to perform for a variety of reasons. Occasionally, one may have an uncooperative or belligerent patient. In these instances, calm and repeated explanations of what is involved and why it is important to the patient's well-being may go far to alleviate the situation. Sometimes, an attempt at anything but the grossest of field tests must be abandoned. In a majority of cases, however, one may have a seemingly cooperative patient, but one from whom it is difficult to obtain consistent data. This shows up as scatter. There are a number of variables that contribute to scatter, and an attempt should be made with each patient to understand and eliminate the factors at play. These "Five Ps of Scatter" may be categorized as follows:

A. Physical
1. Rate of test object movement (kinetic):
   Hold velocity constant for any eccentricity, about 5°/sec; slower in the central zone.
2. Duration of test spot (static):
   Hold duration constant; choose durations of one second or more, or use timed shutter.
3. Luminance and hue of test and background:
   Hold constant; avoid natural light; use constant voltage transformer; don't turn lights on or off (or open doors) after starting the test.
4. Size and reflectance of test object:
   Do not clean or change test objects of same theoretical size during a given test (applies to nonprojection test techniques, such as tangent screen).
5. Time interval between stimuli:
   Keep varying intertest interval within a small range. Avoid very long or very short intervals.

B. Pharmacological
1. Pupil size:
   Do not instill any drops just before fields. All glaucoma medications should be taken well in advance. If it is desired to dilate pupil for perimetric exam, long-acting agents are preferable, and one should wait until the pupil size is stable.

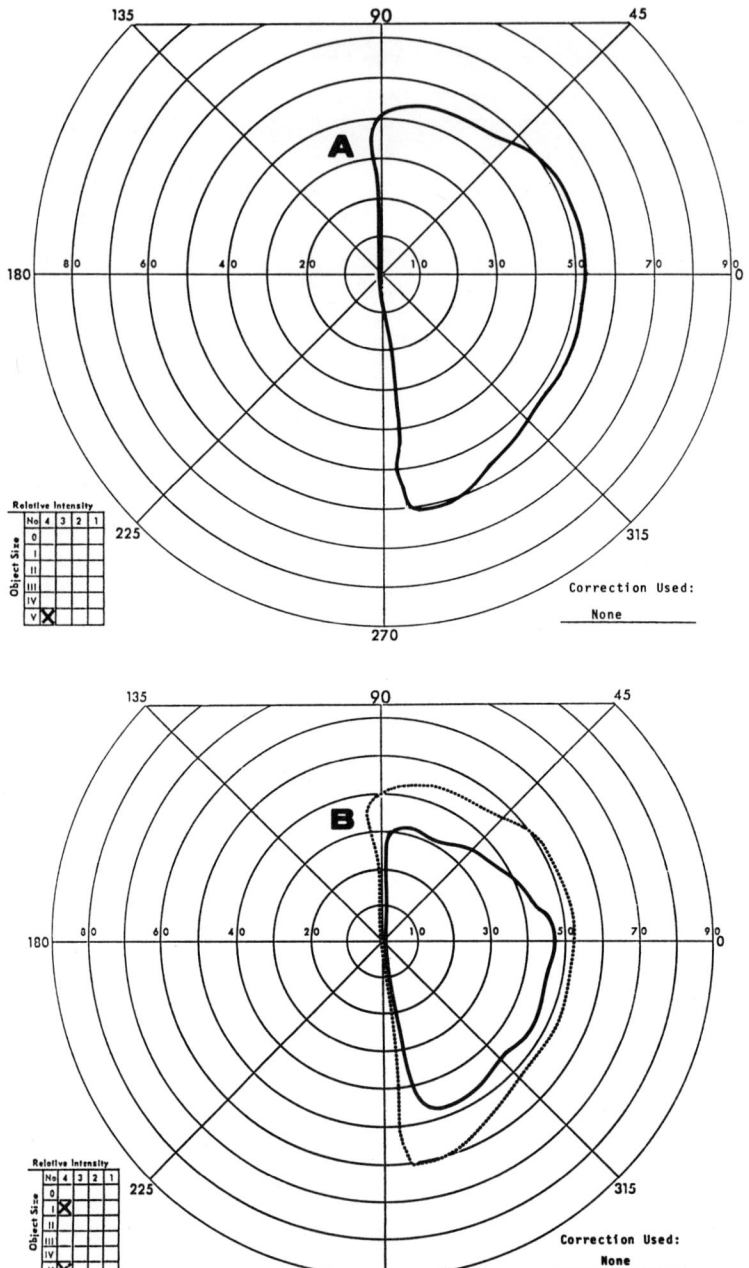

Figure 5-12 Step-by-step example for testing a visual field by the preferred technique. In figures A through L, a solid line is the new isopter. A dotted line corresponds to the last previous isopter. (The left eye is tested in all cases.) (After Lynn JR: Testing the visual field in glaucoma, in Symposium on Glaucoma: Transactions of the New Orleans Academy of Ophthalmology. St. Louis, CV Mosby Co., 1975.)
A Outlining the outer limits of the field with the V-4-e (i.e., the highest value) target should be done early when a large field defect is present. Note no corrective lens was used. **B** An intermediate isopter (the I-4-e) falls 5° to 15° inside the prior isopter and confirms the hemianopsia. Again, no correction is used.

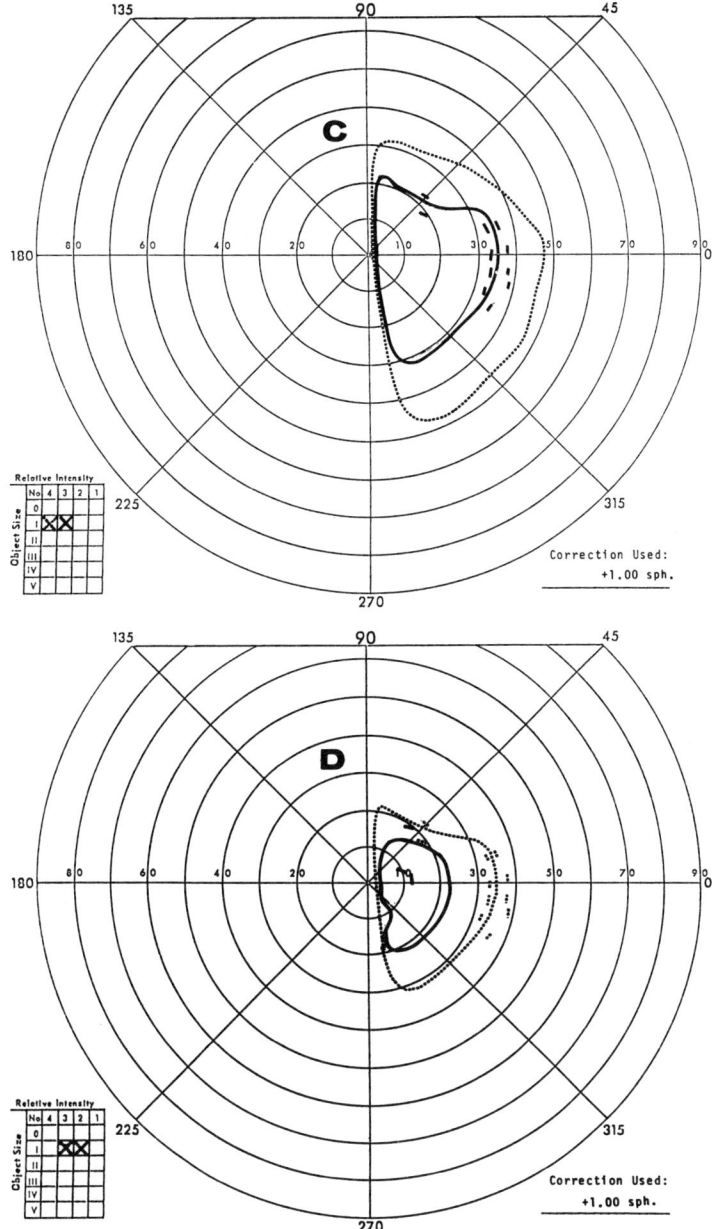

C A correction of +1.00 sphere is placed before the patient, and the first paracentral isopter (with I-3-e) is plotted. Note the appearance of moderate scatter. **D** A second paracentral isopter is plotted using the I-2-e target. Again, scatter is noted. Since scatter in the central isopters alone suggests an improperly corrected refractive error, the refraction in this case was checked and found to be +1.75 sphere.

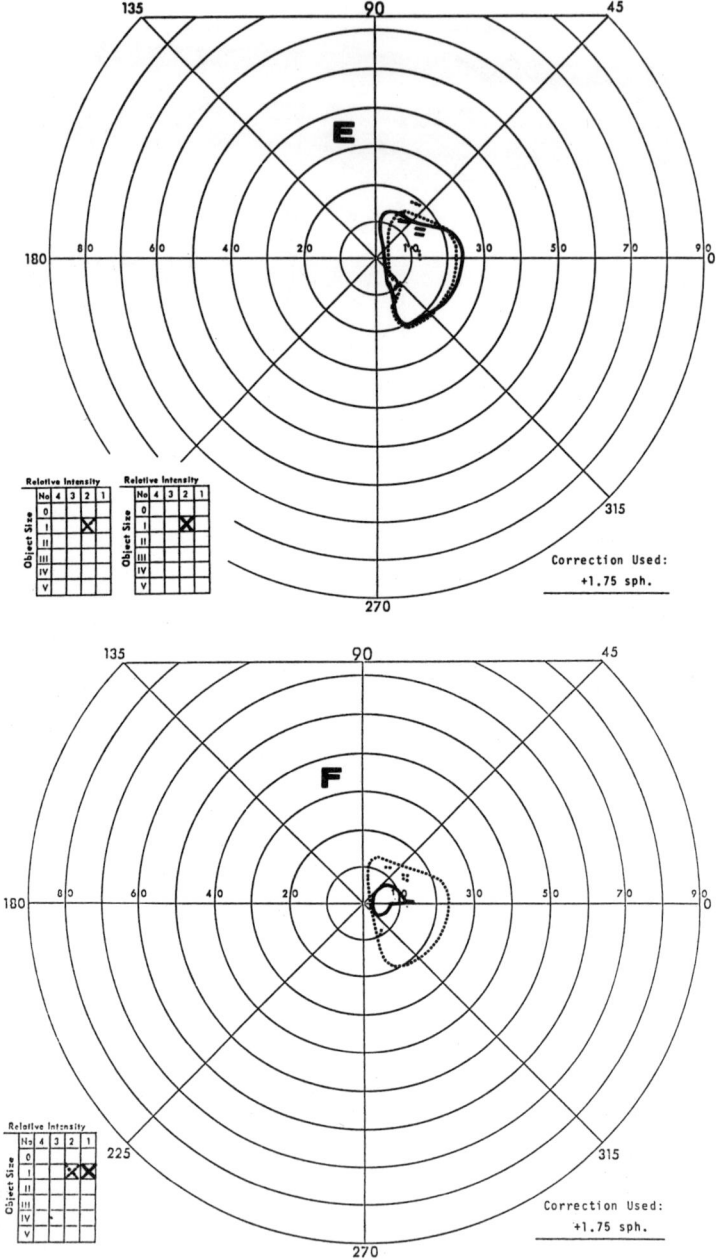

E The I-2-e test is repeated with the new correction, and the scatter observed is less.   **F** The isopter plotted with the I-1-e shows an inferior nasal deficiency. This, plus the wide separation between isopters, suggests that the area should be explored with an intermediate strength isopter, such as the I-2-c.

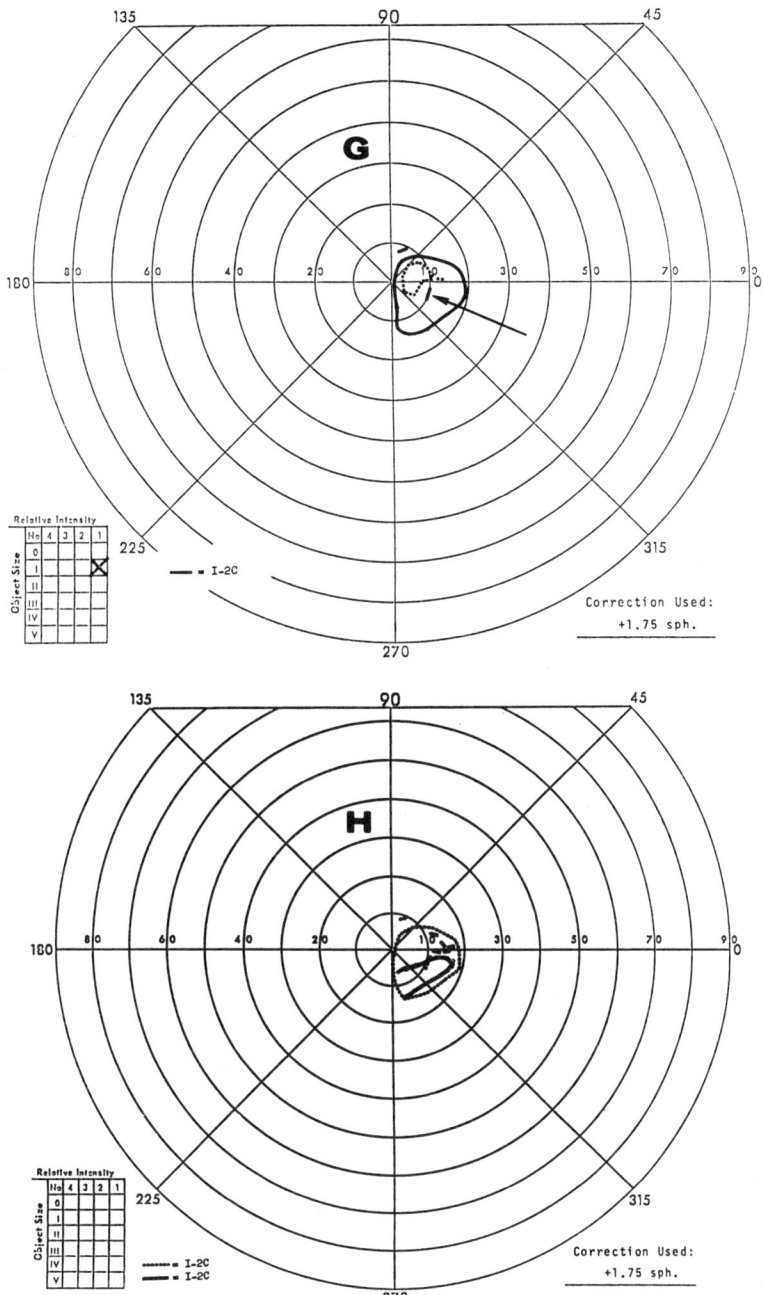

G An isopter is plotted with the I-2-c target and for the most part falls smoothly between the I-1-e and the I-2-e. The isopter is unexpectedly penetrated inferonasally by a few test probes (arrow). This local scatter, coupled with the concavity seen in the I-1-e isopter, suggests the presence of a paracentral scotoma in this area.   **H**   An arcuate defect is plotted, utilizing the same target as in G.

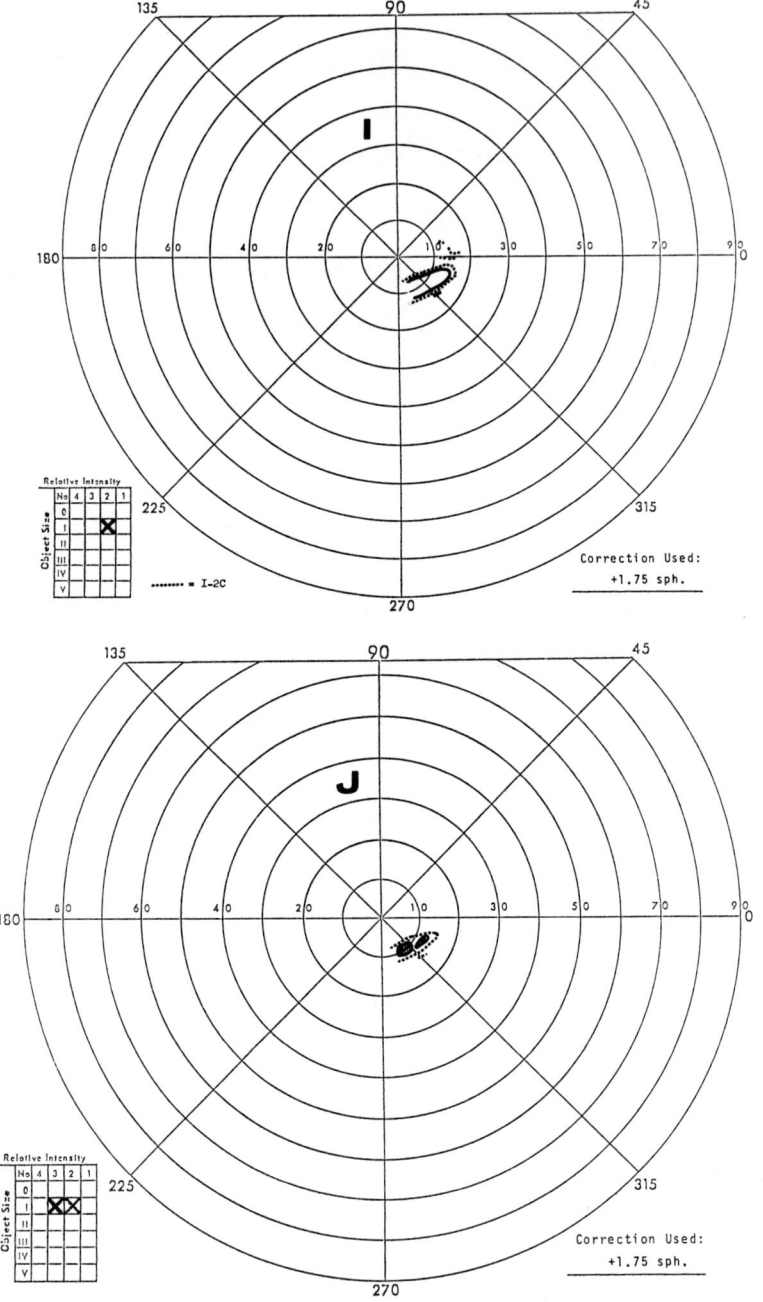

I The arcuate defect is explored with a brighter test (I-2-e, used in Step E) and found to be of moderate density. **J** The densest nuclei are outlined utilizing the I-3-e test object (first used in Step C).

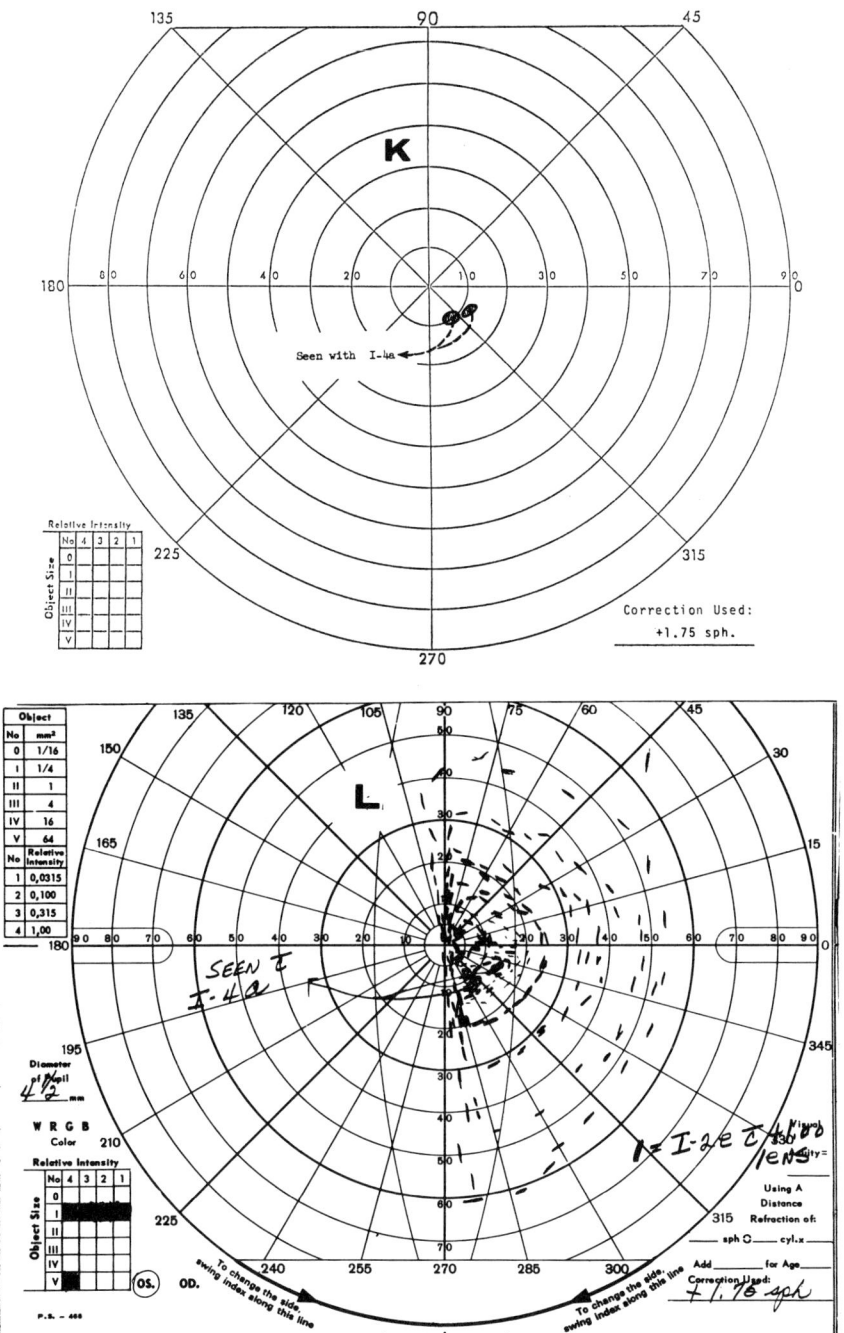

K The depth of each nucleus is determined by static testing. **L** The actual finished field. Naturally, each isopter is coded with a different color pencil, but this cannot be appreciated in print. Note that we do not obscure the raw data by drawing isopter lines. Since "real" fields such as this are confusing, all other fields in the book will be redrawn, and only one or two essential isopters will be shown for clarity.

2. Corneal disturbance:
Do not instill drops, check tension, or perform gonioscopy just before fields. (It is acceptable to allow patients to wear well-fitting contact lenses if they are past the adaptation period.)

C. Physiological
1. Refractive error:
Use large-glass small-rim trial lenses. Refraction used only for central field; expect 25° limit with aphakia and 40° with moderate myopia. Aphakes and persons with high astigmatism may wear contact lenses, but trial lenses, to correct for the test distance, are usually necessary in addition. One may omit lenses on young myopic patients whose distance Rx is −3.25 D or less. Refine initial lenses (see Preparing to Test, Steps 7 through 9) with plus and minus 0.50 diopter spheres.
2. Dark adaptation:
Usually choose photopic background; adapt patient for five minutes during selection of lenses and orientation. If using dim background, the patient should wait at least 30 minutes in the dark before testing begins.
3. Excessive blinking:
Instruct the patient to blink only if necessary, and then only immediately after spot presentations.
4. Accommodative spasm:
Younger and more nervous patients may have a change in accommodation during test. This is usually manifest by the complaint that the fixation target is fading. Refine refraction. If this fails in extreme cases, dilate the patient repeatedly with a long-acting mydriatic so that the last drop is administered at least one hour prior to commencing perimetry.

D. Psychological
1. Learning:
   a. Size, brightness, rate of movement, and duration of test object:
   Orient patient; don't record first four test responses or initial response after changing test objects.
   b. Pattern or order of test object locations:
   Keep attention global by random position. Projection devices are an aid here.
   c. Interval between tests:
   Vary the interval between tests within a range that allows the patient to blink after any test, but do not wait so long that the patient becomes tired, anxious, or bored.
   d. Knowledge of results:
   When you recognize an improbable response, ask the patient where he or she saw the test, then tell the patient whether he or she really saw it or not.
2. Fatigue:
Don't let the patient wait too long between tests. When you're busy, ask the patient to sit back and rest for a minute. Allow the patient brief rests either when requested or when the patient's performance appears to deteriorate.
3. Fixation:
Orient the patient initially; check fixation and correct early; keep test presentations apparently random; remove test as soon as it is seen. Always move test from nonseeing to seeing.

4. Distractions, interruptions:
   Locate the perimetry room away from traffic and be sure it has a door that can be closed. If interruptions do occur, ask the patient to rest.
5. Anxiety:
   a. Concern about performance coupled with reason for unusual and trying test:
      Reassure the patient that she or he is doing a good job.
   b. Prolonged and repeated testing of one area in visual field:
      Avoid testing the same area more than one or two times without presenting the test elsewhere.
   c. Large time interval between tests that are seen:
      If the patient repeatedly does not see the test object as expected, discharge his or her concern about the excessively delayed responses by returning to a previously seen zone. Use larger test objects to find the only area where smaller test objects would have a chance of being seen.
   d. Purposeful or inadvertent suggestion:
      Avoid slowing the test at expected borders, don't record slow reaction times as scotomas, avoid wiggling the test object.
   e. Emotional illness:
      Don't assume spiraling fields mean psychiatric disease without organic pathology. This can also be a sign of changing dark adaptation.
6. Criterion effect, response, and approach to threshold:
   Design the test so that the patient is forced to report a target's location rather than whether or not he sees it (forced-choice indication). If the field appears unexpectedly constricted, demonstrate to the patient that she or he really can see over a larger area by trying confrontation or fingercounting; then retest.

E. Pathological
1. Focal scatter in a quadrant:
   Suspect either a narrow rim around a scotoma or an unexpected small defect in the periphery of an isopter. A flat slope may also be responsible. Static testing in such an area may be helpful.
2. Central scatter:
   In retrobulbar neuritis, one may see the "sieve effect." A grossly inadequate refraction or a cataract may also cause some central scatter.

The factors above influence scatter within a single session. Managing these factors may be sufficient for diagnostic fields, but for quantitative fields, such as are necessary for a glaucoma patient, one must also attempt to minimize variation from session to session. Some sources of variation cannot be controlled but only documented (e.g., developing cataract). Variables that cause intersession scatter are listed below.

1. Scatter factors:
   Apply the same techniques each time. All light bulbs age, incandescents faster than fluorescents; with the Goldmann Perimeter, recalibrate the background before each field since dark skin, hair, or clothing reflect less light which would result in more contrast. With a tangent screen, keep clean, measured test objects and avoid chalk marks on the screen.

2. Refractive media:
   Measure the best visual acuity each time; note and compensate for any intervening change in refractive error. If the isopters are worse with new refraction, try the original perimetry lenses.
3. Pupil size:
   With each field test, measure the size of each pupil in controlled light. Before miotics are started, perform a field test while the pupil is large to record changes to date. Soon after miosis, repeat fields for a new base line.
4. Mental status:
   Note attention and reactions on each field; if the patient is unreliable, utter words of encouragement and allow rest ad lib. Repeat fields on a subsequent visit before deciding whether or not the patient is impossible to test.
5. Data determining isopter:
   Obtain enough points to outline and recheck an isopter, i.e., record all responses except those obviously due to examiner error, known blink, or false alarm. Avoid testing directly along vertical and nasal radii, where change is likely in disease processes.

One final word about scatter: You cannot eliminate all of it. Hence, if you find, in reviewing your technician's handiwork, that the fields are perfect examples of the perimetrist's art, with smooth, ovoid isopters, unsullied by even a hint of scatter, then you have an important clue that your fields are falling victim to the most nefarious force of all: a biased perimetrist. This bias is likely to come from the perimetrist's trying too hard to please his or her supervisor, or from being too sympathetic with the patient and thus wanting the visual fields to look good. The alert supervisor should thus look for the following sorts of errors:

1. slowing the test velocity at expected isopter boundaries
2. oscillating the test object at or near expected boundaries
3. failing to record tests that penetrate the partially plotted isopter, unless such penetration is explained by defective fixation or blinking
4. assuming the reason for an aberrant response is shifting fixation or blinking (without direct observation of this kind of behavior) and thus omitting such responses from the record
5. failing to randomize locations of test presentations
6. failing to randomize the interest interval over a small range
7. overworking to the point of boredom and carelessness by the perimetrist

The cure for most of the above is simply to counsel the perimetrist on the apparent causes of the problem. The last cause is best prevented by assuring a reasonable workload—one the physician would not mind if he or she were the perimetrist—and allowing the perimetrist other duties as a diversion.

6
Additional Techniques and Alternative Approaches to Goldmann Perimetry

The capabilities of the basic Goldmann Perimeter are extended somewhat by three devices. These are the one-dot–four-dot device, the central scotoma projector, and the static perimetry attachment. The one-dot–four-dot device should be a part of every visual field test, especially in those cases in which some question arises whether or not central light sense corresponds to visual acuity or in those cases in which visual acuity is depressed. The central scotoma device is particularly useful to those people who have markedly depressed vision in one eye with relatively good vision in the other, because it allows the patient to fix with his good eye while having the defective eye tested. The static perimetry attachment adapts the Goldmann to the performance of static fields. These devices will be described below. The techniques of utilizing color, flicker fusion, and confrontation are also covered briefly.

ONE-DOT–FOUR-DOT TEST

The projector for the one-dot–four-dot test can be attached in one of two ways, depending upon the model of the perimeter. In older models of the Goldmann Perimeter, there is a bracket just to the right of the lamp housing that holds a cylindrical projector. The projector is inserted into this bracket and a plug from it then inserted into the socket on the body of the perimeter. By flipping a small diaphragm, one can display either a single bright spot projected just to the side of the telescope, or four bright dots arranged in a square. This allows testing among the four dots in the area that is normally occupied by the fixation light.

On the most recent model of the Goldmann Perimeter, however, there is a

180   Principles of Quantitative Perimetry

small plug in the bottom of the lamp housing which may be removed. A different model of the one-dot–four-dot projector slips into this plug and utilizes light from the main lamp to form the dots. By turning a small screw on the back of the device, the spots can be raised or lowered slightly, thus enabling the operator to assure that the vertical alignment is exactly even with the original central fixation spot. A second screw on the front allows the operator to choose between the one-dot or the four-dot pattern (Fig. 6-1).

When this device is in use, the fixation spot is moved 5° to the right side. This necessitates moving the chart slightly to the side in order to maintain registra-

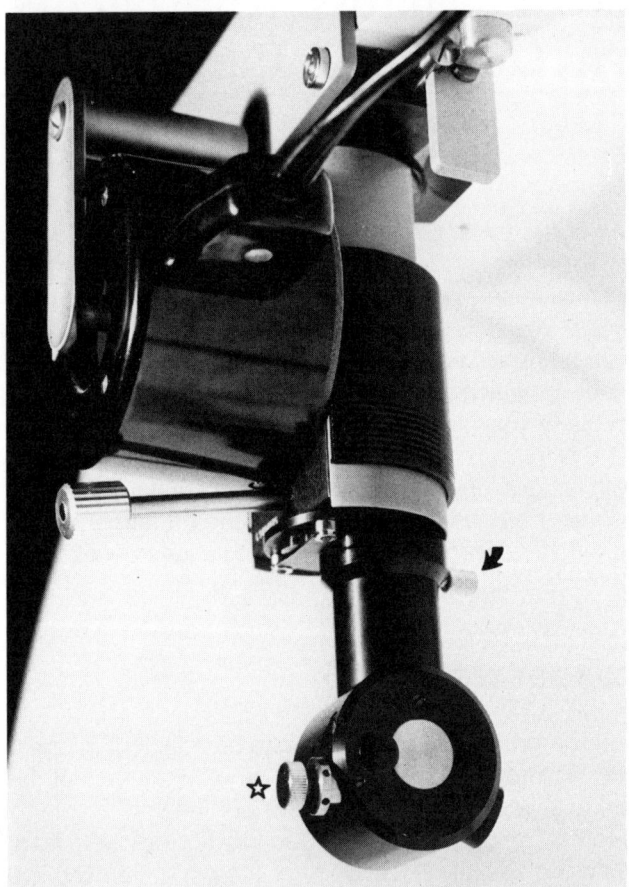

Figure 6-1   The one-dot–four-dot projector installed on the lamp housing of the Goldmann Perimeter. The knurled knob on the long shaft holds the device in place. The small knob at the front (black arrow) selects between one and four dots. The small knob with lock ring to the rear (star) provides adjustment of the vertical position of the spot.

tion. Along the bottom margin of the standard Haag-Streit visual field chart there are four vertical lines (see Fig. 5-4). The line (C) corresponding to the center of the field is somewhat longer than the other three. It is along this line that the chart is usually aligned when doing a standard field. Just to the left of this central line is a short vertical line (B) that corresponds to the proper position for use with the one-dot–four-dot device. When the one-dot–four-dot device is employed, the chart paper should be loosened and slipped horizontally until this mark is aligned with the index notch on the perimeter. The two remaining vertical lines (A) that are furthest from the center are for use with the central scotoma device.

THE CENTRAL SCOTOMA DEVICE

The central scotoma device is to be used primarily on patients with a unilateral absolute or dense relative central scotoma of about 5° or more to either side of fixation. A patient who does not have binocular vision, who cannot recognize the central fixation marks, who has a strabismus of more than 10°, or who has abnormal retinal correspondence cannot be examined with the device. Normal perimetry should be carried out on any patient who has a relatively large central scotoma and who can still recognize the fixation point in the center of the perimeter bowl. Similarly, if a patient is unable to recognize the fixation points with the central scotoma device, it is usually better to attempt normal perimetry without the device by trying to maintain that patient's eye in a good position by frequent encouragement and verbal directions. Because of its limitations, the central scotoma device is seldom used in practice.

The principle by which the central scotoma device works is to keep the eye undergoing examination steady by allowing both eyes to see a circle with hatch marks every 90°. The nontested eye actually maintains the fixation for the pair by looking in a mirror at a fixation target that is projected onto the lateral wall of the bowl. Prior to the visual field examination, the usual checks of visual acuity and refraction are equally important with this device. In addition, one should examine the possibility of heterophorias at near fixation by using any standard method of testing, such as the Maddox wing.

To assemble the device in the perimeter, one loosens the plug from beneath the lamp housing and inserts the plug of the mobile arm in its place. At either end of the mobile arm is one of a pair of saddle bearings that holds the projector. The projector should be placed in the bearing *opposite* the eye that is to be tested. For example, if the tested eye is on the left, the projector is attached to the right saddle bearing (Fig. 6-2). The plug from the projector should be inserted in the socket on the body of the perimeter and power switch turned to the on position. Five luminous points within a circle will be projected onto the middle of the sphere. If they should not be laterally centered, a pin that is provided with

182   *Principles of Quantitative Perimetry*

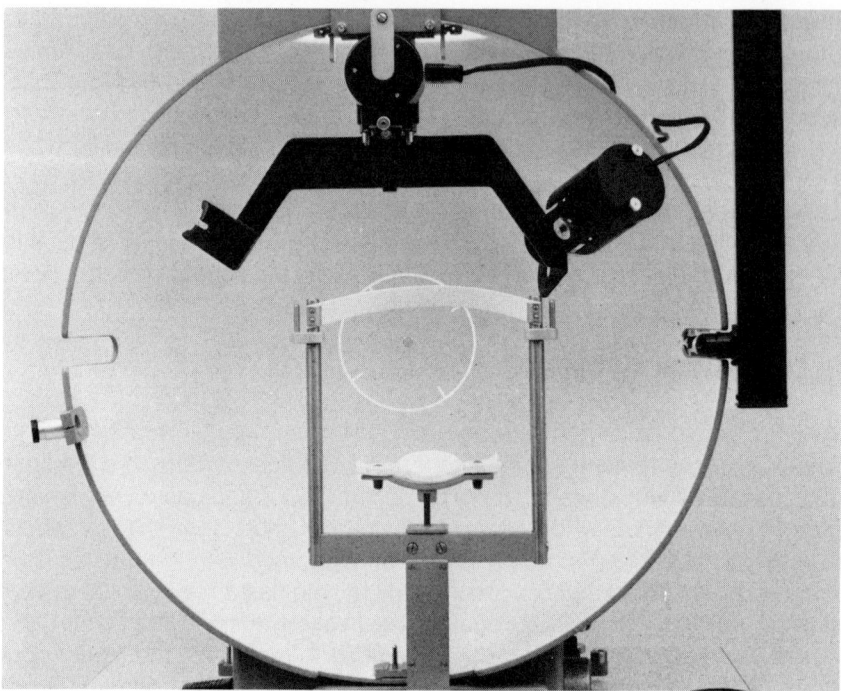

Figure 6-2   The central scotoma device partially installed on the Goldmann Perimeter for testing the left eye. The arm with the projector in the right saddle bearing is shown with the projected pattern properly centered.

the accessory kit is inserted into a small hole in the center of the cam head of the mobile arm. This pin is then used to turn the cam until the five points are properly centered (Fig. 6-3).

Once this adjustment has been accomplished, the arm is deviated 15° *toward* the side of the eye to be tested. The mirror plate is then attached on the *same* side as the projector. It should be oriented such that the opening for the small semiopaque mirror is above the large, trapezoidal ordinary mirror. The semiopaque mirror should be inserted in the mirror plate so that the white dot on its border is just opposite the white dot on the side of the mirror plate toward the patient. A black cover is placed over the side of the trapezoidal mirror *away* from the patient (Fig. 6-4).

The projector beam should pass through the superior semitransparent mirror. This will result in two circles being projected on the perimeter bowl. The first is projected through the semitransparent mirror and is approximately 15° in radius and 15° eccentric from center in the direction of the eye to be tested. The other is reflected from this same mirror and is projected on the periphery of the sphere

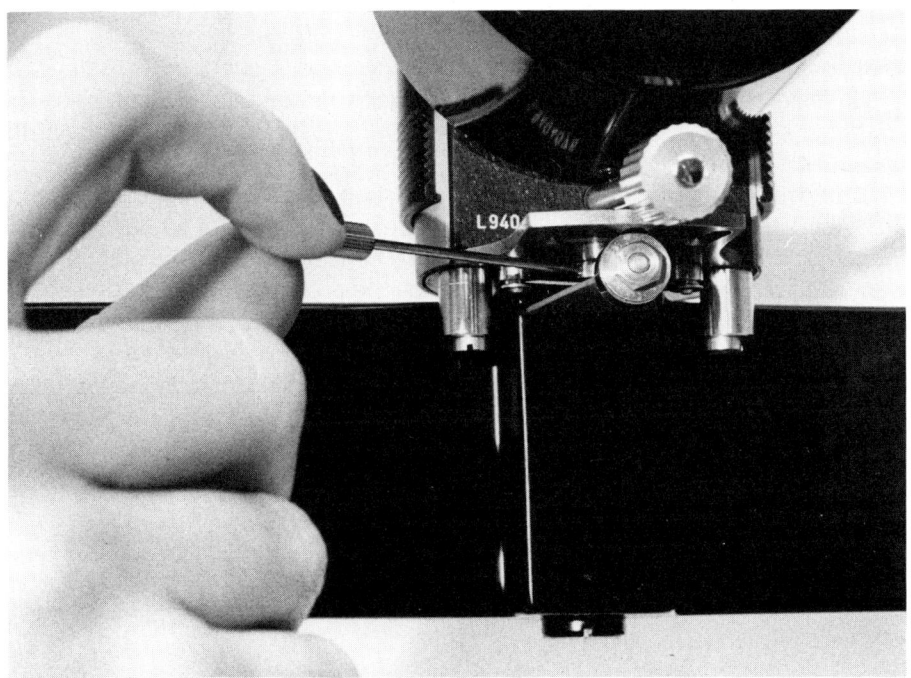

Figure 6-3   Method of lateral alignment of central scotoma device.

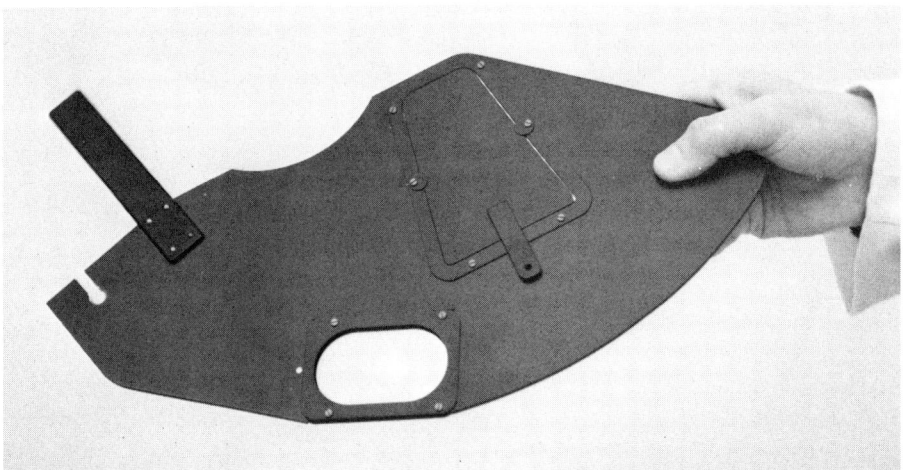

Figure 6-4   The mirror carrier plate showing the side that is away from the patient. The trapezoidal mirror is covered and the small half-silvered mirror is inserted.

184   *Principles of Quantitative Perimetry*

on the side of the fixing eye. This second circle can be seen only by the fixating eye via the ordinary mirror on the mirror plate (Fig. 6-5). The patient is then placed at the machine and the eye to be examined is centered as usual. The visual field chart should be moved 15° towards the eye to be examined. This distance corresponds to one of the outer vertical lines on the bottom of the visual field chart (A in Figure 5-4).

If any heterotropia exists, a rotary prism is then placed before the fixating eye, and the appropriate refraction is placed before the eye to be tested. If it is necessary to use the prism, it may be more convenient to use a standard trial frame to hold the lenses. The diaphragm on the projector is then turned so that the circle on the lateral wall of the projector disappears and leaves only the five-pointed cross, which is at the circle's center, visible to the fixating eye. At this point, the circle only is seen by the eye. The rotary prism is then adjusted until the five points appear to be in the center of the circle. This allows the correction of a moderate degree of heterotropia. Once this has been accomplished, the diaphragm on the projector is then turned to allow the fixating eye to view the circle also; the two circles may now be seen with binocular vision. Testing of the visual field then proceeds as in ordinary perimetry.

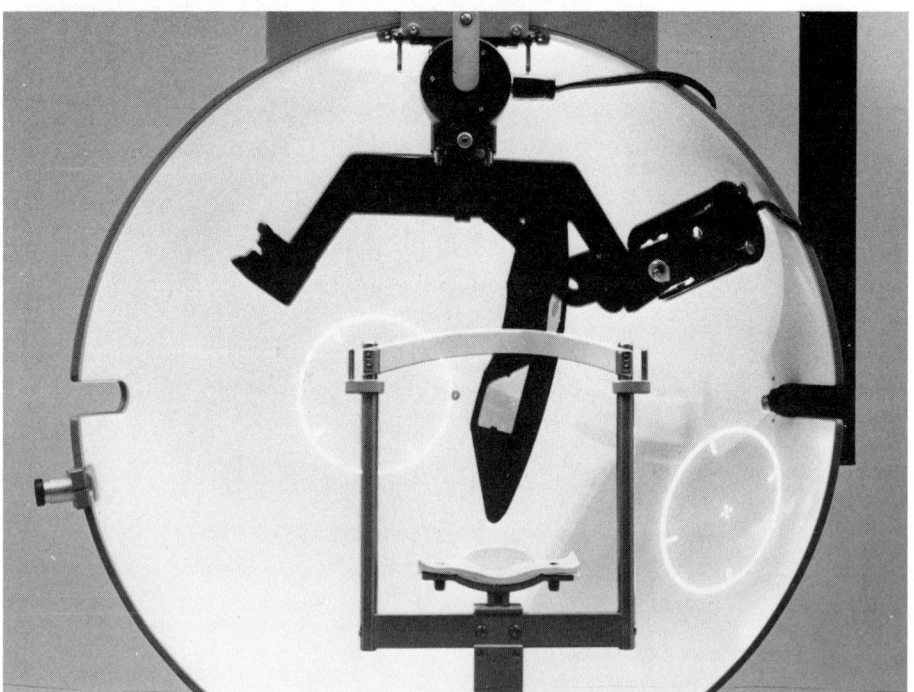

Figure 6-5   The central scotoma device complete and ready to test the left eye.

Additional Techniques and Alternative Approaches 185

STATIC PERIMETRY DEVICE

The Goldmann Perimeter may also be utilized for static perimetry. The static perimetry device consists of a plexiglass plate with holes drilled every 15° about the circumference of a circle, and a meridional arm pivoting at the center of this circle with chartholder and pantograph adaptor. The meridional arm can be rotated so detents on the arm will snap into the holes on the plexiglass plate and thus allow the meridians that are multiples of 15° to be checked by static perimetry. A special chart (Fig. 6-6) is utilized, and this is held in place by clips beneath the meridional arm. A plastic device with stimulus values marked in varying colors along it extends perpendicular to the meridional arm for use in conjunction with the test chart.

To use the device, the plexiglass plate is clamped in place over the chart screen of the Goldmann Perimeter by the clips along the side of the chartholder. Once this is done, the machine is calibrated in the usual manner and the normal pointer of the Goldmann Perimeter is removed from the pantograph arm by loosening the knurled screw, and the new pointer, which attaches to the static perimetry device, is screwed into place. A pin on this pointer fits into a hole on

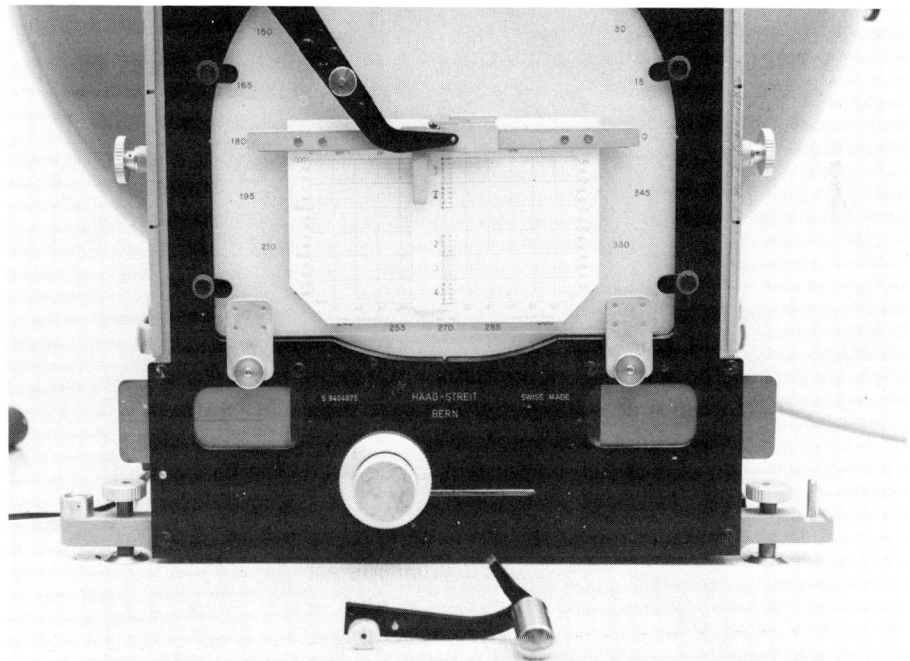

Figure 6-6 The static perimetry device installed on the Goldmann Perimeter. The usual handle (lying on table) has been replaced by the special pointer of the device.

186   Principles of Quantitative Perimetry

the meridional arm's pantograph adapter. The meridian to be tested is selected, the detents on the meridional arm lifted, and the arm rotated until it is aligned with the appropriate meridian. Placing a chart in the holder completes preparations for the test. To move to a different eccentricity along a given meridian, the operator simply grasps the pointer where it joins the meridional arm of the static perimetry device and moves it along the meridional arm until the desired eccentricity is reached. When it is necessary, the pointer is disengaged from the arm, which is then swung through the arc below the chartholder as usual (see Chapter 5), then reattached as before (Fig 6-7).

There are two techniques that are commonly employed for static testing. The classic method is to approach each threshold from some point *below* threshold. If the test is not seen, then it is made brighter by one step. A two-seconds wait is required to allow the retina to recover from the local adaptation phenomenon before the test is presented again. If it is still not seen, the spot is again brightened until the patient signals that he sees it, thus signifying that threshold has been reached. One then moves the pointer to a different eccentricity, and the test begins anew.

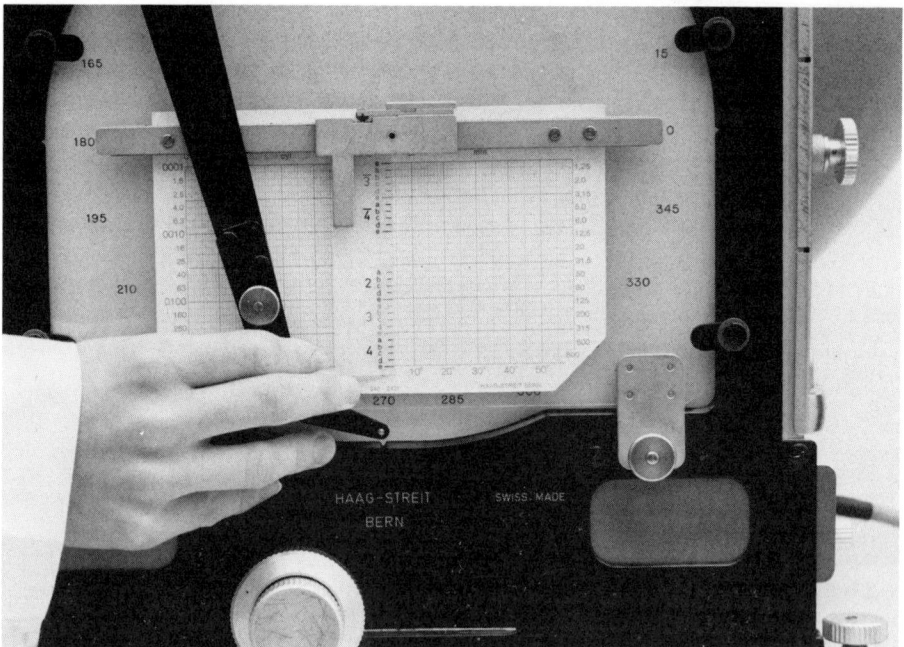

Figure 6-7   Method of changing sides of meridian with static device. The pointer is removed from the arm and swung through the arc below, just as in the usual case.

In our laboratory, a slightly different technique is sometimes utilized. Here one utilizes data from a previously performed kinetic field to gain a rough idea of what one may expect from the thresholds during the static test. These approximate thresholds are penciled in with an ordinary lead pencil. One then begins to test along the selected meridian at threshold. If the spot was seen, a mark for that brightness is made in red, and upon the next testing of that spot, the spot is tested four steps dimmer. If the spot was not seen, a green mark is made opposite that stimulus strength, and upon the next testing of that location, the spot is made two steps brighter. Once one has a stimulus interval bracketed by a red and green mark, one simply tests the intervening interval by a spot of intermediate stimulus value and continues in this fashion until two stimulus values are determined one step apart, one of which is seen, the other of which is not seen. One of the key points of this technique, however, is that one does not test the same spot twice in a row, but tests several other locations before returning. This allows a different spot to be tested each time, and eliminates the need to wait between each presentation of a stimulus for recovery from the local adaptation phenomenon. Although this procedure is somewhat tedious, it can speed up a bit the testing of a static field. It is basically this technique that is utilized in the automatic perimeter developed by the authors.

COLOR PERIMETRY

Conventional color perimetry is a topic about which neither author has a great deal of enthusiasm, since their major interest lies in quantitative techniques. Nevertheless, one should recognize that perimetry with colored test objects, particularly red, is of great use in *diagnostic* fields. Defects that can be discovered on the tangent screen with a red test object would often elude the examiner unless they were sought very carefully with very small, white test objects. The comparison of the saturation and hue of a test object presented at various points in the visual field can be valuable and adds one more clue to the location and the etiology of the lesion. The physiological rationale for using colored test objects as well as the more modern approaches of monochromatic perimetry are discussed in Chapter 2.

In the normal eye, a colored test object essentially is the same as a smaller, dimmer, white test object. Therefore a 2/2000 white test object and a 30/2000 red test object on the tangent screen plot approximately the same isopters. Another way of stating the same thing is that with test objects of the same size, the red isopter will be smaller than the white isopter. Blue targets plot a slightly larger isopter than their red counterparts of identical size. In numerous disease states, however, the isopter plotted with a given colored target seems to be affected more than the isopters plotted with targets of other colors, especially white. Cuts develop in the colored isopter in places where the white isopter for an equivalent stimulus value target remains full. This phenomenon is called by some authors "disproportion" and by others "photochromic disharmony." Disproportion with red may be seen in glaucoma, in optic nerve diseases, in chiasmal lesions, and in other afflictions throughout the nervous system. Disproportion between red and blue targets is seen in the case of retinal detachment involving the macula when a patient shows an acquired tritanopia. With targets of identical size, the blue isopter shrinks more than the normally smaller red isopter and causes a true physiologic interlacing of the red and blue isopters in the area of the retinal detachment. Some authors have claimed that examination with the blue test object is more sensitive than other colors for picking up macular lesions. Nevertheless, in the hands of most clinical perimetrists, reliance is placed upon the red and the white test objects alone without resorting to other colors.

The logic of using a colored test object rests on the assumption that one particular region of the visual spectrum is lost prior to others in some disease states. The problem here is that the test object also reflects other colors of the spectrum that are capable of stimulating a visual response. Thus, one can define four possible thresholds for a patient undergoing conventional color perimetry: (1) sees movement; (2) sees an object, no color; (3) sees an object, wrong color: (4) sees an object, the correct color. Normally, the last of these thresholds plots the smallest isopter and is more commonly employed. This endpoint is somewhat different, and more subjective, than that of merely reporting the visualization of an object as is done in white-light perimetry. This tends to make color fields exhibit a little more scatter than their white-light counterparts. Also, the necessity of using colored objects is questionable, since Lynn reports that in some eighteen years as a clinical perimetrist, he has never seen a defect found by color that was not also plottable by careful perimetry with small, white test spots on the Goldmann Perimeter. Nevertheless, for diagnostic fields on the tangent screen, colored objects are useful.

Differences in the apparent saturation of the color are frequently significant, even though no diagnostic defect can be plotted perimetrically. In the cases of central scotomas, or suspected hemianopsias, a valuable ploy is to exhibit in all four quadrants a large red test object barely eccentric to fixation. The patient is asked to compare the saturation and hue of the test objects at each location. The pattern of the desaturation (e.g., hemianopsia) is just as diagnostic as a change in the geometry of the isopters.[2] This may be valuable in those instances where standard white-object perimetry yields equivocal results in patients suspected of pathology of the visual pathway, particularly with chiasmatic lesions. A particularly elegant way of accomplishing this is championed by Max Chamlin.[1] He has a large felt-covered paddle with two red test objects on its surface. The paddle is moved up and down the hemianopsia line so that each

Additional Techniques and Alternative Approaches 189

object remains an equal distance to either side. The subject is asked to report differences in hue.

Other forms of "saturation perimetry" are still in their infancy. One attempt to quantify the values involves using two projected spots, one fixed and central as a reference, the other a movable test. The task here is to adjust the brightness of the test until the saturation of the test and reference object appear equal. Another form of this test apparently being pursued by both Cornsweet and Lueddeke involves using a colored flickering light of a set frequency and adjusting intensity downward until the light appears constant. Obviously, much more work needs to be done before these techniques can be evaluated accurately.

FLICKER-FUSION PERIMETRY

Flicker-fusion perimetry has been discussed in Chapter 2, and only brief comments need be given here. The test essentially involves the measurement of the frequency at which a flickering light no longer appears fused but is seen to flicker. Defects correspond to low values of their critical flicker frequency. Although flicker perimetry may have some advantages in cases where the refractive medium is poor (such as cataracts), it is not favored by most ophthalmologists for several reasons. First of all, it requires equipment not normally found in the ophthalmologist's armamentarium. Second, it produces an output different in form from any that the ophthalmologist is accustomed to seeing. Nevertheless, when properly used, the technique is capable of providing valuable information.

CONFRONTATION FIELDS

The confrontation field is the minimum visual field. It can be done with nothing more than the examiner's fingers, although using hatpins, which the examiner can keep conveniently pinned to his lapel, adds a degree of refinement to the technique. It may be useful for screening patients in whom no defect is necessarily suspected, and it is also useful for examining patients at the bedside or under other conditions where the visual field equipment is not present. It is particularly useful with patients who have a difficult time cooperating completely in other forms of the field test.

The test is best performed by having the patient look into the eye of the examiner. The patient fixes on the examiner's eye, and the examiner brings in the test object from the periphery along a path equidistant from the patient's eye and the examiner's eye. Essentially, the test consists of the examiner comparing his visual field with that of the patient. Obviously, this works best if the examiner has a normal field. With practice, one can recognize field cuts of moderate size and can plot blind spots in rough fashion. The test is obviously not quantifiable and falls prey to difficulties from a "busy" background such as walls covered with figured drapes, bookcases, or pictures.

One useful modification is the "finger-count field." In this test, the examiner holds up several fingers in various parts of the subject's peripheral field and asks the patient to count them. Once again, the subject should fixate his gaze on the examiner's eye, and the examiner compares the subject's field with his own. Patients with a scotoma or field cut in certain areas will be unable to count fingers in that area, whereas they will be able to do so in a comparable, unaffected area.

Finally, the absolute minimum confrontation test consists of covering one eye of the subject and asking him to fixate on the examiner's nose. The subject is then asked to compare the way he sees each eye or ear. The examiner can then hold up each of his hands a short distance to either side of his head and ask for a comparison of how clearly each hand is seen. This is useful mainly in the case of hemianopsias of either the bitemporal or homonymous variety.

REFERENCES

1. Chamlin M: Methodology and techniques in visual field studies. Surv Ophthalmol 13:97, 1968
2. Frisen L: A versatile color confrontation test for the central visual field. Arch Ophthalmol 89:3, 1973

Additional References

Goldmann Perimeter 940, Instructions for Use. Haag-Streit Ag, Switzerland

Reed, H, Drance SM: The Essentials of Perimetry—Static and Kinetic. London, Oxford University Press, 1972

7
Principles of Interpretation of the Visual Field

GENERAL CONSIDERATIONS

The ultimate goal in the performance of visual fields is to provide information that is valuable to the physician for the care of his patient. If this information is to be both useful and reliable, the field must be performed with care and thought on equipment that is properly maintained. Yet, no matter how much care is put into the performance of the visual field, no matter how fine a perimeter, and no matter how skilled the perimetrist, without proper interpretation, the testing of the visual field is a sterile exercise. In order to interpret the visual field accurately, the physician must know the anatomy of the visual pathways and their blood supply from the retina back to the cortex. A knowledge of the pathophysiology of ailments affecting these pathways, particularly those that affect the retina or the optic nerve, is indispensable. It is the purpose of this chapter to discuss the basics of the interpretation of visual fields, the applied anatomy of the optic pathway, and finally the role of clinical findings in aiding diagnoses.

Before a field can be interpreted, three things must be decided about it: (1) Is it valid? (2) Is it sufficient? and (3) Is it comparable to previously done fields? Let us discuss each of these points in turn.

Validity

In examining a field for validity, the physician should decide whether or not the techniques employed by the perimetrist were adequate for testing those aspects of visual function that should have been tested. Obviously, the minimum requirements become increasingly stringent as the type of field done ascends from Stage I to Stage IV, but poor technique is inexcusable at any stage.

One common technical error is to collect data points directly along the vertical or nasal horizontal midlines instead of on either side of them. Such a practice can cause hemianopic offsets or nasal steps to dissolve into a sea of scatter. Valuable diagnostic information is lost as a result.

This is not to say that all scatter is bad; on the contrary, there should be a small amount of scatter, which indicates that the patient has cooperated. Fields that show absolutely no scatter must be regarded with suspicion, for this may indicate a bias on the part of the perimetrist to eliminate scatter. This bias can cause artifacts in the field, since the perimetrist may slow the test velocity near expected isopter borders or fail to record points that don't agree with what has been already plotted.

Another clue to the validity of the field is obtained by checking how well the central light sense correlates with the recorded visual acuity. A dense central scotoma in the field and a recorded visual acuity of 20/20 are incompatible findings.

A careful perusal of the blind spot can yield much valuable information concerning the field's validity. If no blind spot can be plotted, poor fixation or lack of an occluder on the fellow eye should be suspected. The position of the blind spot is of importance. While it is true that it is found closer to center than its normal 12°–15° in aphakia or high hyperopia (and at a further distance in high myopia), a horizontal displacement of the blind spot in a person with a normal refractive error may signal the presence of a central scotoma and eccentric fixation (Fig. 7-1). Rotary displacement of the blind spot may signal extraocular muscle problems, such as paresis of the cyclovertical muscles, particularly the superior oblique.

Other findings can suggest a field of dubious validity. Intertwining of isopter lines can suggest poor fixation, inconstant test spot velocity, varying status of light adaptation, malingering or hysteria. Certain defects can be due to an artifact, such as the nose, the lids, or the lens holder. Failing to patch one eye is another frequent error (Fig. 7-2). Pertinent additional information includes whether or not the test was conducted in a manner known to produce valid diagnostic isopters, that is, was the patient tested with his refraction considered, appropriately dark-adapted, and properly oriented. It is also helpful to know if this was the patient's first visual field.

Sufficiency

The question of sufficiency is simply the question of whether enough tests have been made in enough places to provide the desired information. For the Stage I field, a relatively few points may suffice, whereas a Stage IV field may

Principles of Interpretation of the Visual Field

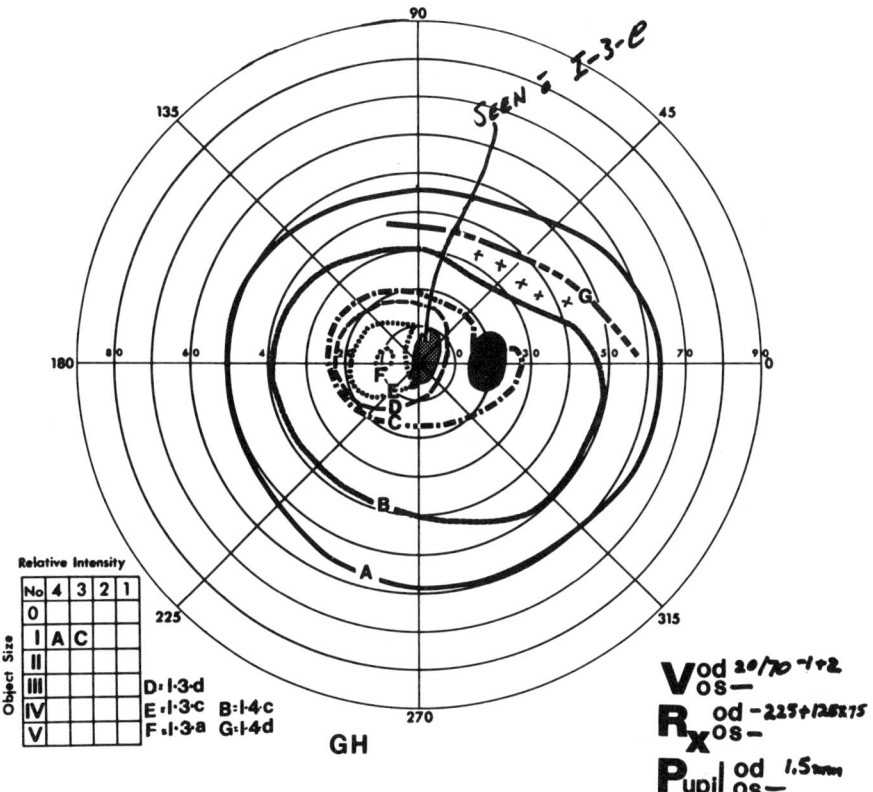

Figure 7-1 An illustration of several elements that go into making the field valid and sufficient. The visual acuity, refraction, and pupil size are recorded, and the vision is compatible with a central scotoma. The position of the blind spot is abnormally far temporal, a finding that tips the examiner to the fact that the scotoma is really a central scotoma with eccentric fixation, as opposed to a paracentral scotoma. Another good point is the presence of isopter "G" and static tests (crosses) through a suspicious area superotemporally. The area is suspicious because of the concavity in isopter B. The field can be improved, however. A partial isopter should be plotted inferotemporally between isopters "B" and "C," since the separation there amounts to 30°. In addition, the left eye should be tested unless this is a follow-up field for a known disorder.

require a few hundred. A simple principle is that information is obtained *only* about the point where the test spot "lands" on the island of vision. Flying over an area with a subthreshold test gives no more information about defects than flying above a fog-enshrouded countryside in an airplane gives about the number of lakes present below. If the examiner wishes to test the area 30° nasal to fixation, he or she must find a test that is first seen at 30°; not two tests, one seen at 25°, the other at 35°. Enough data points must be plotted on the isopters to determine their true configuration. Along with this, the number of isopters is

194   Principles of Quantitative Perimetry

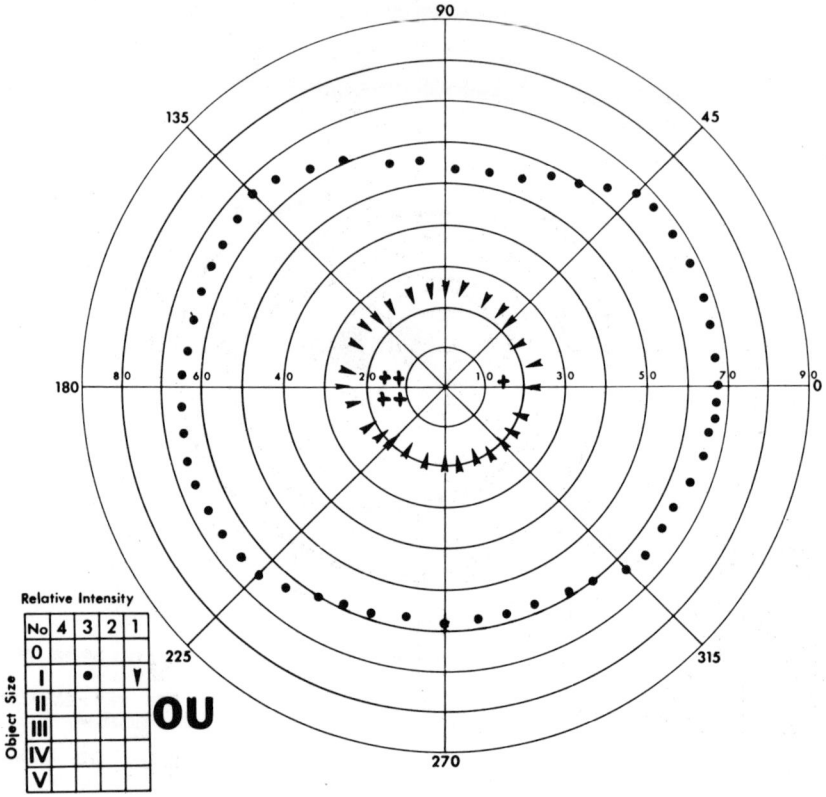

Figure 7-2   A common error in the performance of fields is the failure to patch one eye. Here, the isopter is more nearly symmetrical about fixation, and the blind spot cannot be found. Another common problem is failure to remove the corrective lenses for isopters beyond 30°. In this instance, a "u-shaped," completely dense scotoma (often with a "tail" due to the handle on the lens) provides the clue.

important. If there are large areas between isopters, pathology may be missed. The authors have seen fields on glaucoma suspects in which no testing was done in Bjerrum's area! Generally, for a field that is to be used to follow a patient, an isopter should preferably be present every 8 to 12 degrees. Any scotomas found should have been probed with static tests so their depths are determined accurately. Areas where a concavity of a peripheral isopter is plotted should be checked by turning the head if the nose is a possible limiting element, or by plotting an extra isopter or two inside and outside the concavity to decide whether the defect contains a scotoma.

In those cases in which central light sense correlates poorly with vision, a central scotoma check should be made. For example, if a perfectly normal central light sense is plotted, say for example I-1-c, and a very low visual acuity, such as a 20/400, for example, is recorded, the interpreter should suspect that either the field is not valid, that it is insufficiently done, or that the visual acuity is in error. The one-dot–four-dot projector or the central scotoma device, both of which are available with the Goldmann Perimeter, may be utilized to check the central field.

One of the biggest errors here is failing to test both eyes. Obviously, if the fellow eye is unable to perceive light or has very poor light projection, a visual field is not appropriate. However, visual acuities of even hand motion are probably not valid reasons for not testing the visual field (see Fig. 1-33).

Comparability

The final question is whether the field is comparable to previously done fields. This may not be a necessary consideration if the field is for diagnostic purposes only, and no need is anticipated to follow the patient in the future. However, for patients in whom comparability is important, pupil size, refractive correction, and visual acuity *must* be recorded on all fields. Ideally, there should be no major change in any of these items insofar as possible. In those cases in which a glaucoma patient has been put on miotic therapy, it is important to obtain a field just before starting miotics and just as soon afterwards as the pupil and the refractive state stabilize. The same is true of lens extraction in such patients. This permits current fields to be compared with earlier and later fields.

The cautious interpreter will also wish to be certain that the technique of testing remains the same. Obviously, fields are *not* comparable if done on a Goldmann one time and an Autoplot the next. However, even on the same instrument gross differences in the rate of movement of the test object, the randomness with which the stimuli are presented, the psychological approach of the perimetrist, and the stage of perimetrist experience can all influence the outcome of a field test. Secondly, the first field (or two!) of the patient himself is not likely to be as reliable as later fields. It has been stated that perhaps the best approach is to discard the first visual field. Although the authors do not wholly concur with this, relatively less emphasis is placed on the patient's initial field than on succeeding fields. The calibration of background intensity should be recent and correct. Far more important, the calibration of the test spot with respect to the background should be performed with the patient seated before the perimeter prior to *each* testing period.

INTERPRETATION

Once the examiner is satisfied that the fields are technically adequate, he must then decide if the field is normal, and if not, where the lesion lies. The lesion should be localized as accurately as possible along the course of the visual pathway from the retina to the cortex. This may require correlation with other signs and symptoms. Other information that can be gleaned from interpretation includes an estimation of the activity of the lesion, which can be determined from the slope of the isopter lines in the neighborhood of the defect (see Chapter 1) or, in the event of multiple tests, from the change seen from session to session. If possible, a diagnosis should be made. Finally, the field should be compared carefully with prior fields to see if there has been a progression or regression of the disease process. This is best done by laying the fields on a table in chronological order and comparing each against the other, isopter at a time. Such a technique enables the examiner to spot trends in which the change from session to session seems insignificant but which clearly show progression when viewed over the course of several exams.

A. General Approach
1. Estimate validity, sufficiency, and comparability.
2. Any offset at the hemianopsia line? If so, lesion not likely to be retinal in origin.
3. Defect definitely limited to one eye? (If yes, go to B.)
4. Is defect limited to right or left half of the field in either eye?
5. Is the temporal part of both fields involved, no matter how unequally? (Yes implies lesion at chiasm.)
6. Are the defects present in homonymous locations? (If the answers to 4, 5, and 6 are definitely no, go to B.)
7. Is the defect more dense above or below? (If the answer to 5 is yes, upper field defect suggests pituitary tumor, lower defect suggests craniopharyngioma.)
8. Is there macular sparing?
9. Are the defects congruous?
10. Ignoring the hemianopsia line itself, is the slope in the area of defect shallow or steep?
B. Interpretation of Defects Caused by Prechiasmal Lesions
1. Offsets at the hemianopsia line suggest the lesion is located in the optic nerve or papilla rather than retina. Glaucoma is possible.
2. Unilateral defects (always suspect that bilateral defects are being overlooked) are often diagnosed by ophthalmoscope. Look for lesion in fundus at location that is same distance *above* horizontal line through disc and macula as the defect is *below* a horizontal line through the blind spot and fixation point.
3. Bilateral defects (always suspect that true hemianopsias are being unrecognized) often signify a generalized disease process or intoxication.

Table 7-1 A sequential guide to interpretation.

Orientation with Ophthalmoscopic Findings

One of the first difficulties in interpretation is correlation of defects in the field with lesions in the fundus. This is because the field, as seen by the examiner, is reversed superiorly to inferiorly but not from right to left. Thus, a lesion in the superior left field of the patient will be found in the inferior left retina. The reason for this is a source of never ending confusion to the neophyte perimetrist, but perhaps may be clarified as follows. The image that is focused on the retina is inverted both vertically and horizontally. Therefore, a defect lying in the temporal retina is projected into the nasal field and similarly, the superior retina is projected into the inferior field. If the examiner imagines himself standing behind the subject, peering through the back of the subject's eyeball, he will note this relationship to be true. Things on the right side of the field fall on the left of the retina, and conversely. However, the usual ophthalmoscopic approach is for a person to view the subject from the *front* of the retina, *not* from the back. Here the examiner's right and left are reversed with relationship to that of the subject. This right-to-left reversal, due to the examiner facing the subject, negates the right-to-left reversal in the optic image. Since the examiner does not reverse himself from superiorly to inferiorly, the vertical reversal is not countered, and the superior-to-inferior inverse remains with the field. If the examiner thinks not in terms of right and left, but rather nasal and temporal, then reversal does seem to occur in the horizontal plane. Things that are temporal to fixation in the field, are nasal to the macula in the retina (See Fig. 7-3).

THE NORMAL FIELD

A normal field contains a number of more or less ovoid, smooth isopters, not quite so extensive nasally as temporally. A young, healthy individual with normal visual acuity should be able to see at least the I-1-c isopter centrally, out to perhaps 5°–8°. The I-1-e isopter usually surrounds the blind spot, extending out to around 25° temporally, and perhaps to 15° nasally. The I-4-e isopter may go out as far as 50° nasally, and 70° temporally. By age 60, each isopter has approximately shrunken to the size occupied by the just dimmer standard isopter in the 30-year-old. The extent of various isopters in normals may be seen in Figure 1-13. Although there is some variation in these figures, they can be used as a rough guide. On perimetric devices, such as the Goldmann Perimeter, one may occasionally see an isopter that should just enclose the blind spot, such as the I-1-e, closing nasal to it. However, in these cases a small island is usually found just temporal to the blind spot where the I-1-e can again be seen. This is a normal variant. Absence of this small temporal island is evidence of some constriction of this isopter.

If the field is not normal, then one must decide whether the abnormality lies in one eye or in both eyes. If the defect is truly uniocular, and does not represent a

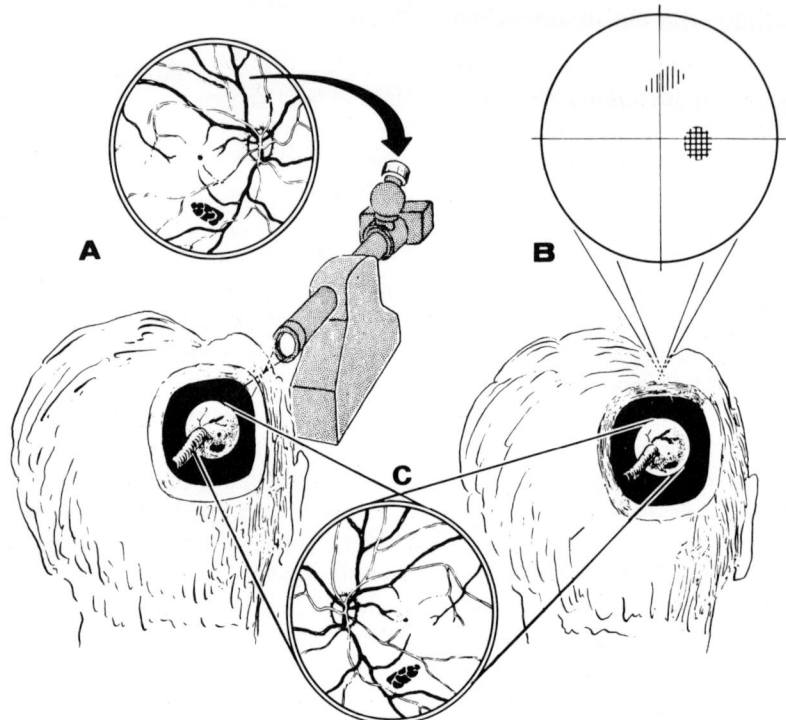

Figure 7-3 The relationship of the view of the fundus, the visual field, and the actual fundus. The actual fundus pathology, as seen from the back of the eye, is seen enlarged in C. In A, the examiner views from the front and sees a noninverted image. Although the examiner agrees that the lesion is inferotemporal to the disc, it would be to the examiner's left and the patient's right. This is because the examiner and the patient face one another. In the visual field, the light rays cross in the pupil, and the visual field can be considered to be similar to an inverted image of the fundus. Here objects in the inferior fundus project onto the superior field. Similarly, objects in the nasal fundus (i.e., the disc) project onto the temporal field (the projection of the disc is the blind spot).

missed binocular defect, then by far the most likely thing is that the defect lies in the retina or optic nerve. If the field shows defects binocularly, then it may show bilateral uniocular defects, or it may show defects typical of chiasmatic or postchiasmatic lesions.

UNIOCULAR DEFECTS

This group of defects comprises the largest number of patients that will be seen by the average ophthalmologist. Glaucoma, optic nerve disease, retinal disease and, on occasion, disturbances of the refractive media all may cause uniocular field defects. The majority of these defects, however, are a direct consequence

> *Cataract*—central constriction and scatter with nearly intact periphery. Eccentric posterior subscapsular plaques rarely cause peripheral cuts.
>
> *Diabetes*—focal scotomas correspond with local infarcts, hemorrhage and proliferans, though the disease ultimately leads to retinal detachment (see below). Associated with vascular occlusion and ischemic optic neuropathy (altitudinal hemianopsia).
>
> *Hypertensive Vascular Disease*—like diabetes—has small local scotomas, vascular occlusion and ischemic optic neuropathy.
>
> *Retinal Detachment*—when not yet total, shows a fairly sharp line, neither vertical nor horizontal, between normal and detached. Detached retina associated with shallow-sloped relative cut that is proportional to the extent of the peripheral detachment; macular detachment may be associated with postoperative relative central scotoma.
>
> *Senile Macular Degeneration*—central scotoma.
>
> *Uveitis*—corresponds to choroidal lesions; see also cataract.
>
> *Glaucoma*—seven characteristic features:
>
> 1. arcuate scotomas (Bjerrum scotomas), connected to blind spot twice as often as not
> 2. nasal step of Rönne or nasal contraction
> 3. temporal and/or central island(s) of residual vision
> 4. vertical step or offset at the hemianopsia line
> 5. paracentral scotomas, dense or relative, initially small
> 6. ring scotomas (double Bjerrum)
> 7. generalized concentric contraction
> 8. baring or elongation of blind spot
> 9. fan-shaped defect extending temporally from blind spot

Table 7-2 Visual field changes in seven leading causes of blindness in USA.

of the anatomy of the fibers of the innermost neural layer of the retina or its extension into the optic nerve.

A simple logic underlies the anatomy of the nerve fiber layer. Each nerve fiber follows the shortest path from the point of origin to the optic disc, constrained only by three rules:

1. No fiber may cross the macula.
2. Those fibers arising most peripherally with respect to the disc run in the most peripheral (or deepest) portion of the nerve fiber layer, farthest from the center of the eye.
3. Those fibers that arise most peripherally in the retina enter most peripherally in the optic disc.

This system results in a radiating fan-shaped arrangement of the fibers in the nasal hemiretina which gradually gives way to gracefully curving arcs about the macula in the temporal retina. The fibers from the upper and lower temporal quadrants divide along the horizontal temporal radius from the macula to form the *horizontal raphe.* Fibers that arise superior to the horizontal raphe sweep superior to the macula and conversely, an anatomical fact that bears the responsibility for the nasal step defect sometimes seen in fiber bundle damage. (See Figures 7-4 and 7-5.) Fibers arising from the macula itself run directly nasally to form the *papillomacular bundle.*

The nerve fibers enter the disc in an arrangement reminiscent of their origin in the retina. This area of the anatomy is open to discussion, and the conflicting views have been discussed by Lynn[10] and are illustrated in Figure 7-6. Once the nerve fibers have plunged through the lamina cribrosa, they acquire a myelin sheath and the fibers that serve the macula move toward the center of the nerve. Fibers from the temporal retina move laterally, and those that originate nasally move medially. Similarly, the fibers segregate themselves into a superior-inferior organization in the nerve exactly corresponding to that of their

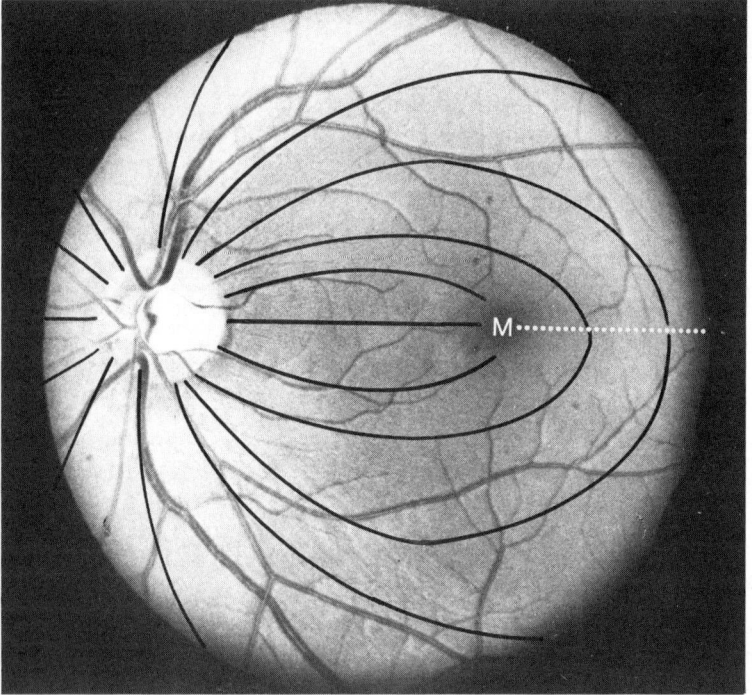

Figure 7-4 The topography of the fiber pathways in the retina. Fibers arising in the nasal retina run directly to the disc, but those arising in the temporal retina must arc gracefully around the macula (M). Those fibers arising superior to the horizontal raphe (white dots) pass above the macula; those arising inferior to the raphe pass below.

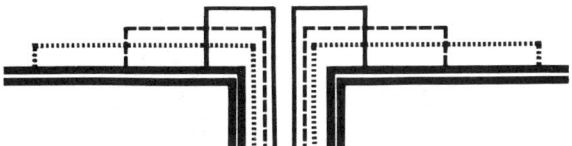

Figure 7-5 The cross-sectional arrangement of nerve fibers in the retina. Those fibers arising nearest the disc course most superficially in the retina and enter the disc most centrally. Conversely, the more peripheral their origin, the deeper in the retina they lie and the more peripherally they enter the disc.

origins in the retina. This arrangement then rotates slowly (right eye, counter clockwise; left eye, clockwise) as the fibers approach the chiasm.

From the foregoing description of the anatomy of the prechiasmal optic path, one can make several predictions about lesions of this area. Any lesion that interrupts the fiber bundles at the disc, such as characteristically appears in glaucoma, will likely form defects that follow normal fiber paths in the retina. In the nasal field (temporal retina), these would be scimitar-shaped field defects, whereas temporally they may radiate in a straighter, fan-shaped pattern. Also, since the nerve fiber layers are arranged with those fibers serving the most peripheral retina the deepest, it is possible to have only a portion of an individual fiber bundle interrupted. Therefore, a peripheral involvement of a given fiber bundle may be seen. An example of this is seen in glaucoma where small, isolated paracentral scotomas eventually coalesce to form a typical arcuate scotoma.

Secondly, those defects caused by lesions anterior to the disc should be predictable by ophthalmoscopy. Visual field defects caused by lesions in the retina itself will depend in no small part on the type of lesion. Thus, in a retinal detachment, where the retina near the border of the detachment may be yet alive but have a decreased function due to its relative anoxia, the field defect will show a gradual slope into its scotoma (which may not be absolute), whereas an area of retinoschisis, which splits the neural path through the retina at the outer plexiform layer, will cause an absolute scotoma that has an extremely sharply sloped periphery. Diabetic retinopathy, maculopathies, and other such lesions will have the shape and size of the scotomas determined by the insult itself. An early choroiditis may involve only the deeper layers of the retina initially, resulting in a localized scotoma. As the lesion progresses, the outermost fibers of the nerve fiber layer may be affected, resulting in the appearance of a second, more peripheral defect. Indeed, such observations provide a clinical demonstration of the anatomy of the nerve fiber layer in man.

The blood supply to the retina may also be the culprit responsible for a variety of fan-shaped visual field defects. These defects respect by and large the distribution of the occluded vessel. (See Chapter 8.) Either the retinal or the

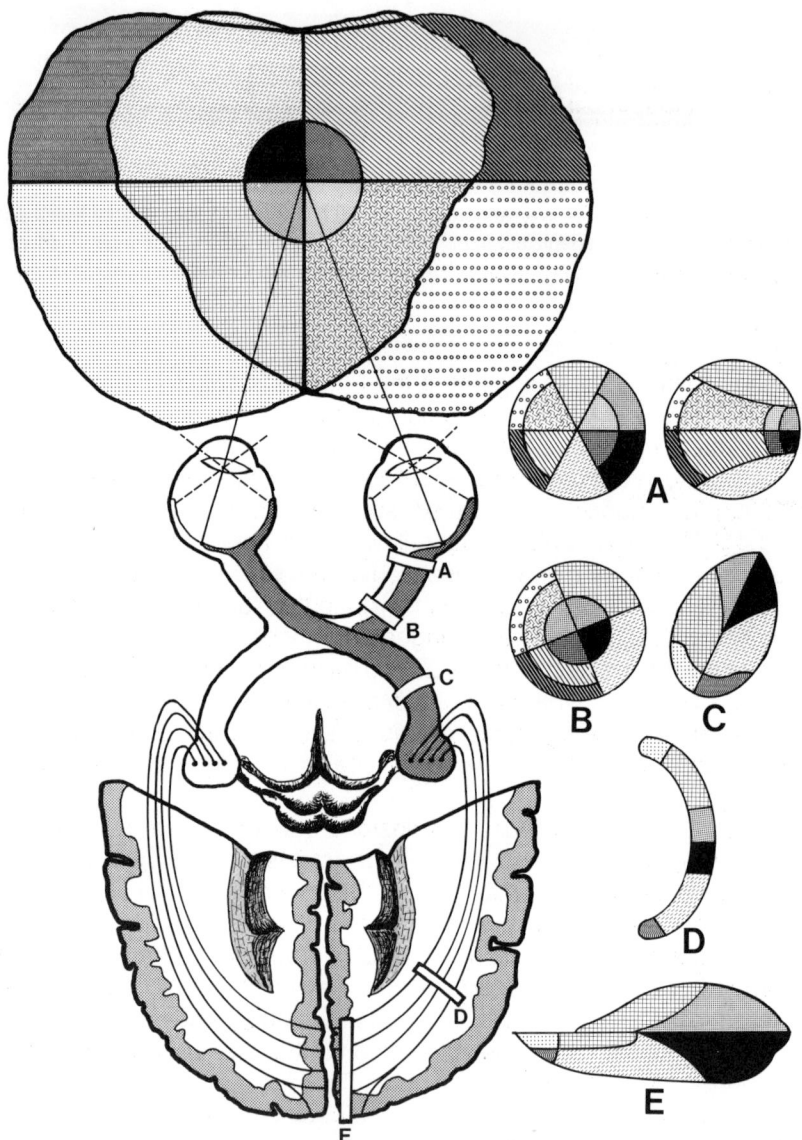

Figure 7-6 The distribution of fibers carrying information from various parts of the visual field as a function of location in the visual pathway. The optic disc is represented in A. The circle on the left represents one classical scheme; the one on the right represents an alternative scheme. B represents the posterior part of the optic nerve; note that the macular fibers are now central. C represents the optic tract; now only fibers from the appropriate half of the visual field are present. D is the optic radiation. The macular fibers are central, while those from the inferior field are superior, and conversely. E is the occipital cortex; the macular representation is near the posterior pole, while the peripheral field is represented anteriorly.

choroidal circulation may be at fault. The former is responsible for nourishing the inner retinal layers, whereas the choroid supplies the photoreceptors and the macula. Defects in the branches of the central artery or vein are responsible for sector-shaped defects* in the visual field, whereas abnormalities of the choroidal circulation are involved in irregularly shaped defects due to a variety of pathological conditions, perhaps the most common of which is neovascular proliferation through breaks in Bruch's membrane, as seen in a variety of conditions. The choroidal circulation connects with the pial arterial plexus about the optic nerve and contributes to the circulation of the optic disc. It may also furnish terminal branches (cilioretinal arteries) to the retina.

The optic nerve head and its blood supply are worthy of special note. Current theories on the pathogenesis of the glaucomatous visual field defects all implicate this region, either because of its special circulation pattern, which predisposes the nerve fibers to ischemic injury, or because of the possibility of collapse of the collagenous scaffolding of the lamina cribrosa, thus interfering with axoplasmic flow in these fibers. The truth probably lies in some combination of these views.

Hayreh[6-9] has divided the disc region into three parts (Fig. 7-7). These are:

1. the surface nerve fiber layer
2. the prelaminar region
3. the lamina cribrosa region

The surface nerve fiber layer consists of compact optic nerve fibers as they turn to enter the nervehead. This layer receives its blood supply mainly from branches of the retinal arterioles, and the surface capillaries are continuous with those of the surrounding retina.

The prelaminar region is distinguished by the nerve fibers being arranged in bundles and surrounded by glial channels. These channels are formed by spider cells, a specialized astrocyte. This region is sometimes referred to as the anterior (or glial) part of the lamina cribrosa. This region receives its blood supply from centripetal branches from the peripapillary choroidal vessels as well as from vessels in the lamina cribrosa. There are usually no contributions from the central retinal artery.

The lamina cribrosa region, also known as the scleral part of the lamina cribrosa, is the region where the nerve actually penetrates the sclera. The

---

*The central retinal artery enters the eye at the optic disc and divides into superior and inferior branches that again branch into nasal and temporal branches. The superior and inferior temporal retinal arteries branch dichotomously as they sweep around the macula in a wide arch roughly reminiscent of the nerve fiber anatomy. They end along the nasal raphe.

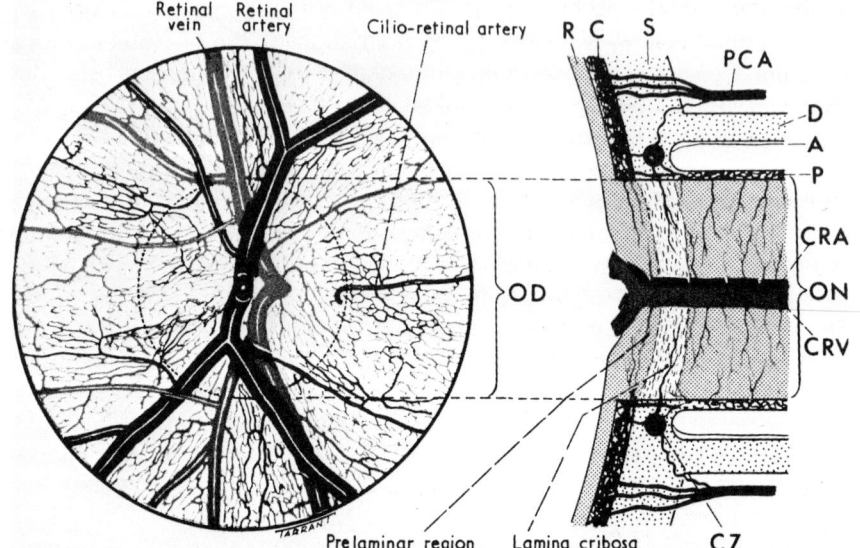

Figure 7-7 The blood supply to the optic nerve head, according to Hayreh. Note the prelaminar region derives its blood supply from the peripapillary choroid, not the central retinal vessels. OD is the optic disc; ON, optic nerve; R, retina; C, choroid; S, sclera; PCA, posterior ciliary artery; D, dura; A, arachnoid; P, pia; CZ, circle of Zinn and Haller; CRA, central retinal artery; CRV, central retinal vein. (With permission, from Hayreh.[8])

lamina cribrosa shows bands of dense connective tissue interspersed with glial elements. These connective tissue bundles form oval openings that are aligned to form canals in the normal eye.

The blood supply to the lamina comes from penetrating branches of the short posterior ciliary arteries. Uncommonly, an arterial circle, the circle of Zinn and Haller, may be present, but this structure enjoys a fame far out of proportion to the frequency of its anatomic occurrence. Although this portion of the nerve seldom receives branches from the central retinal artery, the immediately retrolaminar portion of the optic nerve did receive such branches in 75% of the specimens that Hayreh examined.

The capillary bed of all portions of the nerve head is continuous with the retinal capillaries anteriorly and the retrolaminar optic nerve posteriorly. This interconnection of the capillaries permits the vessels that are exposed to high intraocular pressure to shunt their flow into a low pressure (i.e., retrolaminar) system. The optic nerve head and the peripapillary choroid are thus the most susceptible to elevated intraocular pressure where the rest of the choroidal and the retinal circulation are relatively immune to raised intraocular pressure. Collapse of the prelaminar and peripapillary circulation is seen whenever the intraocular pressure and the diastolic blood pressure are within 10 mmHg of each other. Although it seems clear that ischemia is the initiating event, other mechanisms may contribute to field loss once damage occurs. Emery et al[3] have also shown collapse of the scleral architecture, which raises the possibility of the interference with axoplasmic flow as another contribution to the glaucomatous field defect, along with ischemia. Other mechanisms, including defects of the astroglia,[1] have been proposed, but none universally accepted.

The classical field defect resulting from lesions in the retrobulbar portion of the optic nerve is the central scotoma (Figs. 1-32, 1-41). Although insults to the nerve may result in arcuate defects (as does damage to the disc), most give rise to central or centrocecal scotoma. This is particularly true of inflammatory disease but also occurs in compression from tumors.

An altitudinal hemianopsia (see Figs. 1-35 and 1-36) may occur with ischemia, tumors, or other lesions of the optic nerve, as it may from glaucoma. Those resulting from anterior lesions of the nerve more commonly involve the inferior field, while those from glaucoma tend to favor the superior field. Unfortunately, there are enough exceptions in each direction to render this rule somewhat impotent. (Diseases of the optic nerve are discussed in more detail in Chapter 8.)

BILATERAL FIELD DEFECTS

A special problem arises in those patients who have bilateral defects anterior to the chiasm. One such typical patient is the glaucoma patient. Bilaterality may also be seen in various optic neuropathies, whether due to a generalized disease process or to intoxication. Nevertheless, in the absence of a clearly definable etiology for bilateral defects, the suspicion that these are unrecognized true hemianopsias should initiate a careful search for offsets along the hemianopsia line.

There are certain specific patterns of defects that are usually recognizable as prechiasmal. These include arcuate scotomas, a generalized contraction, altitudinal hemianopsias, ring scotomas (really two adjoining arcuate scotomas), individual small scotomas (which may be incomplete arcuate scotomas), juxtacecal or centrocecal scotomas, central scotomas, a residual temporal island of vision, and the so-called "sieve effect" seen very frequently in optic neuropathy. Nasal and vertical steps may also be prechiasmal patterns, although the likelihood of a postchiasmal lesion exists in the case of a vertical step. A final word of caution is that arcuate defects can uncommonly be caused by chiasmal lesions.

BINOCULAR FIELD DEFECTS INVOLVING CHIASM

If a visual field has a binocular defect that cannot be readily explained on the basis of bilateral pathology, the question is then whether the lesion lies at or behind the optic chiasm. The chiasm itself has a very special anatomy, which at once lends itself to damage by a variety of pathological processes as well as to pathognomonic field defects. Anatomically, the chiasm is an x-shaped structure formed by the junction of the optic nerves which lies in the interpeduncular extensions of the cisterna basalis. Each optic nerve enters the anterior arms of the "x" and the optic tracts emerge from the posterior arms. Functionally, it serves to allow the nerve fibers from each nasal hemiretina to decussate to the opposite side, while the temporal fibers follow a direct ipsilateral path.

Its position is somewhat variable. In approximately 79% of the cases, it lies in close relationship to the diaphragma sellae. In 4% of the cases it is further posterior (postfixed), and in 17% of the cases it is further forward (prefixed) to some degree. The position is determined by the lengths of the intracranial portions of the optic nerve and the angle at which they approach each other.

The optic chiasm has a number of important anatomical relationships. It lies just inferior to the third ventricle and hypothalamus, and just superior to the pituitary body and sphenoid sinus. The anterior communicating and anterior cerebral arteries pass anteriorly while the internal carotid arteries pass laterally. Posteriorly it is crossed by the posterior communicating arteries and, in most cases, the infundibulum. Therefore, the chiasm has ample opportunity to be damaged by tumor (craniopharyngioma, pituitary adenoma) or aneurysm of any of the arteries in relationship to it.

The temporal fibers pass along the outer portions of the chiasm maintaining much the same relationship as in the optic nerve. The upper fibers lie dorsomedially, while lower fibers lie ventrolaterally. The more peripheral the origin of the fibers, the closer they lie to the surface of the chiasm.

The nasal fibers cross as a widely spread bundle. The upper fibers lie dorsally and cross posteriorly, while the lower fibers lie ventrally and cross anteriorly. This arrangement may be remembered by the mnemonic, "The Optic Snowplow," since the blade of a snowplow tips backward with its top edge posterior to the lower edge. The macular fibers likely cross posteriodorsally.

The inferior crossing fibers may swing as far as 3 mm anteriorly into the contralateral optic nerve before resuming a posterior course. This forms "The Genu of the Chiasm" or the "The Knee of Wilbrand." Thus, posterior optic nerve lesions may damage the genu, thereby causing contralateral defects. The superior fibers enter the ipsilateral optic tract to form a similar, but much smaller, loop.

The general characteristics of the field loss produced by parachiasmal lesions should be predictable from the anatomy, but the chiasm is so compact, so variable in position and attacked by pathology that is itself so highly variable, that any generalization will likely prove false in a significant percentage of cases. Perhaps the safest generalization is that the field defects have a high degree of variability in their form, symmetry, and mode of progression, even when only a single underlying disease is considered. Other useful rules are that (1) pressure from above and behind tends to produce inferior bitemporal defects; (2) pressure from below and anteriorly tends to yield superior bitemporal defects (Fig. 7-9); and (3) pressure from the sides (i.e., two lesions) tends to result in a binasal defect (see Figs. 7-8 and 1-34). If the involvement is anterior and asymmetric so that only the genu is involved, the resultant damage may be a typical "optic nerve" type of field defect (e.g., blind eye, central scotoma, etc.) on the side of the lesion, coupled with a superior temporal quadrantic loss in the periphery of the field of the fellow eye (Fig. 7-10). The famous "Junction Scotoma of Traquair" belongs to this group of defects. Homonymous defects (i.e., confined to the right or left field of each eye) are not features of chiasmal lesions but rather implicate a more posterior location of the morbid process. Finally, although chiasmal lesions generally cause field defects that respect the midline, this is by no means absolute, since the compactness of the structure permits damage to fibers serving both sides of the visual field. Crossing of the midline is in fact a typical form of progression of such lesions, even though they may have respected the midline earlier. These features are illustrated in Figs. 7-9, 7-10, and 7-11 and summarized in Table 7-3.

The variability of the lesions affecting this area makes their clinical detection difficult. The detection of a high percentage of early chiasmal lesions requires a combination of careful perimetry and a suspicious clinician. We feel both the central and peripheral field should ideally be examined by whatever techniques are available. Particular attention should be given to associated complaints in these patients. Loss of visual acuity is a frequent presenting complaint. Some may notice a decline in peripheral vision, difficulty in driving, or other symptoms related to the field defects. Optic atrophy is unreliable and occurs late. Headaches of a mild nature are common, and they are rarely severe or associated with increased intracranial pressure (an exception is craniopharyngioma). Other symptoms include diabetes insipidus, endocrinologic disturbances, and change of mental status. Patients with suggestive fields or symptoms deserve a thorough neurological and neuroradiological examination.

Finally, remember that asymmetry is the rule in chiasmal lesions, and even if the *complaint* is unilateral, it is advisable to do bilateral visual fields, at least initially. Do enough isopters, and maintain a high level of suspicion. Otherwise, you may be unpleasantly surprised to see how many cases of "optic neuritis" eventually prove to have a pituitary tumor.

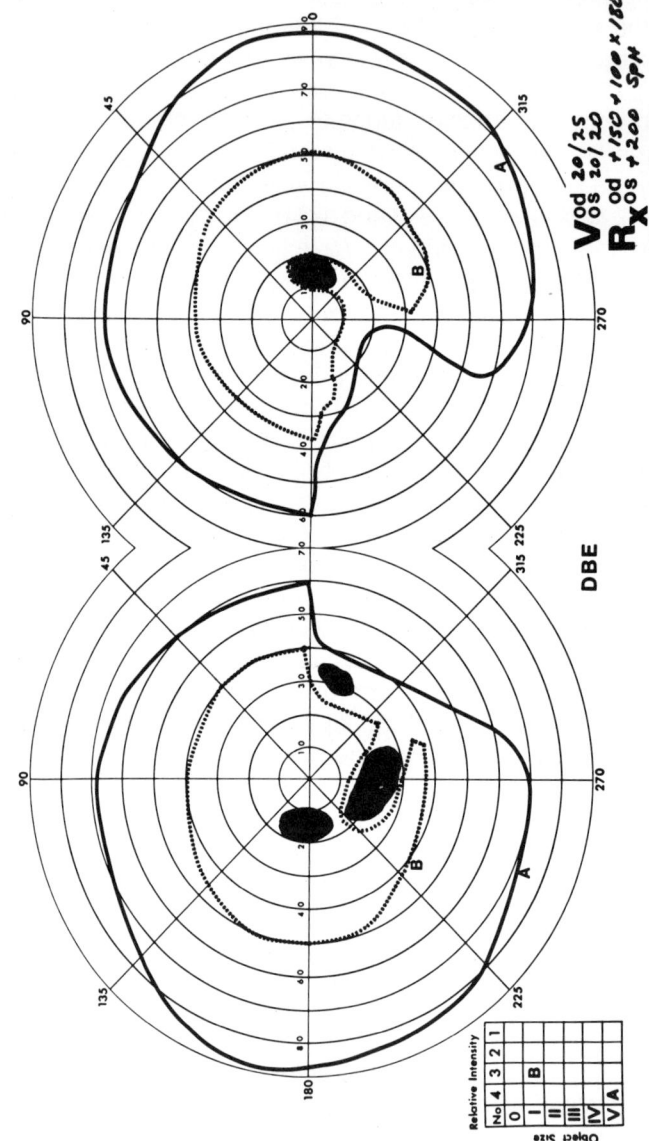

Figure 7-8 Binasal defects due to drusen of the disc. If only the peripheral isopters were examined, this case would appear as a binasal hemianopsia. Drusen are among the most common causes (some say that they are the most common cause) of binasal hemianopsias.

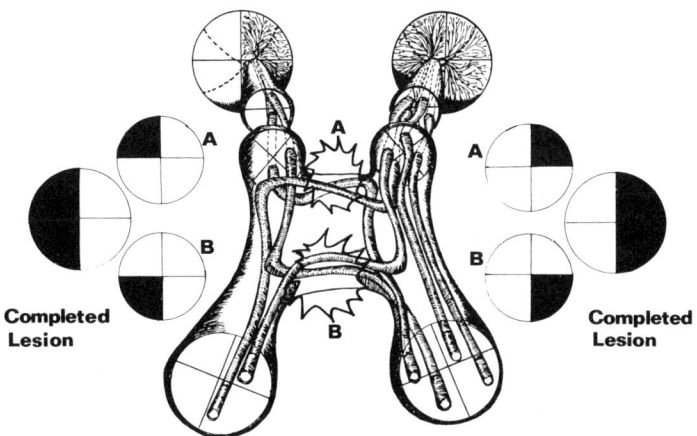

Figure 7-9 Patterns of chiasmal compression affect the patterns of visual field loss. Lesions that attack the chiasm anteriorly and below (A) cause superior bitemporal quadrantanopsias. Those that approach the chiasm from above and behind (B) first cause inferior bitemporal quadrantanopsias. In either case, a complete bitemporal hemianopsia develops as the lesion progresses to bisect the chiasm.

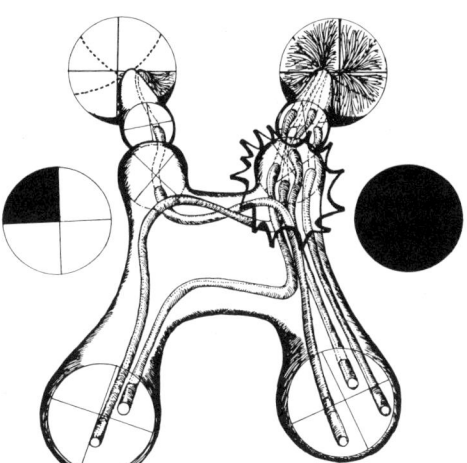

Figure 7-10 Anterolateral compression of the chiasm causes damage to the ipsilateral optic nerve and the fibers from the contralateral optic nerve that swing forward in the genu of the chiasm. Thus, one sees field defects typical of optic nerve damage (such as a blind eye, central scotoma, etc.) in the ipsilateral eye, coupled with a superior temporal quadrantic defect in the fellow eye.

210 *Principles of Quantitative Perimetry*

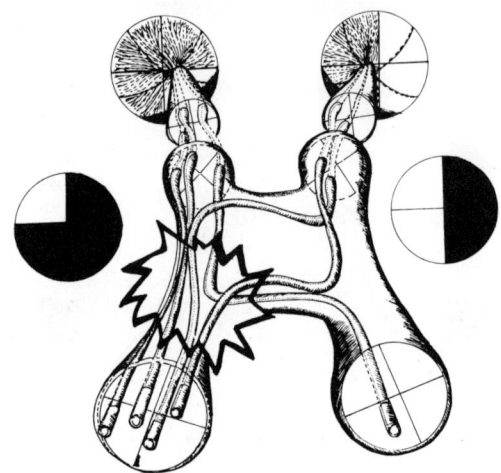

Figure 7-11 Posterolateral compression of the chiasm causes a typical tract lesion (a homonymous hemianopsia contralateral to the lesion) coupled with an inferior temporal quadrantanopsia in the ipsilateral eye. Such lesions are uncommon.

POSTCHIASMAL LESIONS

The hallmark of the postchiasmal lesion is the homonymous hemianopsia (see Fig. 1-31). Once the chiasm is passed, the organization of the nerve fibers is based not so much on nasal or temporal retina but on right or left visual field (see Fig. 7-6). Therefore, any interruption of the postchiasmal pathways will be confined to the half of the visual field subserved by these fibers. The retina of each eye to the right of the macula, and hence the left visual field, is served by the right side of the brain including the right optic tract, lateral geniculate body, visual radiation, and occipital cortex. Similarly, the right visual field is served by the left side of the brain. Thus we have a rule: The lesion lies opposite the field defect in postchiasmal lesions. Other concepts aid in the localization of lesions along the retrochiasmal pathway. The most important of these are congruity, specific patterns of the defect, and associated signs or symptoms due to damage to related structures.

The concept of congruity was introduced in Chapter 1, but it merits further discussion here. In essence, it means similarity of form of field defects in that portion of the field served by binocular vision. The far temporal periphery of each eye's field is seen uniocularly only. The concept of congruity has no meaning in this area, nor is a field defect that extends over both the binocularly seen field and uniocularly seen field necessarily incongruous simply because it appears dissimilar to that seen in the fellow eye because of the extension into

Pressure from:	Pattern of Field Loss:	Comment:
Midline below	Superior temporals, then lower temporals, then lower nasals, then superior nasal quadrants.	Found in pituitary tumor. Exact pattern varies with position of chiasm (whether prefixed, postfixed, or normal) and growth pattern of tumor.
Midline above	Inferior temporal, then superior temporal, then lower nasal, then superior nasal quadrants.	Found in craniopharyngioma. Note both here and above the superior nasal quadrant is last to be affected.
Anterolateral	Central scotoma or any other uniocular field defect (including blind eye) on side of tumor and upper temporal defect in fellow eye.	A junctional scotoma found in pituitary tumor, meningioma, or aneurysm of carotid or of anterior cerebral artery.
Posterolateral	Homonymous hemianopsia on side of field opposite lesion plus inferior temporal defect in the eye on same side as lesion.	Many variations exist. This exact pattern is seldom seen. Resultant lesions depend upon whether damage predominantly involves tract or chiasm. Found in tumor and aneurysm.

Table 7-3 Patterns of chiasmal compression. In practice, chiasmal lesions cause some combination of the four patterns described here. Chiasmal defects are notoriously variable in form, partly because of variability in the pathology and partly because of variability in the position of the chiasm. Chiasmal lesions may either be due to direct compression or to interference with blood supply.

	Optic Tract or LGB	Temporal Lobe	Parietal Lobe	Occipital Lobe
Congruity is:	Minimal	Moderate	Noticeable	Marked
Macula is:	Often split	Usually split	Usually spared	Often spared
Slope is:	Related to activity	Related to activity	Related to activity	Steep with stroke; otherwise, activity
Portion of field involved is:	Unpredictable	Superior quadrant	Inferior quadrant	Unpredictable
Associated signs and symptoms:	Endocrine changes, Wernicke's hemianopic pupil. May see optic atrophy in lesions involving LGB or very anterior optic radiation, may see hemiplegia, numbness or dysthesia of opposite side. Aphasia is possible.	Delusions of peculiar tastes and odors. Formed visual hallucinations. Auditory hallucinations if dominant side involved.	OKN decreased only with movement toward lesion; extinction of objects in field opposite lesion on double simultaneous stimulation; conjugate ocular deviation on forced lid closure. Various forms of aphasia or apraxia in parietotemporal lesions.	Formless visual hallucination. Denial of blindness (Anton's syndrome).
Frequency:	Rare	Common	Uncommon	Common

Table 7-4 Homonymous hemianopsia: associated findings with various locations of lesions.

the uniocular field. Only the binocularly seen parts must be comparable. Secondly, the concept can apply only to retrochiasmal lesions, since none other is truly homonymous. Lastly, in complete hemianopsias, the concept has no meaning, since the lesion simply corresponds to a complete severance of the contralateral visual pathway at any point behind the chiasm. In those lesions to which the concept is applicable, the congruity increases the farther posteriorly the lesion is located. Cortical lesions are typically perfectly congruous, while optic tract lesions are much less so.

The remaining two parameters that aid in localization are strongly influenced by the regional variations in anatomy. In the case of characteristic defect patterns, the separation of the fibers in the pathway and the variation in blood supply are the important considerations. The associated signs and symptoms depend entirely upon what other structures of importance are in the area.

In the case of retrochiasmal lesions, it must be understood that certain signs and symptoms are due to the hemianopsia per se and have no localizing value. Although the visual acuity in such patients is typically undisturbed (in contrast to patients with chiasmal lesions), the patient may complain of difficulty in reading. If the hemianopsia is to the right of fixation, reading is slow, while if the defect is to the left, the line may be read without difficulty, but the patient may be unable to find the start of the next line of print. Another common complaint is that they bump into objects on the side of the hemianopsia. The patient may "fill out" an object seen in his good field into his blind field, then complain of double images or afterimages when he discovers it is no longer there. The cause for this is not clear.

In the case of the optic tracts, the anatomy is such that there is a paucity of both characteristic patterns and damage to associated structures. The optic tracts run posteriorly from the posteriolateral arms of the optic chiasm, around the cerebral peduncles and end at the lateral geniculate body. Although they lie in the vicinity of a number of important anatomical structures, only the posterior cerebral artery is likely to damage the tract due to aneurysm. The other important relationships include the internal capsule, the lentiform nucleus, and the limbic constituents of temporal lobe, including the uncus and hippocampal gyrus, but concomitant damage to these structures is comparatively rare. One distinguishing point is that pupillary afferent fibers travel in the tract, exiting just before reaching the lateral geniculate. Therefore, pupillary abnormalities may be seen with tract lesions, but not with more posterior pathology (Wernicke's Hemianopic Pupil). Unfortunately, this rather nice story is sullied by two facts. The first is that clinically testing for this sign is unreliable; the second is that Harms[4,5] as well as others[2] have reported pupillary abnormalities with isolated cortical lesions. Although the significance of these findings is not completely clear anatomically, they do serve to diminish further the value of a hemianopic pupil as a localizing sign.

| | Tumor | Vascular | | | |
| | | Ischemia | | Hemorrhagic | Trauma |
		Carotid	Basilar-Vertebral		
Speed of field loss	Gradual	Sudden	Sudden	Sudden	Sudden
Macular sparing	Usually split	Usually spared	Usually spared	Split	Usually split
Awareness of defect	Usually unaware	Usually unaware or partially aware	May be unaware, partially aware or deny blindness (Anton's syndrome)	Partially aware	Acutely aware
Hallucinations	Moderately common, especially with temporal-parietal lesions	Common with late scarring	Common with late scarring	Common with late scarring	Common with late scarring
History	May be none	Transient ischemic attacks	Transient ischemic attacks	Hypertension, heart or lung disease	Trauma

214

Associated findings	Signs of increased intracranial pressure, such as papilledema. May see compression of posterior cerebral arteries in cases of uncal herniation with sudden onset of hemianopsia. May have elevated spinal fluid protein. Convulsions frequent.	Ipsilateral amaurosis fugax with hemiplegia and heminaesthesia of contralateral side.	Dizziness, confusion, cranial nerve palsy, dysarthria, dysphagia, hemiplegia and hemianesthesia, nystagmus, internuclear ophthalmoplegia, pain in homolateral eye. Make association with subclavian steal syndrome.	Sudden onset of headache, confusion, progressing to coma. May have nausea or vomiting, acute seizures. May complain of scintillating scotoma in A-V malformation. Usually has blood in CSF.	Depends on site of lesion. May have multiple areas of damage along visual pathway. May have profound changes in neurological status with subdural hematoma. Convulsions occasional.
Usual site	Temporal	Uniocular (prechiasmal)	Occipital	Parietal	Variable

Table 7-5 Homonymous hemianopsia: associated findings with various etiologies of lesion.

216   *Principles of Quantitative Perimetry*

Lesions of the lateral geniculate body (LGB) similarly lack a large number of distinctive features. The LGB serves as a relay and association station in the visual pathway. It is here that the axons from the ganglion cell layer of the retina end and the geniculocortical neurons begin. In human beings, the LGB appears as a folded oval structure on the posteriolateral aspect of the pulvinar at the termination of the optic tract. It is this peculiar folded shape that gives it the name "geniculate," meaning "kneelike." The LGB receives its blood supply from the anterior and posterior choroidal arteries.

On cross section, the nucleus is divided into several laminae of grey matter separated by bundles of white matter (Fig. 7-12). Each lamina contains multiple interneurons that richly arborize within the lamina and may cross to other laminae. The most complex visual function is projected into the area with the most laminae. The portion of the LGB subserving macular function has six layers. In that part that is concerned with the central (binocular) fields, Laminae IV and VI and also III and V fuse medially and laterally, reducing the number of laminae to four. In that portion of the LGB that deals with the extreme periphery of the visual field (i.e., the uniocular fields), laminae I, IV, and VI and also laminae II, III, and V fuse to form only two laminae.

The exact manner in which the retinal fibers project upon the lateral genicu-

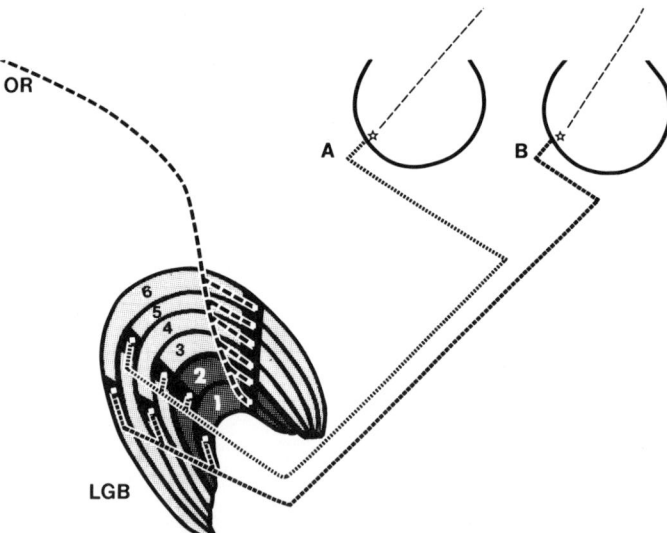

Figure 7-12   A schematic representation of the anatomy of the lateral geniculate body (LGB). The LGB is divided into six laminae. Laminae 1 and 2 (dark shading) contain larger cells than the remaining four layers. Fibers from the contralateral eye (B) end in laminae 1, 4, and 6, whereas those from the ipsilateral eye (A) end in laminae 2, 3, and 5. Fibers forming the optic radiation arise from all six laminae.

Principles of Interpretation of the Visual Field 217

late body in human beings is not completely certain. However, it is known that crossed retinogeniculate fibers terminate in Laminae I, IV, and VI, whereas uncrossed fibers terminate in Laminae II, III, and V. The axons that project onto the cortex are derived from all six layers.

Clinical examples of lateral geniculate body lesions are extremely rare (Fig. 7-13 and 7-14). Since the upper retina is represented on the medial LGB, the macula in the central portion and the lower retina in lateral LGB, one would anticipate homonymous upper hemianopic field defects with lateral LGB lesions, and so on. Obviously, a complete homonymous hemianopsia would result with complete destruction of the LGB. If the neighboring thalamus is involved, contralateral dysesthesias may be present. Should the nearby internal capsule be damaged, some degree of hemiplegia may result, usually of the lower extremity. Since lesions involving the midbrain may result in stupor, field studies cannot be obtained in all such patients.

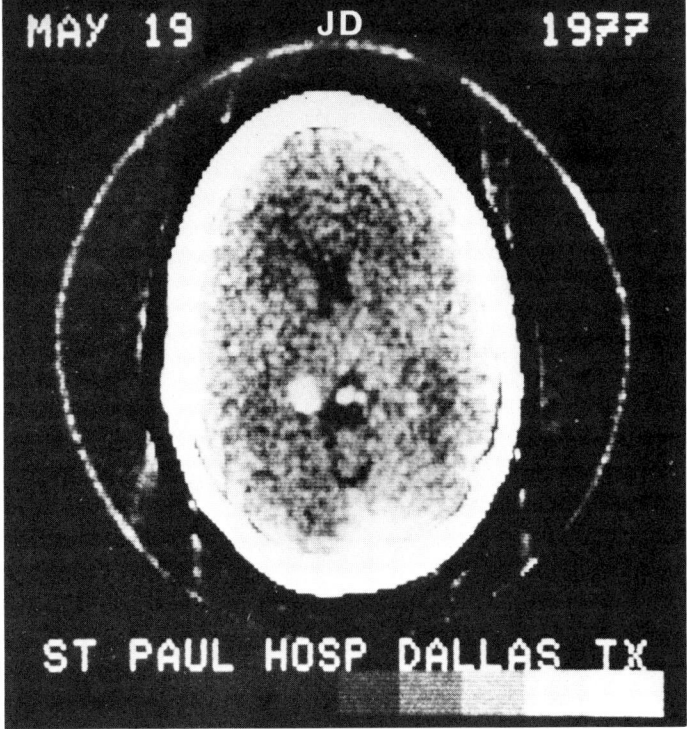

Figure 7-13 Computerized axial tomogram of a 28-year-old woman, showing a calcified mass which the radiologist thought involved the lateral thalamus. A calcified pineal gland can also be seen in the midline. The patient had a right homonymous hemianopsia (Fig. 7-14) which, like her neurological exam, had been stable for years.

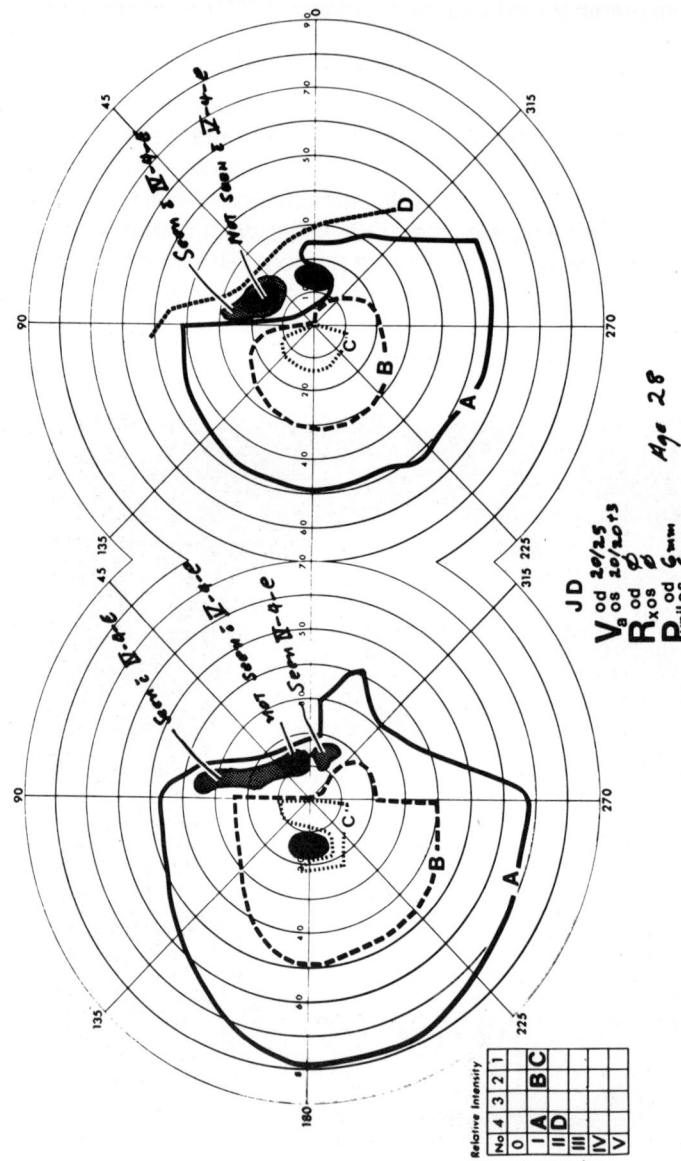

Figure 7-14 Visual field of the patient seen in Figure 7-13. This is probably one of the few examples of a field defect due mainly to a lesion of the lateral geniculate body, although some damage to the anterior optic radiation undoubtedly is also present.

The first opportunity for a real variety of specific patterns of visual field defect as well as definitely helpful associated defects comes with the next step down the visual pathway, the optic radiations,* or more formally, the geniculocalcarine pathway. There is the opportunity for at least three distinct perimetric and clinical syndromes as the radiation passes in turn through the internal capsule, the temporal lobe, and the parietal lobe.

The first chance for a recognizable syndrome occurs as the axons comprising the radiation arise from all six laminae of the LGB and course dorsolaterally in a compact bundle through the posterior arm of the internal capsule. The fibers at this point pass through an area that takes them just posterior to the main sensory radiation and the internal auditory radiation in the internal capsule. (See Figure 7-15.) This area is usually supplied by the anterior choroidal artery, and occlusion of this vessel is associated with a syndrome of hemianopsia, hemiplegia, and hemianesthesia, especially of the lower extremity.

The second clearcut perimetric syndrome is a result of the fiber pathway through the temporal lobe.

Upon emerging from the internal capsule, the dorsal fibers (which subserve the inferior field) course directly posteriorly, but the ventral fibers sweep into the temporal lobe in a wide curve lateral to the lateral ventricle. (See Fig. 7-18.) This is most marked in the fibers carrying information from the inferiormost retina. Their axons may loop forward as far as the anterior tip of the inferior horn of the lateral ventrical to form the "Loop of Meyer." The fibers then swing posteriomedially, passing beneath the inferior horn of the lateral ventrical in relation to the hippocampal gyrus prior to rejoining its superior fellows in the external sagital stratum. It should be noted that Meyer's loop is not always so pronounced and may be absent in some individuals. However, it provides the anatomical basis for the superior homonymous quadrantanopsia noted in those individuals who are unfortunate enough to suffer temporal lobe lesions.

The superior homonymous quadrantanopsia is nearly pathognomonic of temporal lobe lesions, and its progression is even more so. If the lesion involves only the tip of the temporal lobe, a very narrow wedge-shaped scotoma immediately adjacent to the superior midline will result, the so-called "pie-in-the-sky" defect (Fig. 7-16). As the lesion encroaches further and further posteriorly, the wedge widens, just as if someone sliced additional pieces from the pie. Finally, a complete quadrant is lost. This relatively slow progression results from the widespread separation of the fibers of Meyer's loop, which serve only the superior field. This is not the case with the fibers responsible for the lower quadrant of the field, and progression from a superior homonymous quadrantanopsia to a complete homonymous hemianopsia is relatively rapid.

---

*Eponymously, the "Radiations of Gratiolet."

220 *Principles of Quantitative Perimetry*

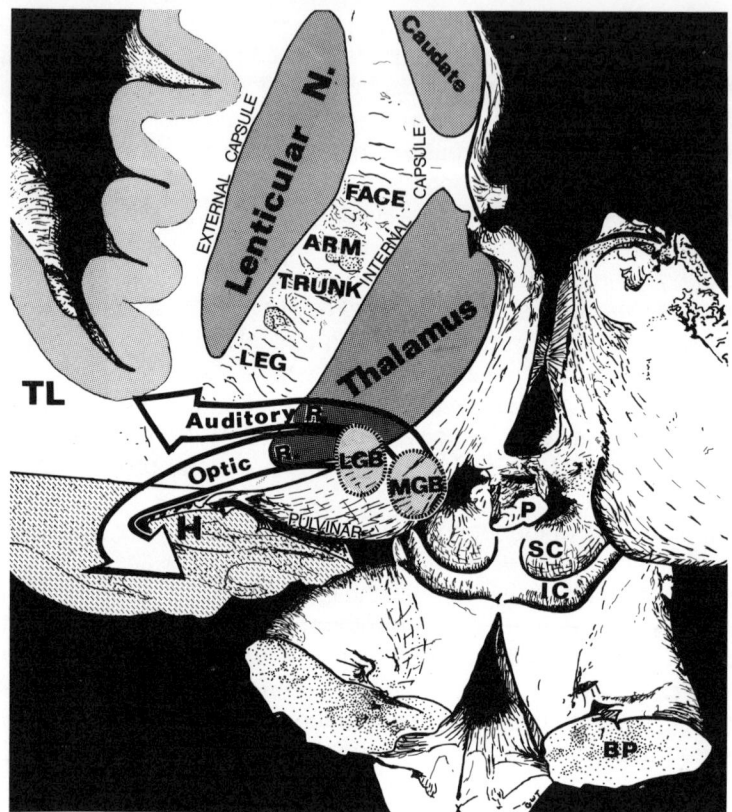

Figure 7-15   The anatomy of the anterior optic radiation and lateral geniculate body. Note the important relationships of the sensory modalities in the internal capsule and the auditory radiation to the optic radiation. TL is the temporal lobe; H, hippocampal gyrus; P, pineal gland stalk; SC and IC, superior and inferior colliculus, respectively; BP, brachium pontis.

The final member of this trilogy of recognizable patterns of field loss is due to vascular (usually ischemic) lesions of the optic radiation as it passes through the parietal lobe. The fibers representing the contralateral and ipsilateral retina run in closely associated parallel bundles without obvious intertwining. Fibers from the upper and lower retina occupy the upper and lower portions of the optic radiation respectively and are widely separated by the macular fibers which are the most central (Fig. 7-6). Those fibers serving the most peripheral field are similarly most peripheral in the optic radiation. This separation permits fairly definite quadrantanopsias to form. The formation of quadrantanopsias is aided by the nature of the blood supply to the parietal portion of the radiation. The dorsal fibers are supplied by the middle cerebral artery, whereas the ventral fibers are nourished by the posterior cerebral artery. Thus, either superior or

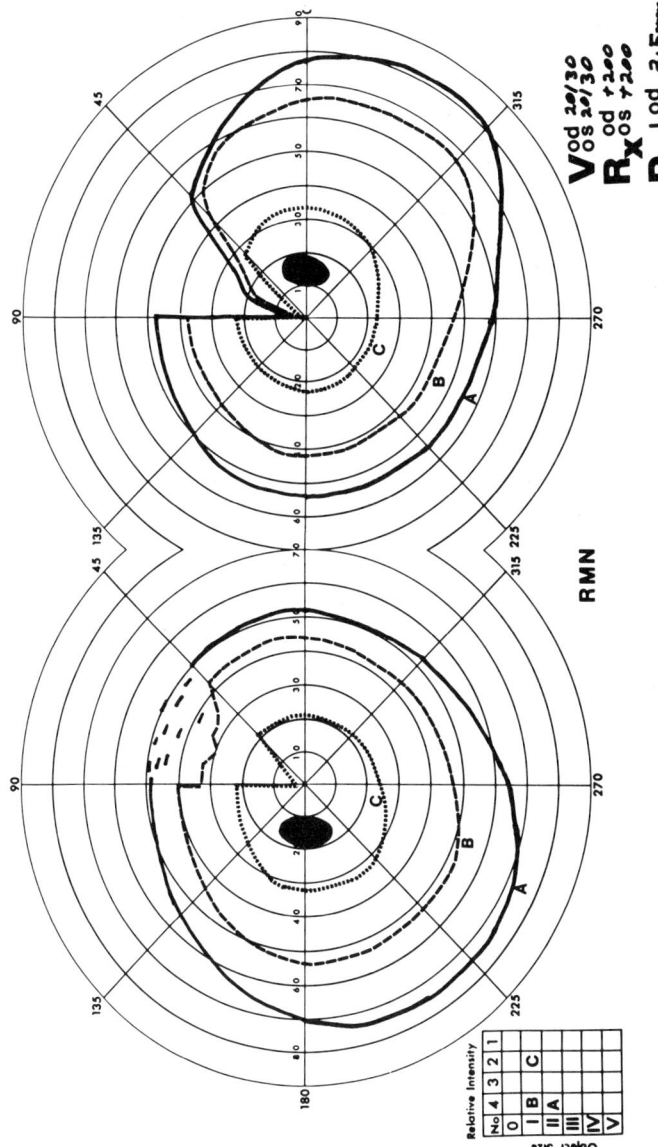

Figure 7-16 "Pie in the Sky." A right superior quadrantic field defect typical of a left temporal lobe lesion.

inferior quadrantanopsias are possible, but inferior quadrantanopsias are far more common for an anatomical reason. Because the predominant blood supply to the occipital lobes comes from the posterior cerebral artery, complete hemianopsias are likely when this vessel becomes diseased. Therefore, in contrast to the superior homonymous quadrantanopsia of the temporal lobe, an *inferior* homonymous quadrantanopsia is the hallmark of the parietal lobe lesion, or at least those with a vascular basis. (See Fig. 7-17.)

The pictures of the associated findings seen with parietal and temporal lobe lesions are quite similar and tend to merge into one another. Abnormal optokinetic nystagmus (OKN) (diminished response with rotation *toward* the side of the lesion),* astereognosis, conjugate deviation of eyes to the side *opposite* the lesion with forced lid closure,† and lack of visual attention, particularly in lesions of the non-dominant hemisphere, frequently accompany parietal lobe lesions.‡ Formed hallucinations and photopsias can occur with temporal and parietal lobe lesions. Convulsions may also be seen, sometimes with focal signs, such as deviation of the eyes in the direction opposite the side of the lesion.

Certain temporal lobe lesions may cause assorted symptoms that permit precise localization of the lesion. One is the uncinate fit in which the patient complains of disagreeable odors or taste and which may be accompanied by chewing movements. It is associated with lesions of the inferomedial temporal lobe. This area is called the uncus and is superficial to the amygdaloid nuclei, one of the basal ganglia that receives olfactory information. Another such symptom is peduncular hallucinations that are brightly colored, kaleidoscopic lights caused by lesions involving the medial temporal lobes and midbrain.

Expanding lesions in this region may also be responsible for the herniation of the hippocampus through the tentorium, which consequently results in compression of the brain stem. If the posterior cerebral arteries are compressed, total blindness may result and mask a preexisting hemianopsia. Patients with the problem are frequently quite old, with altered levels of consciousness, nystagmus, oculomotor palsies, dysarthria, respiratory distress, and internuclear ophthalmoplegia. One particularly valuable, and occasionally the only, sign of this occurrence is mydriasis. It is unilateral and typically (but not invariably) on the side of the lesion.

One group of symptoms seen with parietotemporal disease deserve special

---

*Asymmetrical OKN may also be seen in lesions of the thalamus, and absent OKN may be either a normal variant or seen in lesions of the pons. Asymmetrical OKN is *not* due to the hemianopsia itself.
†This sign may occur in rare normal individuals or with some lesions of the brain stem.
‡Other rare, or poorly documented, signs of parietal lesions include metamorphopsia, teleopsia, macropsia, and micropsia.

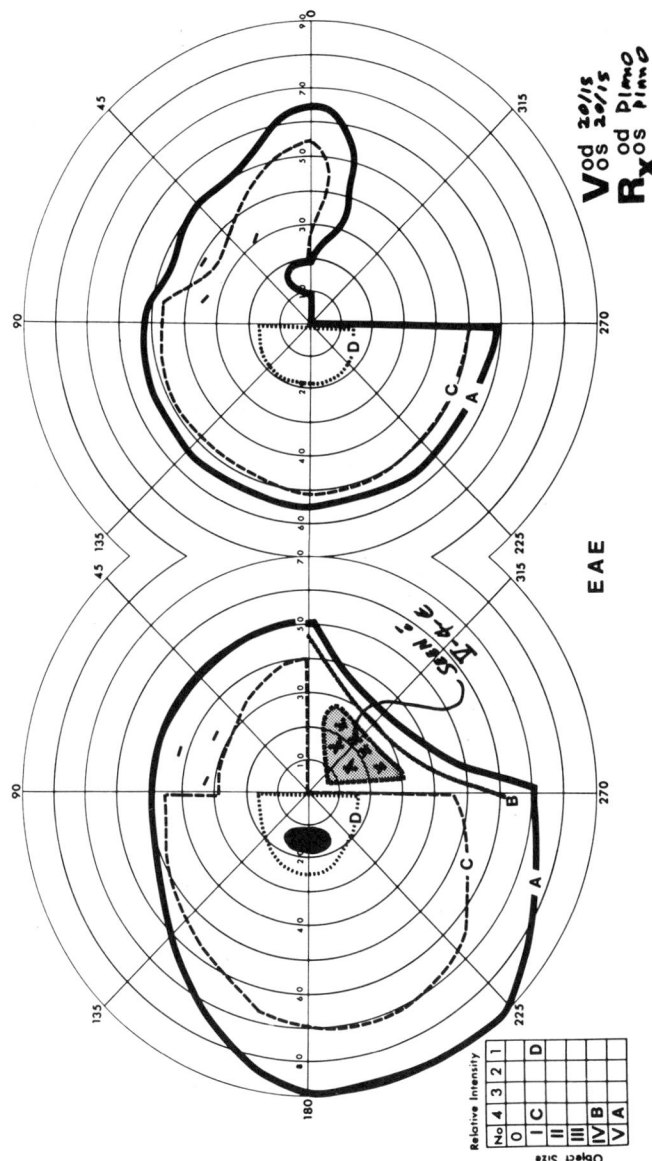

Figure 7-17 A right inferior homonymous quadrantanopsia thought to be due to an ischemic infarct in the left parietal lobe.

comment: the aphasias. The angular gyri are responsible for visual cognitive functions, and thus lesions of this region on the dominant side give rise to a potpourri of functional disturbances (alexia, agraphia, etc.) collectively known as visual agnosias. Gerstman's syndrome consists of agraphia, the inability to perform simple calculations, the inability to recognize one's own anatomy as one's own, and confusion between right and left. It frequently is accompanied by homonymous hemianopsia. It is due to lesions in the region of the dominant angular gyrus.

Lesions on the nondominant side give rise to a different form of agnosia termed topographic agnosia. Such patients may lose their way in familiar surroundings, or have difficulty in drawing geometric figures. Such patients may have difficulty in operating machinery due to confusion in the arrangement of the controls or may have difficulty in dressing.

Bilateral parietotemporal lesions are uncommon, but when present may present in the context of several syndromes. Bilateral parietal lesions produce Balint's syndrome, an unawareness of objects and persons in their surroundings which a normal person would easily recognize. It is coupled with a defect of voluntary eye movements, although random movements are full. Deep bilateral temporal lesions may produce a global visual agnosia, where the patient is unable to identify objects by sight but can by use of the other senses.

The termination of the optic pathway is the visual cortex,* also referred to as the striate cortex (Fig 7-18). It derives this name from a white line (the "white line of Gennari") formed by a plexus of medullated nerve fibers running through the gray matter.

The striate cortex is situated largely on the medial aspect and posterior pole of the occipital lobe, with a small extension to the lateral surface of the lobe. The striate cortex is deeply grooved by the calcarine fissure, and much of the cortex lies buried within its cleft. The visual cortex is absolutely indispensable to form vision since there are no alternative cortical pathways. Complete visual function, however, requires the assistance of the extrastriate cortex.

The point-to-point representation of the retina is only roughly maintained at the visual cortex with the macula receiving the lion's share of the cortex. At the fovea, 1mm^2 of cortex subserves 2 minutes of visual angle while at only 5° eccentricity, 1mm^2 of cortex serves 18 minutes of visual angle, a ratio that goes much higher in the far retinal periphery. Altogether, the macula projects onto about half of the available cortex.

The more central retinal fibers are projected more posteriorly, whereas the

---

*The striate cortex corresponds to Area 17 of Brodmann. The neighboring prestriate area, Areas 18 and 19 of Brodmann, which account for the remainder of the occipital cortex, are probably concerned with visual patterns, associations, and perhaps motor functions.

Principles of Interpretation of the Visual Field 225

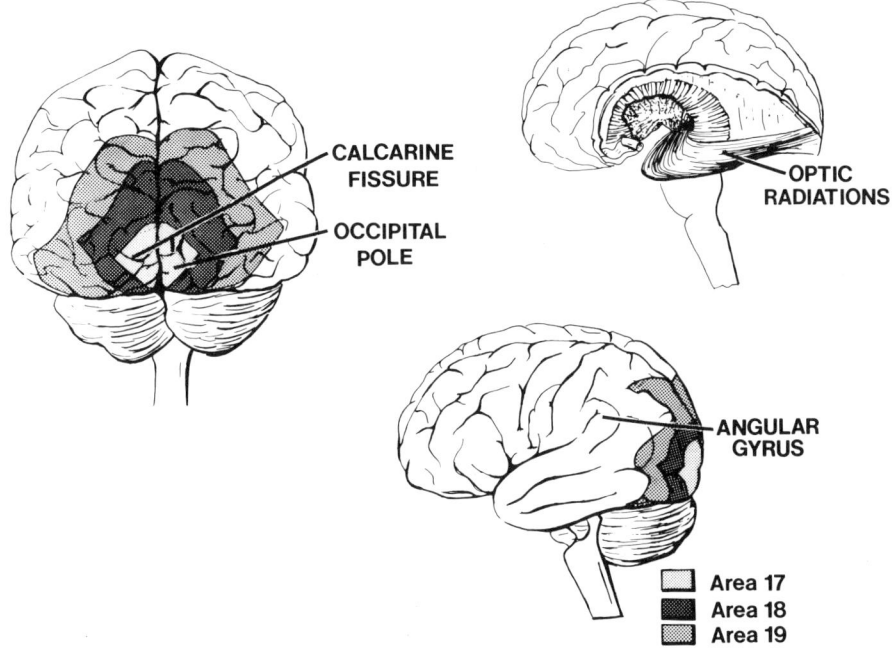

Figure 7-18 The anatomy of the optic radiations and the visual cortex. The occipital lobe contains the striate cortex (Area 17) and the parastriate and peristriate cortices (Areas 18 and 19). The angular gyrus is an important landmark since lesions near it may cause aphasia as well as visual field defects.

more peripheral fibers are anterior. Thus, the uniocular fields occupy a position on the far anterior tip of the striate area. Along the posterior calcarine fissure, fibers from the upper retina are superior to the fissure, whereas lower retinal fibers project inferior to the fissure. Anterior to the parietooccipital fissure, however, both superior and inferior retina are projected inferior to the sulcus.

By and large, the only thing seen either perimetrically or clinically in patients with a limited lesion of the striate cortex* is an exquisitely congruent hemianopsia (Fig. 7-19). Should the lesion be on a vascular basis, the vertebrobasilar system is frequently involved and thus appear all the symptoms of basilar artery insufficiency, such as vertigo, nystagmus, diplopia, internuclear ophthalmoplegia, perioral numbness, and a host of other dysfunctions that are related to impairment of the cranial nerve nuclei, pyramidal tracts or pathways to and from

---

*Note that lesions in the parastriate cortex, still a part of the occipital lobe, may be associated with problems of voluntary gaze, nystagmus, or similar findings.

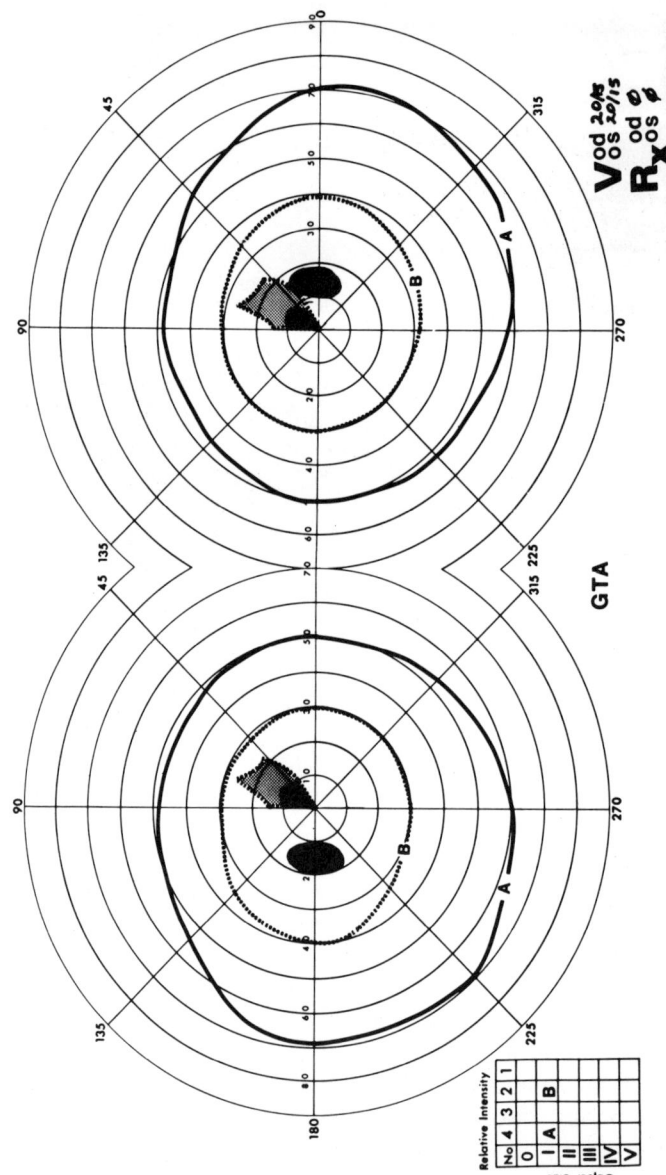

Figure 7-19 A typical visual field defect due to a traumatic occipital lobe lesion. These defects usually involve the central field and are exactly congruous.

the cerebellum. Frequently, the patient will have numerous transient prodromal episodes of blurring or blackouts before the final insult.

Unformed visual hallucinations(photopsias) may occur, but true hallucinations are rare. The entity of denial of blindness, or Anton's syndrome, is not rare with cortical blindness, either as a hemianopsia or total blindness. Persons with Anton's syndrome resort to a magnificent variety of confabulations to alibi their inability to see. The signs that accompany the hemianopsia of parietal lesions, such as abnormal OKN or conjugate deviation of the eyes on forced lid closure, are not seen with cortical lesions unless the lesions are large enough to insult areas outside the striate cortex as well.

Lesions of the posterior pole, be they neoplastic or traumatic, characteristically involve fixation. In the case of trauma, bilateral homonymous defects may be produced, resulting in a central scotoma if the lesion crosses the midline far posteriorly. More anterior lesions spare fixation but produce a constricted field. If both supracalcarine cortical areas are damaged, an inferior altitudinal hemianopsia may be produced. The corresponding superior altitudinal hemianopsia of cortical origin is virtually never seen since its production almost surely entails fatal damage to the venous sinuses.

Neoplastic lesions of the region have been known to mimic other types of disease. Tumors may cause field defects that appear suddenly, perhaps due to vascular interference, and thereby mimic a vascular lesion. Unlike the vascular etiology, the neoplasm enjoys a relentless progression following its debut. Meningiomas of the falx may produce a bitemporal field defect if they are far enough forward to damage only that portion of the cortex serving the uniocular fields.

No discussion of the visual field defects produced by lesion of the posterior visual pathways would be complete without a discussion of macular sparing. The question of macular sparing has been the subject of controversy far out of proportion to its importance. Current evidence states that there is no bilateral representation of the macula on the cortex and no commissures connecting one striate cortex to the other. The other classical explanation, that of dual blood supply to the occipital cortex by the posterior and middle cerebral arteries, is currently in disrepute since most studies show that the visual cortex receives virtually its entire blood supply from the posterior cerebral artery. Finally, one cherished legend, which holds that it is most common with pure cortical lesions, is also untrue. Parietooccipital or even parietal lesions show the phenomenon more frequently. It may rarely be so in temporal lobe lesions also, but never in lesions of the tips of the occipital lobe (i.e., the occipital poles).

Explanations of macular sparing that may still be true are varied. One of the most plausible is that this is a relative sparing only, since the macula is normally the most sensitive part of the field, and that with progression, it, too, is lost. Other possibilities rest on the facts that it is difficult to control fixation in hemianopsias, that the macula has a very diffuse cortical representation, or that it is some other artifact of testing.

SUMMARY

The interpretation of the visual field rests upon the answers to four basic questions: (1) Is the field valid, sufficient, and comparable to previously done fields? (2) Is the defect prechiasmal? Such defects are either definitely limited to one eye or, if bilaterally present, explainable. They tend to cross the midline smoothly, but there are exceptions. (3) Is the lesion chiasmal? Such lesions are usually bitemporal in nature but are notoriously variable. They usually, but not always, respect the hemianopsia line, depending on the nature of the lesion itself. (4) Is the lesion postchiasmal? In this case there should be a true homonymous hemianopsia present. These defects respect the hemianopsia line perfectly in most instances, and the location along the visual pathway can be indicated to some extent by the location of the defect in the visual field, the congruity of the defect from eye to eye, and associated findings. The activity or the nature of the pathology may be indicated by the slope of the visual field, although this depends to some extent upon the type of lesion. Naturally, a steep slope along the hemianopsia line is a reflection of the anatomy of the pathway and not the activity of the disease.

The anatomy of the visual pathway makes it possible to locate lesions along the tract. For example, in the temporal lobe, the typical visual field defect is mainly in the superior quadrants, the so-called "pie-in-the-sky" field defect. The parietal lobe typically has an inferior quadrantanopsia in vascular lesions.

A second means of locating lesions is use of the fact that congruity increases with increased chiasm-to-lesion distance. Lesions of the optic tract show little congruity while in the occipital lobe, lesions involving the cortex show marked congruity. Thus, the more posterior the insult, the more congruous the field defect. Another differentiating feature is that one often sees macula sparing with parietal and occipital lobe lesions, whereas the macula is usually split with lesions further forward in the tract.

Finally, associated signs and symptoms may give an indication of the affected area. Thus, endocrine changes may be present with lesions in the area of the anterior optic tract. Numerous other associations exist.

A wide variety of neurological findings ranging from abnormal optokinetic nystagmus to aphasia may be seen with lesions along the optic radiation as it courses through the temporal, parietal, and occipital lobes in turn. Formal visual hallucinations may be seen with parietotemporal lesions whereas only photopsias are usual in cortical lesions. Anton's syndrome may be seen in cases of cortical blindness. If the lesion extends into the extrastriate cortex, visual cognitive or oculomotor functions may be disturbed.

REFERENCES

1. Anderson D R: Pathogenesis of glaucomatous cupping: a new hypothesis, Symposium on Glaucoma, Trans New Orleans Academy of Ophthalmology. St. Louis, C. V. Mosby Co, 1975
2. Bresky R H, Charles S: Pupil motor perimetry. Am J Ophthalmol 68:108, 1969
3. Emery J M, Landis D, Paton D, Boniuk M, Craig J M: The lamina cribrosa in normal and glaucomatous human eyes. Trans Am Acad Ophthalmol Otolaryngol 78:290, 1974
4. Harms H: Grundlagen, Methodik und Bedeutung der Pupillenperimetrie für die Physiologie und Pathologie des Sehorgans. Albrecht von Graefe's Arch Ophthalmol 149:1, 1949
5. Harms H: Hemianopische Pupillenstarre. Klin Monatsbl Augenheilkd 118:113, 1951
6. Hayreh S S: Anatomy and physiology of the optic nerve head, Trans Am Acad Ophthalmol Otolaryngol 78:240, 1974
7. Hayreh S S: Blood supply of the optic nerve head and its role in optic atrophy, glaucoma, and oedema of the optic disc. Br J Ophthalmol 53:721, 1969
8. Hayreh S S: Optic disc changes in glaucoma. Br J Ophthalmol 56:175, 1972
9. Hayreh S S, Revie I H S, and Edwards J: Vasogenic origin of visual field defects and optic nerve changes in glaucoma. Br J Ophthalmol 54:461, 1970
10. Lynn J R: Correlation of pathogenesis, anatomy, and patterns of visual field loss in glaucoma, in Symposium on Glaucoma, Trans New Orleans Academy of Ophthalmology, St. Louis, C. V. Mosby Co, 1975

General References

Cogan D G: Neurology of the Visual System. Springfield, Illinois, Charles C Thomas, 1970

Walsh F B, and Hoyt W F: Clinical Neuro-ophthalmology. Baltimore, Williams and Wilkins Co, 1969

Last R J: Eugene Wolff's Anatomy of the Eye and Orbit. Philadelphia and Toronto, W. B. Saunders Co, 1972

8
Visual Field Defects in Specific Diseases: Diagnosis of Specific Diseases by Visual Field Testing

The purpose of this chapter is to discuss the visual field findings in a few specific disease states that are not obvious consequences of the anatomical lesion. A tumor of the temporal lobe may interrupt the fibers of Meyer's loop, and very little else needs be said concerning visual field defects to be expected. By comparison, a visual field defect that is due to a glaucoma or vessel occlusion can vary in form depending upon the path the disease process takes, upon the presence of other ocular or systemic disease, and upon a host of other factors. Toxic amblyopias may offer some surprises both with respect to the drugs that cause them and with respect to their clinical course. We wish to discuss illnesses of this sort in this chapter in order to amplify the material presented in the preceding chapter.

GLAUCOMA

Glaucoma represents one of the most important reasons for doing reproducible visual fields. It is one of the few absolute "always" indications for quantitative multiple-isopter kinetic perimetry or multiple-meridian static testing. It is our opinion that the adequate examination of a glaucomatous visual field requires some combination of static and kinetic perimetry. We take a slightly different approach from those championed by Harms and Aulhorn, or by Drance, in that we put relatively more emphasis on kinetic perimetry and then assign the predominant role in exploring the depths of individual scotomas to static perimetry. We differ slightly in our personal preferences of how this is done. Lynn is satisfied with a loose grid of perhaps two to four tests through the defective area, while Tate is happiest with at least one partial static meridian that spans the defect in addition to this grid. Clinically, these differences may seem unimportant since the significant fact is that most authorities agree that (1) some amount of kinetic testing is useful to find defective areas of the field and (2) static exploration is mandatory to determine the "floor" of the scotoma so that progression may be determined at a later date.

The use of visual fields instead of stereo photographs to follow a glaucoma patient deserves some comment. In the authors' clinic, both visual fields and stereo photographs of the disc are used in order to detect and follow the progression of damage from the earliest possible stage in glaucoma patients. We feel that every chronic open-angle glaucoma patient, actual or suspected, should initially have a base-line study consisting of a complete visual field by Stage IV techniques, along with stereo photographs of the optic nervehead. We do not feel that any disc drawing is likely to be a sufficient means of patient follow-up, although it may complement the photographs. It should also be emphasized that disc photography alone is *never* an adequate means of following a patient.

How often the patient should be restudied and by what techniques depends upon the ophthalmologist's assessment of the degree of risk to the patient. A patient with a documented family history of visual impairment due to glaucoma is about 8 to 15 times as likely to develop visual field changes as a similar patient without such a family history. The level of pressure is important, but with reservation. There is no "magic number" for intraocular pressure, one below which the patient is safe and above which he is certain to suffer insult. Patients who are older or who have large optic cups, an asymmetry in the cup/disc ratio greater than about 0.2 between eyes, or vertically elongated cups are all more likely to develop field defects than persons without such characteristics. Finally, the presence of systemic disease, cardiovascular problems, peptic ulcer, and hematologic disorders (e.g., anemia) should all serve to make the physician more cautious as to how he proceeds.

Recently, the group at the glaucoma center at Washington University has pointed out that the presence of the histocompatibility antigens HLA-B12 and HLA-B7 on the patient's leucocytes make the eventual development of visual field loss more likely.[3,31,32] In contrast, the presence of antigens HLA-A11 and HLA-BW35 seem to protect against field loss.[30] Another observation is that ocular hypertensives who are "epinephrine responders" (i.e., the intraocular pressure is significantly reduced by topical 1% epinephrine) are most likely to eventually develop field loss than a similar group that are not responders.[4]

These findings must be amplified and confirmed, and some workers have privately expressed doubts that the entire story will withstand the scrutiny of a large, carefully analyzed series.

Additional risk factors can and should be sought in specific forms of glaucoma. For example, combined-angle glaucoma carries the additional risks of acute angle-closure attacks in addition to those inherent to chronic open-angle glaucoma. Obviously, the more such "risk" factors one can identify in a patient, the more likely his disease will progress. In a patient with mild ocular hypertension (pressure in the low twenties), no "risk factors" and a negative family history, it is sufficient to repeat the photographs and fields on a yearly basis. At the other extreme, we have repeated the visual field exam within a week on a patient whom we feared was deteriorating rapidly.

As a general principle, we compare the ophthalmoscopic appearance of the disc against the photographs during the intervening visits and take photos only once, or perhaps twice, a year, usually at the time of visual field exam. In the stable, well-controlled patient, yearly fields are frequently adequate so long as the cup/disc ratio is below about 0.5–0.6 and visualization of the entire cup is possible. If there is any evidence of change in the optic disc during an intervening visit, the discs are rephotographed (to permit the comparison of stereo photograph to photograph) and a visual field is repeated. One particularly ominous finding is the presence of small, splinter hemorrhages on the disc.

The concept of relying heavily on the appearance of the optic disc as opposed to the field is not without its limitations. Once the cup/disc ratio (C/D) passes about 0.6, or an undermining of the rim is present, more reliance must be placed on the field exam, since it may be difficult to assess subtle changes in the cup in such cases. This problem grows with the cup/disc ratio, and in our experience, following a patient with a cup/disc ratio over about 0.7–0.8 is quite difficult ophthalmoscopically (Fig. 8-1). It should also be noted that field defects can and do appear at a small C/D or without an obvious change in the appearance of the disc.

The patient who is not in obvious control deserves more frequent fields, since damage to the field may precede the disc changes if the patient suffers relatively short, but large, elevations of pressure. This is particularly true of angle-closure and combined-angle glaucoma. It is common for persons with angle-closure glaucoma to show field changes out of proportion to the appearance of the disc.[11] In all but the most stable of such patients, six months represents about the maximum interval between fields. In practice, we do fields initially at a much closer interval, and gradually we stretch the interval between field exams as the patient goes without damage or shows no evidence of progression of existing damage at a given stable level of pressure (confirmed by occasional diurnal pressure curves).

The classical defects of glaucoma are due to damage of nerve fiber bundles. The arcuate fibers leaving the disc superotemporally and inferotemporally

Visual Field Defects in Specific Diseases

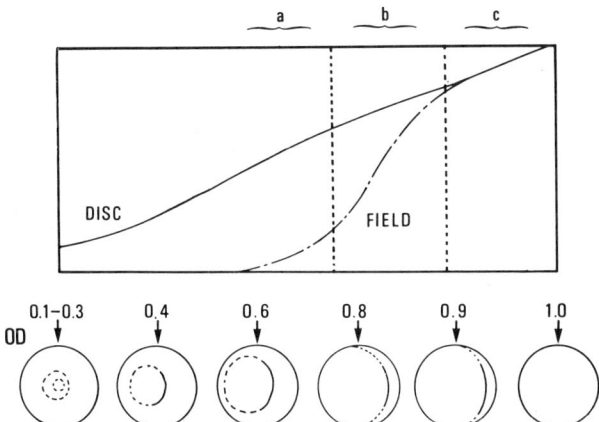

Figure 8-1 Correlation of disc and field changes. The usual relationship of optic disc to visual field changes in glaucoma. Changes in the disc usually precede changes in the visual field. As the cup unfolds temporally, the likelihood of visual field defects increases. The study represented here utilized the Armaly-Drance screening for glaucomatous field defects; presumably a few additional early field changes would have been discovered with a more exhaustive approach. One should always remember, however, that the reverse, though uncommon, is possible. Field defects can progress without significant change in the disc (more common with large C/D ratios) and defects may appear with small (even C/D = 0.1 or less) cup sizes. (With permission, from Read and Spaeth.[28])

seem most susceptible to damage by elevated intraocular pressures, although any of the nerve fibers may be involved. Fibers from the nasal side of the disc are involved around 4% of the time.[2, 21, 11] Multiple visual field defects that result from this one basic cause have been described. Examples include enlargements of the blind spot, baring of the blind spot, arcuate scotomas (with a huge variety of aliases), nasal steps, ring scotomas, or central island of remaining vision, as well as others. The classification of defects of the glaucomatous field lacks uniformity. Some authors choose to split them into many morphologic groups whereas others lump them into fewer categories based on their pathology. We choose to take a middle road and propose the following set of classes:

1. contraction defects and field cuts, including general concentric contraction and nasal contraction of the field (nasal step of Rönne)
2. arcuate scotomas, including ring scotomas (a double arcuate scotoma) and paracentral scotomas
3. nonclassical defects, including sector defects in the temporal field and offsets in one or more isopters along the hemianopsia line

Aulhorn and Harms have done a great deal of work on the frequency of specific visual patterns in glaucoma patients.[2] These results are shown in Figure 8-2. General concentric contraction was the most frequent finding. The second most frequent finding was a central island of residual vision, the end

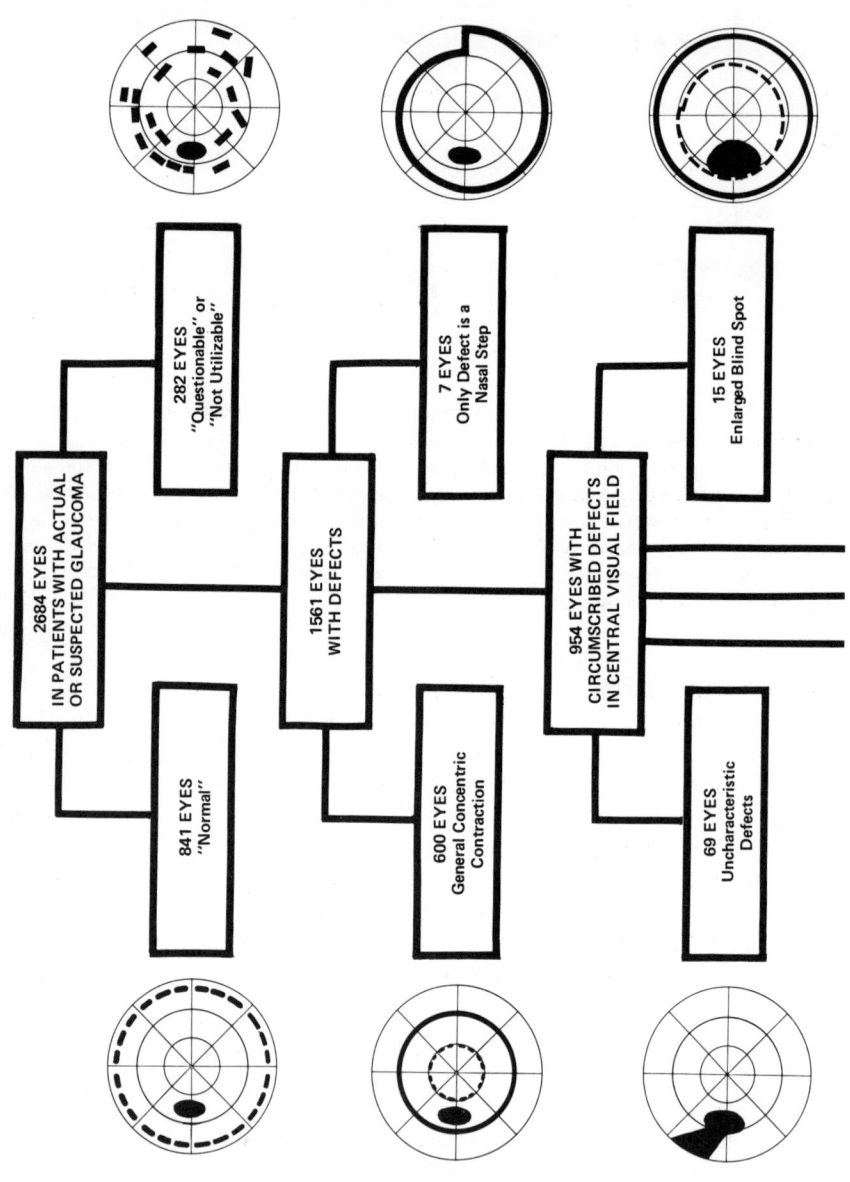

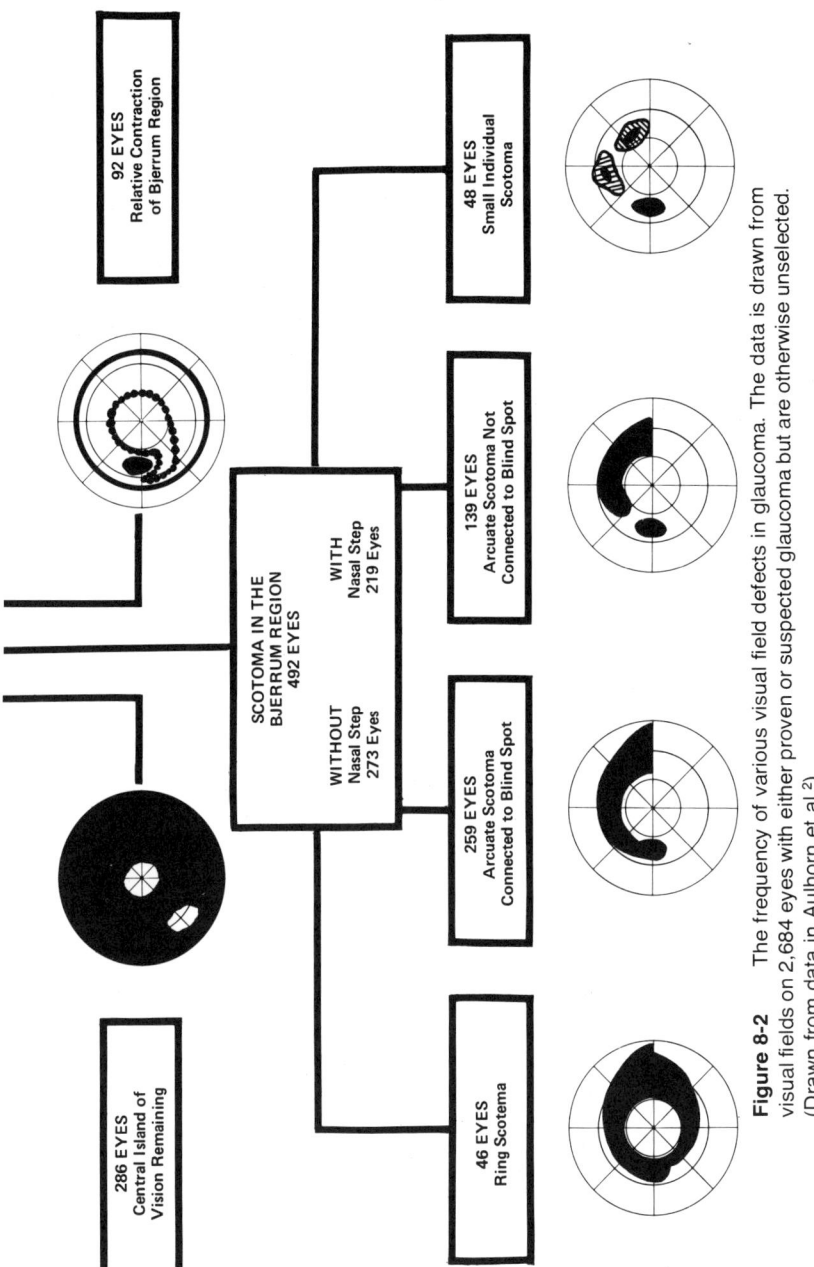

Figure 8-2 The frequency of various visual field defects in glaucoma. The data is drawn from visual fields on 2,684 eyes with either proven or suspected glaucoma but are otherwise unselected. (Drawn from data in Aulhorn et al.[2])

result of the onlaying of many arcuate scotomas. This finding has little diagnostic significance, since by the time it appears, there can be no doubt as to the nature of the disease. A temporal island of vision frequently accompanies a small central island; or the temporal island may itself be the final remainder of vision.

Contraction Defects

Generalized concentric contraction is found very frequently in glaucoma patients (about 38% according to Aulhorn and Harms), but it is not typical of glaucoma alone. Drance (Fig. 8-3) has shown that, with increasing age, normals may show concentric contraction of the visual field which may be caused by pupillary miosis, early cataract formation, circulatory disturbances, and aging itself—all in addition to glaucoma. The fact that concentric contraction may accompany glaucoma is, in the authors' opinion, without doubt (Fig. 8-4), but the demonstrated nonspecificity of concentric contraction does destroy some of

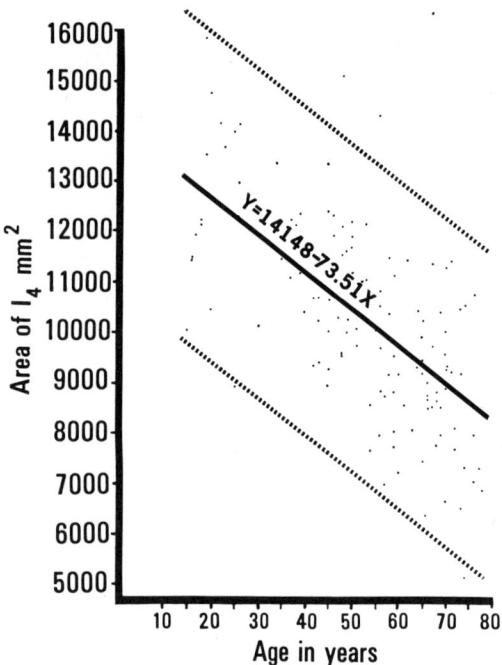

Figure 8-3 The change in size of the visual field with age alone. The ordinate is the area of the I-4-e isopter in square millimeters. The abscissa is the age in years. (Drawn after data of Drance from a discussion section in Aulhorn et al.[2])

its diagnostic usefulness. Armaly[1] feels that concentric contraction may be accepted only as a retrospective diagnostic criterion of glaucoma, and then only under specific circumstances. He will accept concentric contraction only if there is a definite expansion of the visual field after the pressure has been reduced, or if the attempted pressure control was not adequately successful and the visual field develops characteristic nerve fiber bundle defects within a year following the identification of the concentric contraction.

The term "nasal step," first used by Rönne in 1909, signifies a discontinuity in the smooth outer limit of an isopter which occurs at the junction of the upper and lower nasal quadrants of the visual field.[29] A nasal step may thus be thought of either as a form of arcuate scotoma that is completely externalized to become a cut or as simply an asymmetric contraction of an isopter. Aulhorn and Harms[2] feel that a nasal step *alone* is a very unusual finding since it is limited to less than 1% of all patients, although other authors have published data that indicate a correct figure that is somewhat higher,* anywhere from 1.6% to 11%. All the series published to date, however, note that nasal steps occur in association with other defects approximately 25% to 30% of the time. A nasal step may not be present in all isopters. Indeed, it is confined to peripheral isopters only about 2% of the time. Its characteristic form changes somewhat depending upon the part of the visual field in which it is found. When situated close to fixation, a nasal step has more the appearance of an obtuse angle, whereas in the far periphery it resembles an acute angle, reflecting the anatomy of arcuate fibers. The presence of a nasal step is thus an extremely useful collaborative sign, and it should alert the perimetrist to search the central field carefully for associated arcuate or paracentral defects.

Baring of the blind spot is a defect that has been described as an early sign of glaucoma, and indeed it may be. When due to glaucoma, it may be thought of as an asymmetrical contraction of the isopters of the Bjerrum region, usually exposing the superior part of the blind spot. The diagnostic value of this defect must be minimized, however, since *any* normal person can be made to show baring of the blind spot if an appropriate test object is utilized. Baring of the blind spot is due to the fact that the retina superior and inferior to the disc seems to be less sensitive than elsewhere, with the retina just inferior to the disc being the least sensitive of all. The slope in this region is quite flat, and this flatness of the slope can produce a baring of the blind spot[2] (Fig. 8-5). Furthermore, baring of

---

*LeBlanc and Becker[19] found that approximately 26% of their patients had a nasal step, but only 11% had a nasal step without other field defects. Armaly[1] showed about 7% of patients had nasal steps without paracentral defects, although 27% showed nasal steps combined with other defects. Drance[9] states that nasal steps occur as the only field defect of glaucoma in 1.6% of the cases.

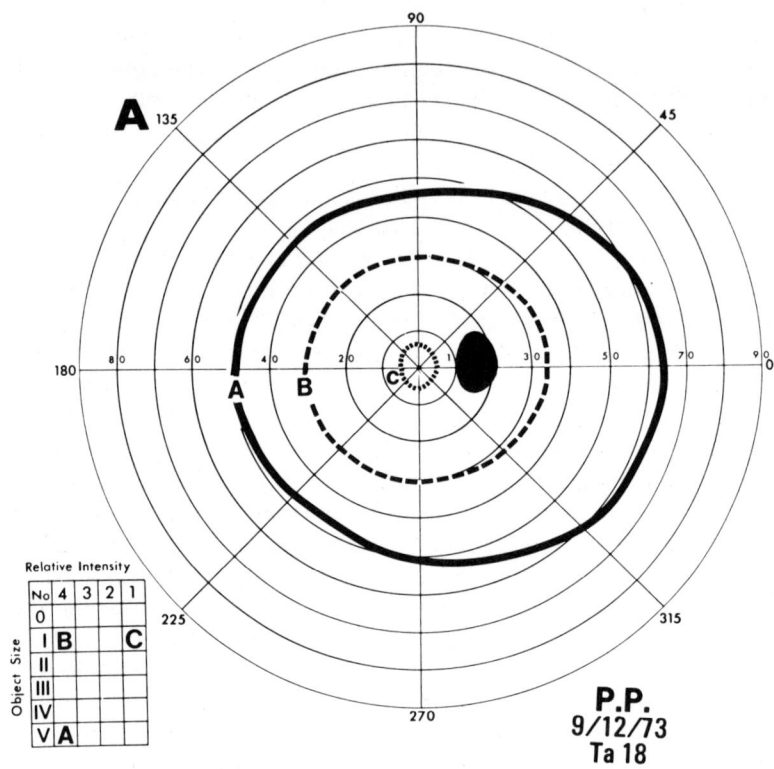

Figure 8-4 Low-tension glaucoma. In A, the visual field of a patient with glaucoma seen in 1973. At that time, his tension was controlled to the high teens and low twenties range with medication. In B, the pressure has been controlled to the low teens by filtering surgery. Nevertheless, field loss has continued. OD shows mainly concentric contraction, but OS (not shown) is reduced to a temporal island. In C, with a pressure of 8 following cyclocryotherapy, the field has reexpanded.

the blind spot can develop with age in perfectly normal individuals. Since isopters normally contract with age,* an isopter that was full earlier can suddenly show baring as it contracts to a critical size;† thus baring of the blind spot is too nonspecific to be of any diagnostic value in glaucoma fields without further investigation, such as static cuts through the area in which baring appears.

---

*As a rule of thumb, the fields of a 60-year-old person are one isopter (i.e., one standard stimulus value) smaller on the Goldmann Perimeter than are the fields of a 30-year-old person.
†This is because the effective stimulus *at the retina* falls to coincide with the retinal stimulus that would have previously produced an isopter with baring.

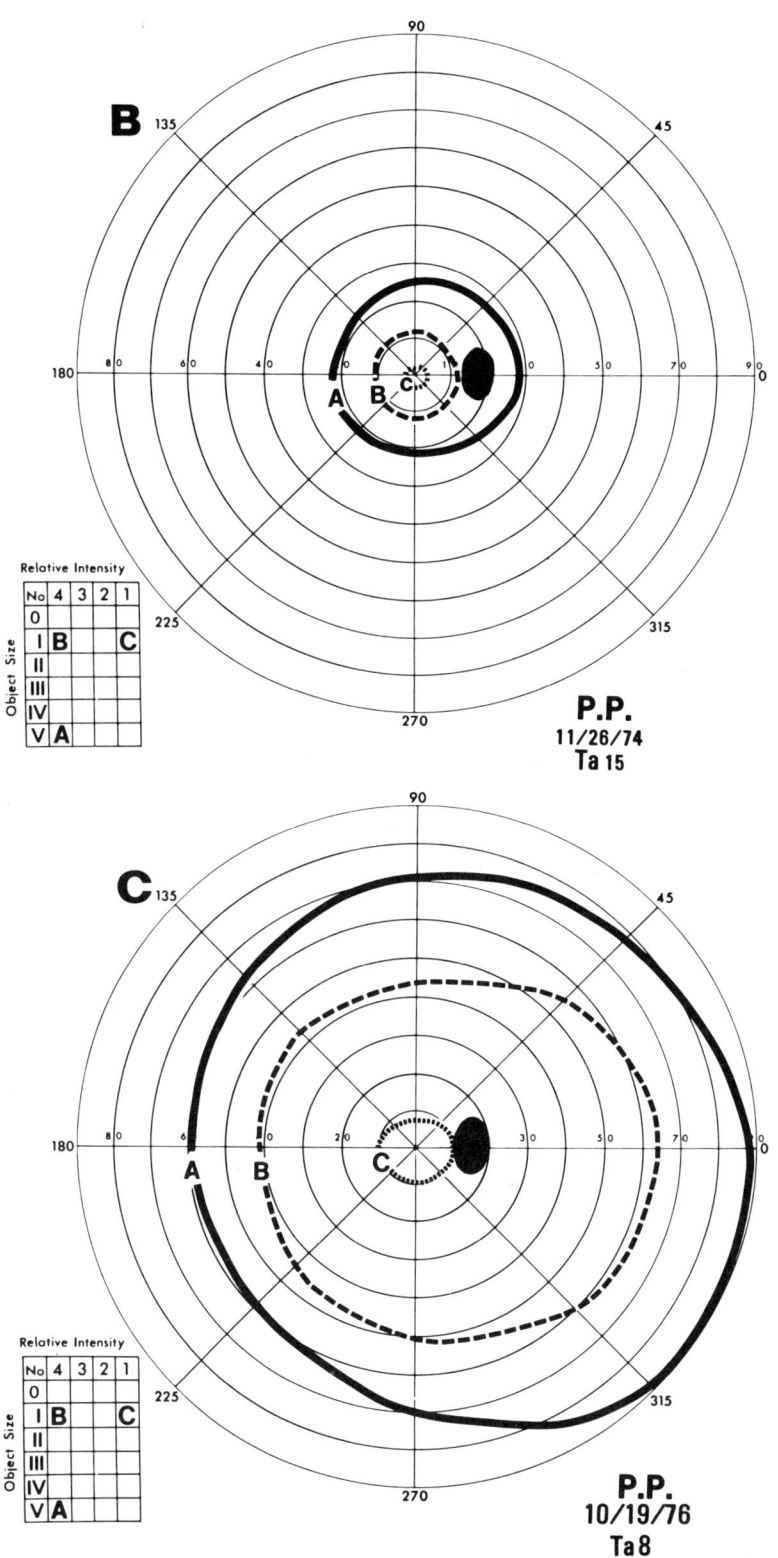

240 *Principles of Quantitative Perimetry*

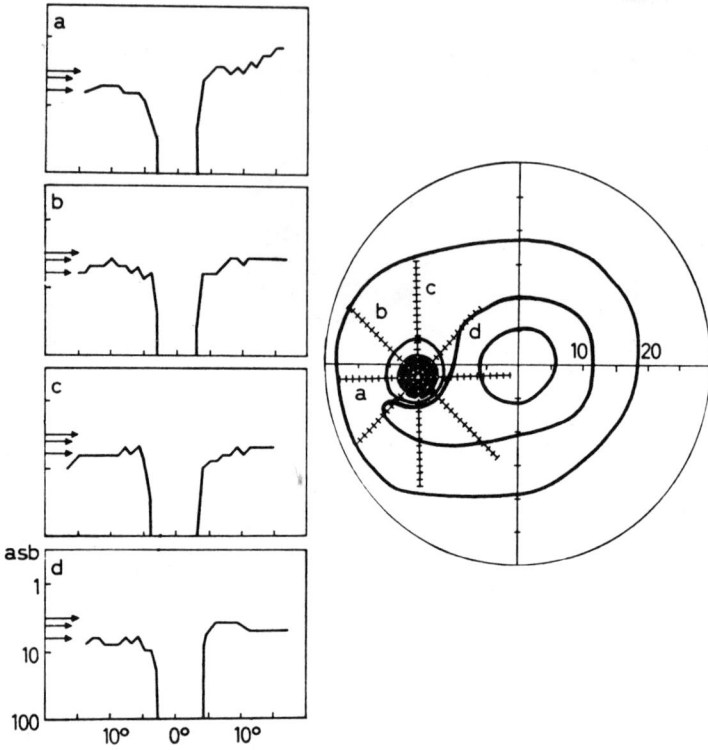

Figure 8-5 The mechanism of baring of the blind spot is exposed. Static perimetry cuts at different meridia through the blind spot reveal a flat slope in all directions from the center of the blind spot, except toward the center of the field. A test point chosen so that it just skims along the surface of this plateau may show either superior baring (as illustrated), inferior baring, or complete externalization of the blind spot depending on very small variations in the sensitivity of the eye, the mood of the patient, and the technique of the examiner. (With permission, from Aulhorn et al.[2])

Arcuate Defects

The arcuate scotoma is *the* classic defect of glaucoma. This scotoma has gone by a variety of names, such as the Bjerrum scotoma, but it is basically due to a defect in the arcuate nerve fibers that enter the superotemporal and inferotemporal areas of the optic disc. It starts as a series of small paracentral scotomas that, according to Drance, are the single most common *early* finding in glaucoma. Paracentral defects in the temporal field are typically in the Bjerrum region, an area 10°–20° from fixation. In the nasal field, their location is more variable. Basically, they may occur at any location where arcuate fibers terminate, which is from a few minutes of arc to 40° or more from fixation. According to Drance, the defects are often absolute when first discovered, but they may be surrounded by areas of less dense involvement. As the defects progress, more paracentral defects may appear and coalesce into a more or less typical arcuate scotoma. Arcuate defects may grow both superiorly and inferiorly, frequently meeting to form a ring scotoma.

One very important point to note is that these scotomas rarely join the blind spot initially. In the Aulhorn and Harms series, which was not selected for early cases, only two-thirds of the arcuate scotomas present joined the blind spot. More recently, Aulhorn has reported the majority of early paracentral scotomas may be found just superior to fixation and just inferior to the horizontal midline nasally (Fig. 8-6). It is important to note that only an enlarged blind spot, which for years was thought to be the beginning of arcuate scotomas, is found in only 1% of the cases with defects (see Fig. 8-2). Thus perimetry of the blind spot alone, without checking the remaining central field carefully, will miss the majority of early glaucomatous defects.

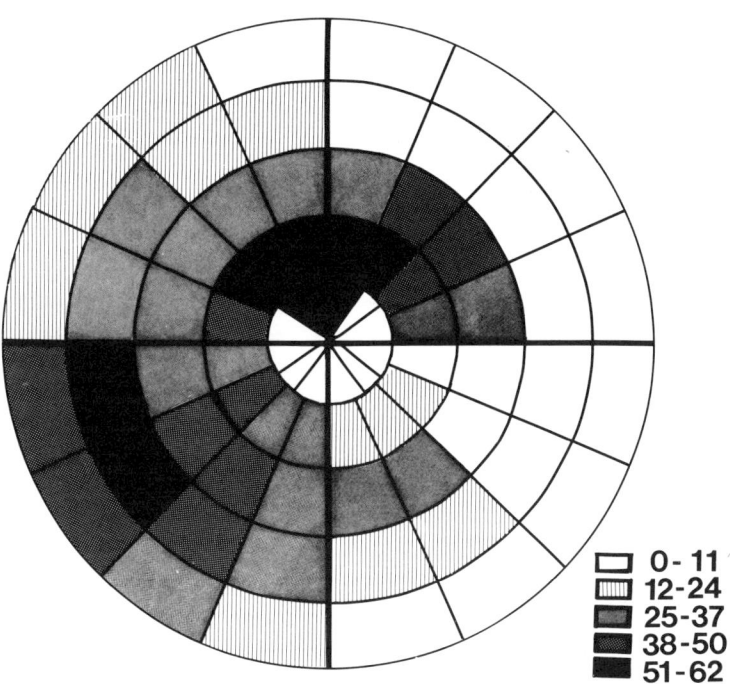

Figure 8-6 The distribution of early visual field defects in 200 patients with glaucoma. Field is drawn as though for right eye. All patients with advanced defects were excluded from the study. Note that the defects predominate just superior and inferotemporal to fixation. (Drawn from data kindly provided by Professor E. Aulhorn.)

Nonclassical Defects

Atypical visual field defects may also be found in glaucoma patients, but such findings in no way detract from the diagnosis. Aulhorn and Harms report about a 4.4% instance of atypical defects[3], and Drance[11] has noted sector-shaped defects in the peripheral field in areas other than the Bjerrum region. These defects may take the form of wedges following the nerve fiber distribution in the temporal field. Thus, the perimetrist's attention should not be limited only to one area of the field.

The final feature that may be present in glaucomatous visual fields is vertical steps or hemianopic offsets. These offsets may also be seen with pathology located more posteriorly along the visual pathway. The presence of any hemianopic offset should alert the perimetrist to the possibility of intracranial pathology. Nevertheless, Lynn[22] has shown that hemianopic offsets may also be due to glaucoma, and he demonstrated that in this case, the vertical step is actually a form of the arcuate defect. Some offset at the hemianopic line may be expected in about 20% to 25% of glaucoma patients. The defective part of the vertical step appears about twice as frequently on the nasal side as on the temporal. When present, these defects are completely incongruous with defects present in the fellow eye.

The vertical offset has probably not been mentioned previously because of a combination of factors. Early thoughts on the pathogenesis of glaucoma, plus a suspicion of the accuracy of perimetry, resulted in such patterns of defect either being discounted or assumed to be coincidental. Moreover, poor technique in performing visual fields must share the blame. Defects in technique, such as collecting data along, rather than to each side of, the hemianopsia line as well as failure to approach the expected isopter at right angles and failure to maintain a constant test velocity can all serve to smooth out such small details in an isopter. The authors therefore feel that the vertical step is a real entity. Drance[11] has also acknowledged the existence of hemianopic defects in glaucomatous fields, but he specifically cautions the interpreter to be concerned about the possibility of neurological defects. The authors completely agree in this caution.

The Progression of Glaucomatous Visual Fields

Glaucomatous visual field defects may progress in one of two ways. They may extend slowly from the edges of existing lesions, with the defect becoming progressively denser and larger. Another way is with the sudden appearance of a new visual field defect of the nerve fiber bundle type. New pathology is most likely to be seen near previous defects, although it may appear independently in a previously uninvolved field. One frequent pattern of progression is where a small paracentral scotoma progresses to form an arcuate scotoma (e.g., superiorly) and then another arcuate scotoma develops inferiorly and results in a classic ring scotoma. This ring scotoma frequently shows nasal offsets because the two arcuate scotomas may not be of equal width. Very often, field continues to be lost, with more and more fibers dropping out above and below the optic disc so that a residual island of vision is the result. Usually, a small central island is left where the visual acuity may be 20/20, as well as a temporal island served by the relatively more resistant fibers leaving via the nasal side of the disc. Offsets may be found frequently along the border of the central island as a result of the asymmetrical development of arcuate scotomas that move ever closer to fixation. The final blow comes when either the central or the temporal island is snuffed out, to be followed sooner or later by the other island, thus leaving the eye in darkness forever.

Frequent Errors in Interpretation of Glaucomatous Fields

There are a number of pitfalls in the study of glaucomatous fields. Refractive scotomas must be suspected and screened for by placing lenses of various powers before the patient, particularly if she or he is myopic. Such patients occasionally have a pale-appearing fundus, usually inferior to the disc.

The second pitfall that one may encounter is the presence of a small pupil. Small pupils are part and parcel of the glaucomatous patient since they result from miotic therapy for glaucoma. Particularly when combined with lens opacities or other clouding of the media, the small pupil may cause profound changes in the visual field which are reversible simply by dilating the pupil (Fig. 8-7). Much of the effect of miotics can be neutralized, however, by the simple expediency of performing field examinations just before and after significant changes of therapy, such as changing drops from pilocarpine to echothiophate, which can regularly be expected to produce pupils with diameters of less than 1.5 mm. Should a question of glaucomatous progression exist, even with back-to-back visual fields as previously advocated above, a visual field should be repeated after dilating the pupil.

Finally, visual system pathology other than glaucoma may be present, including several types that may be masked by very small, hard-to-dilate pupils. Patients with glaucoma are more likely to acquire intraocular vascular occlusions; strong miotics have been implicated in retinal detachment; and glaucoma does not protect patients from developing tumors about the chiasm or elsewhere in the visual pathway. Thus, when glaucomatous fields seem to progress in an atypical fashion, every effort should be made to examine the patient by whatever means are necessary to secure a complete and detailed diagnosis.

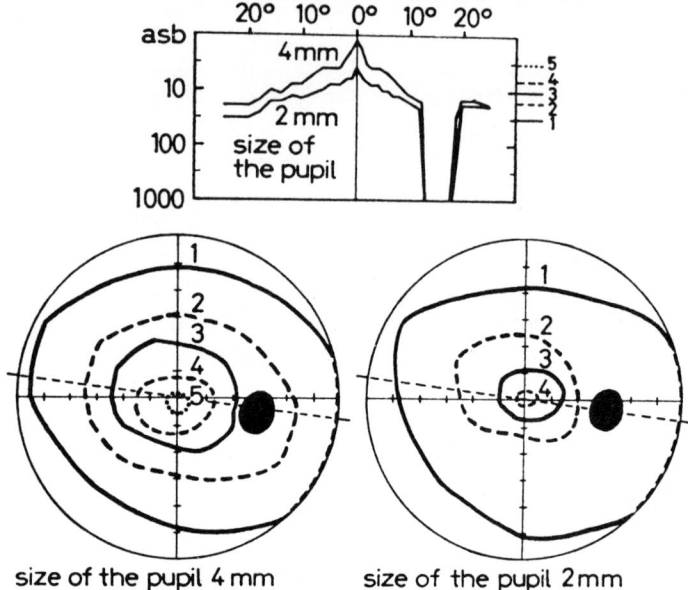

Figure 8-7 The influence of pupil size on field size in a normal eye. The more central isopters (number 2 and above) are more affected than the more peripheral isopter (number 1). Eyes with disease are usually even more profoundly affected than sound eyes. (With permission, from Aulhorn et al.[2])

ISCHEMIC LESIONS OF THE OPTIC NERVE

Vascular supply to the optic nervehead is, on the one hand, a function of the blood pressure in the ophthalmic artery and, on the other, a function of the pressure within the eye. The effective perfusion pressure is ophthalmic artery pressure minus the intraocular pressure. Thus, either a rise in intraocular pressure or a fall in ophthalmic artery pressure can so reduce the perfusion pressure at the optic nervehead that visual field damage may result. Glaucoma represents one side of the coin, and ischemic disease of the optic nerve the other. The ischemic processes represent a wide spectrum of disease, ranging from so called "low-tension glaucoma" to acute occlusion of the ophthalmic artery and ischemia of the retrobulbar portion of the optic nerve. The visual field changes that these lesions may produce vary from those that are identical with glaucoma to total blindness. Depending upon the etiology of the ischemia, the lesion may be stable or it may be relentlessly progressive, in spite of all therapeutic effort.

Low-tension glaucoma is a representative and controversial member of the spectrum of ischemic disease of the optic nerve. Before diagnosing "low-tension glaucoma," the ophthalmologist should be aware that around 10% of the population with glaucoma show elevated pressures only at night. Therefore, diurnal pressure curves should be obtained on all suspected low-tension glaucoma patients. Also, some patients may be falsely diagnosed as "low-tension" because of an abnormal scleral rigidity that can effect Schiotz tonometry readings, a source of confusion in pre-applanation tonometer days. Nevertheless, once all of the "pseudo-low-tension glaucoma" is sliced away, there still remains a core of patients who never elevate their pressures above 22–23 mmHg and yet suffer field loss typical of glaucoma. In one sizable group of these patients, the loss may be static and permanent. According to Drance,[10] most of these patients have suffered some episode of vascular hypotension in the past. These episodes are usually due to hemorrhage, myocardial infarction, cardiac arrythmia, and the like. Assuming that these episodes do not recur, the defect should be nonprogressive.

More severe visual failure may occur if the hemorrhage is severe, particularly if the patient is elderly with a marginal circulation. These patients may suffer visual failure up to several weeks posthemorrhage, the situation being perhaps aggravated by an ensuing anemia. The visual loss is usually bilateral but may be unilateral. One may see a mild disc edema and a few cotton-wool exudates or hemorrhages. The pupil may be sluggish or fixed. Later, optic atrophy begins to develop, and about half such patients progress to blindness. A lucky few achieve a complete or partial return of vision. The visual field loss seen in people whose hemorrhagic episodes are not so severe usually resembles that seen in glaucoma. This fact prompts some to consider posthemorrhagic optic atrophy to be a variant of low-tension glaucoma. The field loss with the others is variable, and usually there is peripheral field loss with large sector defects or arcuate scotomas resulting from the abrupt infarction of nerve fiber bundles. One frequently sees an altitudinal hemianopic type of defect, more often in the inferior field. Therapy in these patients is obviously directed towards the cardiovascular embarrassment and prevention of its recurrence.

The other group of "low-tension glaucoma" patients once again show no markedly elevated pressures but suffer, nevertheless, a steady progression of field loss. Many of these patients have low blood pressure, and ophthalmodynamometry reveals a decrease in the ophthalmic artery pressure. Many of them tend to have a family history of chronic open-angle glaucoma, and some patients even show low-tension glaucoma in one eye and chronic open-angle glaucoma in the other, thereby generating speculation that this form of low-tension glaucoma is a variant of open-angle glaucoma. These patients deserve a thorough workup for problems stemming from their impaired cardiovascular status (e.g., periodic arrythmias or carotid occlusive disease). Central nervous system syphilis may mimic this disorder. Every attempt should be made to lower the intraocular pressure, preferably into the low teens, or even lower. If this is done, frequently such patients will cease losing field (Fig. 8-4). The field defects that are seen are identical in all respects to those seen in other forms of glaucoma.

An acute occlusion of the small blood vessels represents yet another variety of ischemic disease. This entity within the nerve or disc may resemble a papillitis, with edematous segments of the disc being present, complete with hemorrhages. For this reason, this condition is frequently called ischemic optic neuritis. There is usually a sudden onset of a field defect corresponding to those fibers that are affected. Altitudinal hemianopsias are frequently seen. This is usually true of older persons afflicted with maladies such as arteriosclerosis or diabetes. Ophthalmoscopic examination of the peripapillary retina with red free light may later show fiber bundle dropout.

Granulomatous arteritis, such as cranial arteritis or temporal arteritis, is another cause of very severe ischemic visual loss. Usually the patients are in their seventh decade or beyond. The onset of symptoms is often accompanied by headaches and tenderness of the scalp. The patients may also complain of malaise, anorexia, and difficulty in sleeping. The erythrocyte sedimentation rate (ESR) is usually quite high in these patients, although patients with biopsy-proven arteritis and normal ESR have been reported. Prompt treatment with steroids is necessary if vision is to be preserved, for once blindness ensues, it is permanent. These patients may have nerve fiber bundle defects, central scotomas, or altitudinal hemianopsias.

OCCLUSIONS OF THE RETINAL CIRCULATION

Any of the major vessels of the retinal circulation, be they artery or vein, central or branch, may be occluded. On occasion, both artery and vein may be occluded simultaneously. The resultant visual field loss and symptoms of the patient depend upon the exact pattern of the occlusion. The occlusion is always painless. When the artery is involved, the loss of vision is sudden. Occlusions of the venous circulation produce loss of vision that is somewhat more gradual and usually less severe. Central scotomas frequently accompany venous occlusions unless an arterial occlusion occurs concomitantly, thereby limiting the amount of retinal edema present while infarcting a still larger segment of extramacular retina.

Whenever any sort of vascular occlusion is suspected, the examining physician should search for the possible presence of any number of predisposing factors. Perhaps the most common predisposing condition is atherosclerotic lesions that narrow both the arterial and venous lumens with ensuing thrombosis of the vessel. Other pathology may be contributory, and in central retinal vein occlusion, glaucoma is present in over 20% of cases. Hypertension is common. Oral contraceptives may also predispose to thrombosis. With arterial occlusions, conditions that might predispose to emboli, such as mitral valvular disease, cranial arteritis, or carotid insufficiency, must be investigated.

With arterial occlusions, the resultant field defects are characteristically absolute, have an extremely steep slope, and are permanent (Fig. 8-8). Death comes to the retinal ganglion cells once they have been deprived of oxygen for only a few minutes, and thus no recovery occurs, nor is it expected. If the central retinal artery is involved, the entire eye becomes blind with the occasional exception of a small rim of retina about the optic disc that is connected collaterally to choroidal circulation. In some cases, a cilioretinal artery will continue to supply the papillomacular bundle, and a small remaining central island over its area of supply will remain. Alternatively, a cilioretinal artery may be occluded with exactly the opposite result; a large centrocecal scotoma develops while the remainder of the visual field remains intact.

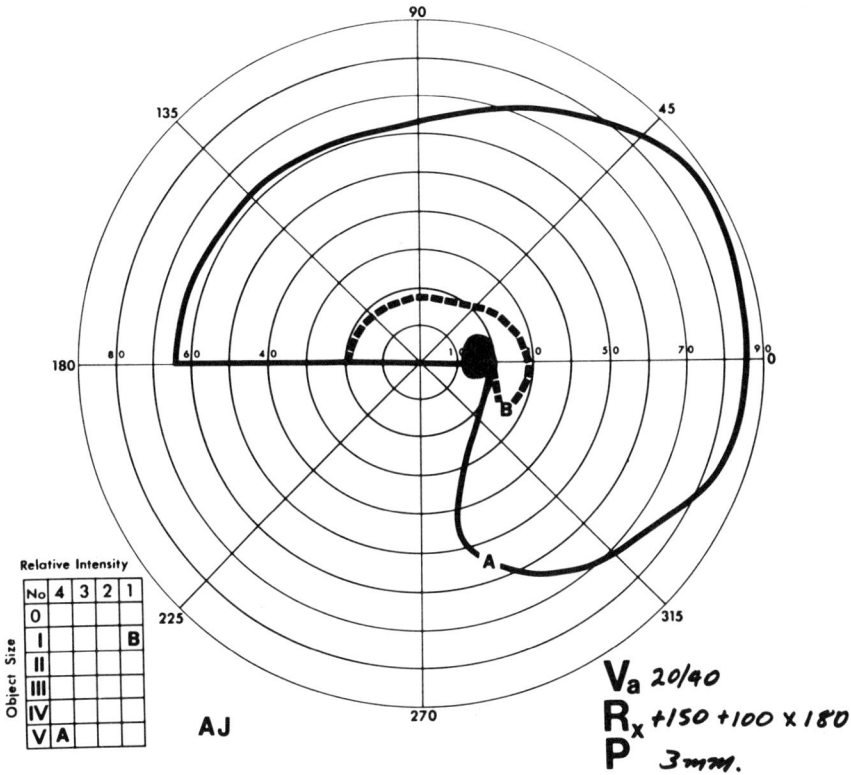

Figure 8-8 Branch artery occlusion of the superotemporal artery. In the absence of a cilioretinal vessel, branch artery occlusions cause an absolute defect with steeply sloping margins. The macula is split by the resulting altitudinal defect.

In acute cases, one seldom needs a visual field to help make the diagnosis since the picture of sludging in the vessels and pale edematous retina in the involved section is characteristic. Later in the course of the disease, however, the characteristic shape and slope of visual field patterns may be of some help in diagnosing old occlusions of branch arteries.

Any of the central retinal artery branches may be occluded, but the superior temporal is most commonly affected. Branch artery occlusion usually occurs at arterio-venous crossings. When the cilioretinal artery is absent, branch artery occlusions that occur sufficiently close to the disc cause a sector field defect that bisects the macula. These can be differentiated from fiber bundle defects on the basis of extent and anatomy.

Retinal vein occlusions are generally less severe than the arterial occlusions. The loss of vision is usually more gradual, requiring several hours or more to develop, or the patient may notice that his vision is poor upon awakening in the morning. There is very little doubt of what has occurred in acute cases because the appearance of disc edema, dilated torturous veins, and hemorrhages scattered in profusion across the involved retina (the blood-and-thunder fundus) is almost unmistakable. With central vein occlusions, one usually sees some peripheral contraction of the visual field as well as a central scotoma (Fig. 8-9). It has been suggested that the central scotoma is secondary to macular edema, which in turn is due to the elevated retinal venous pressure. Any of the branch veins may be occluded. As in the case of arterial occlusions, the superior temporal vessel is most commonly affected (Fig. 8-10). Once the acute episode with edema and hemorrhages has subsided, there may be a great deal of resolution of the defect. If recanalization of the vein occurs promptly, vision may improve dramatically, but in other cases, particularly those involving the central or superior temporal veins, a central scotoma may remain because of damage to the macula. Neovascularization in the area of the occlusion may be present, and this may contribute to a variety of problems including macular edema, macular pucker, and vitreous hemorrhage. Success may sometimes be had by photocoagulating these vessels and clearing unremitting vitreous blood by vitrectomy.

TOXIC AMBLYOPIAS

The number of agents that have been reported to cause a decrease in vision due to a toxic effect on the retina or optic nerve is legion.[12-14] The mode of action of most agents is poorly understood, since very few of these eyes are ever obtained either through autopsy or enucleation. Some toxins, such as chloroquine, may be fairly specific for a certain portion of the retina, whereas other toxic agents, such as arsenic, lead, or ethanol, may be more generalized

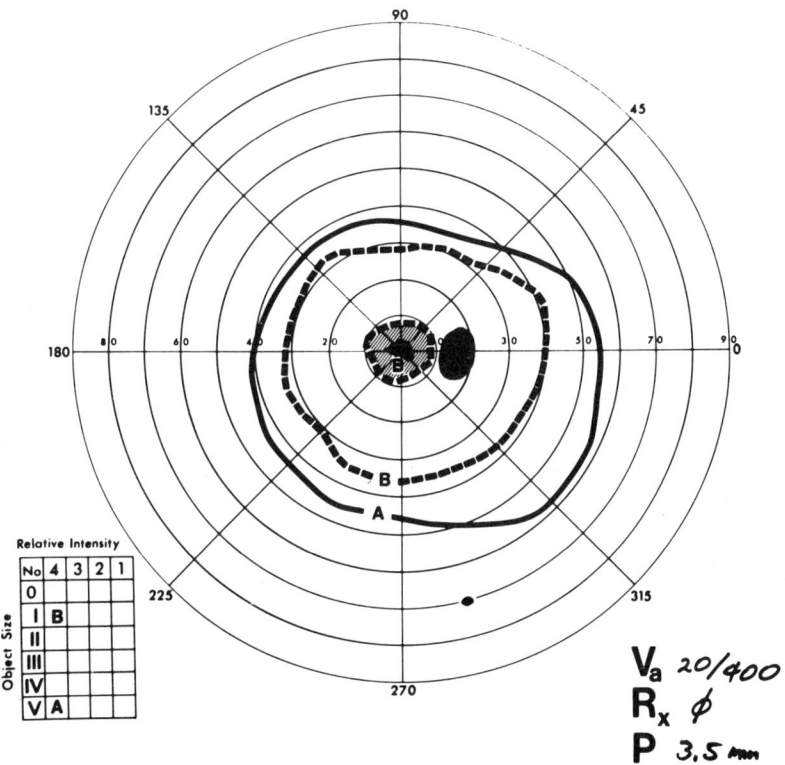

Figure 8-9 Central retinal vein occlusion. Note the constriction of the field and the central scotoma.

and cause peripheral neuritis as well. Proposed mechanisms of action for various toxins include nutritional disturbances, inflammation of the optic nerve, and poisoning of the enzyme systems of the retinal cells.

The toxic amblyopias are classically divided into three groups on the basis of the type of visual field defect seen. Thus, group one includes those toxins that cause central scotomas; group two, those that cause peripheral field contraction; and group three, those that cause both central and peripheral field defects. Toxic agents almost always produce bilateral field loss, although the involvement in one eye may be greater than in the other. One must always remember that exceptions abound and toxins that have been reported to cause mainly central scotomas or peripheral contraction frequently cause both types of defect as the intoxication proceeds. Nevertheless, most toxins do not cause complete loss of sight except in unusual circumstances.

Visual field loss caused by many toxic agents will diminish if the causal agent

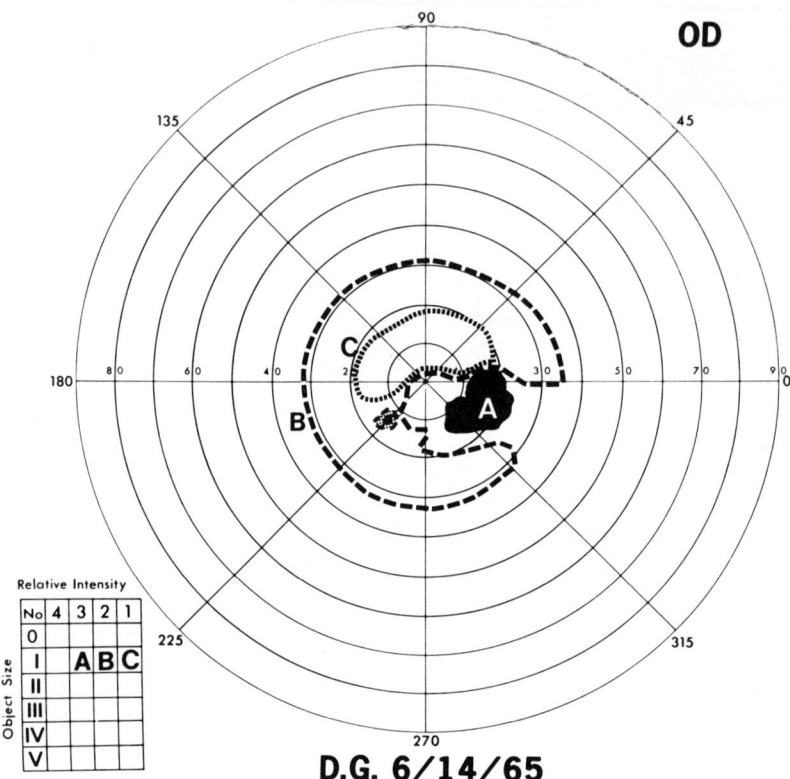

Figure 8-10   Visual field of a patient with a branch vein occlusion in the right eye. As is most common, the superior temporal vein was occluded. This defect gradually resolved.

is promptly eliminated. Thus, the patient with tobacco amblyopia, which is thought to be basically nutritional, recovers on an improved diet, whereas the patient with amblyopia that results from digitalis or sulfonamides generally shows a recovery when the exposure to the offending agent is terminated. Methyl alcohol, however, tends to cause a permanent defect. Most of the agents that have been implicated in the production of toxic amblyopias are listed in Appendix C. Certain classic amblyopias that have been considered toxic, such as tobacco-alcohol amblyopia and ethanol amblyopia, will be discussed in more detail in the section on nutritional amblyopias. Toxic agents, such as chloroquine and its cogeners, will be discussed here.

Chloroquine has been used widely in the prophylaxis and treatment of malaria as well as collagen diseases. Its use was particularly widespread during the conflict in Viet Nam. The typical lesion of chloroquine is a paramaculopathy that causes a donut-shaped scotoma (Figs. 8-11 through 8-13). This may be

Visual Field Defects in Specific Diseases 251

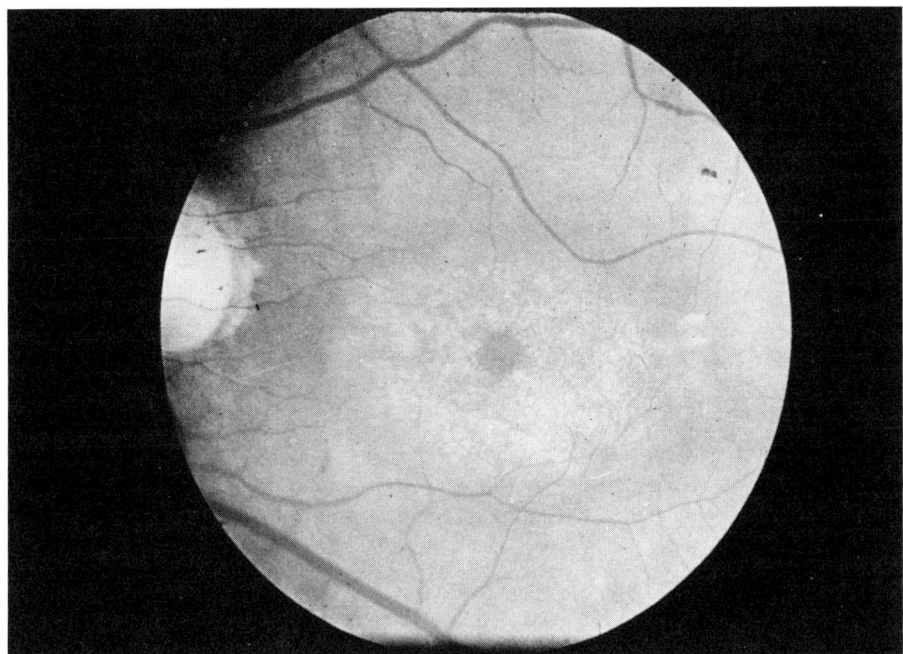

Figure 8-11 Fundus photograph of the left eye of a woman in her late fifties with moderately advanced chloroquine retinopathy. Note the paramacular pigment disturbance.

quite severe and involve the peripheral fields, although typically it causes an early ring scotoma with fixation preserved. Ophthalmoscopy of these patients reveals fine pigment dots around the macula which have a "bulls-eye" or "donut" appearance (Fig. 8-11). These tend to occur fairly late so that a visual field defect may be well established by the time there is visually observable evidence in the fundus that chloroquine toxicity is present. Once the changes have developed, they tend to progress for several years, even though the drug is stopped. It is said that if the drug can be stopped before any ophthalmoscopic evidence of toxicity occurs, the condition is reversible. Detection at this early stage requires extremely careful perimetry and a suspicious ophthalmologist. Static perimetry is helpful, if not essential, in making this diagnosis early.

The initial field defect is a small circular scotoma surrounding the fixation point, a scotoma that initially leaves the central and peripheral field intact. Eventually, the central island disappears, leaving a large central or centrocecal scotoma, with reduction of vision below 20/200. By this time, the chloroquine toxicity is irreversible. Peripheral contraction may also be seen although some vision usually remains.

A second group of drugs, the phenothiazine derivatives, is important because

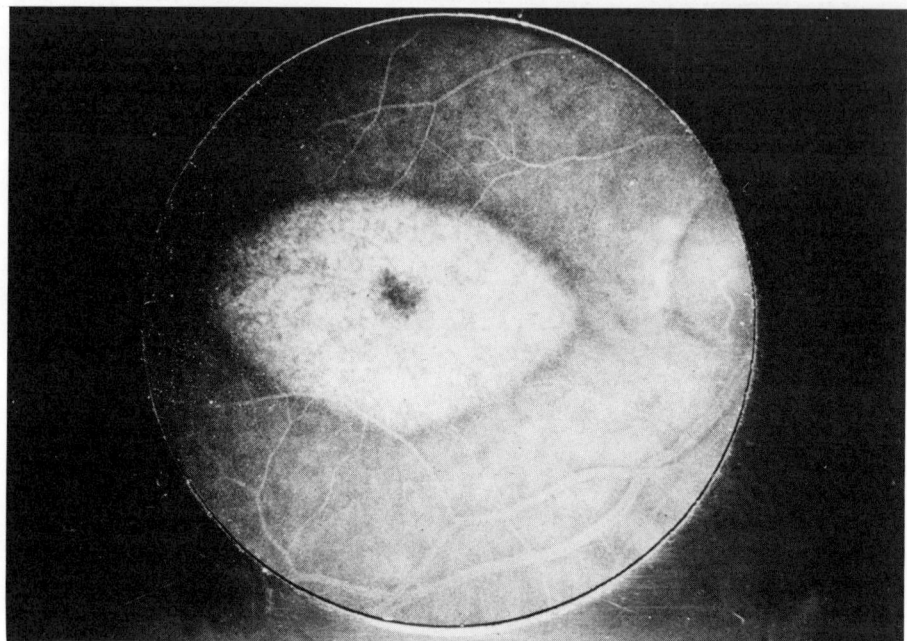

Figure 8-12   Fluorescein angiogram of the right eye of the patient in Figure 8-11.

of widespread use as major tranquilizers. Of this group, the piperidines, an example of which is thioridazine, are most likely to cause retinopathy. Dimethylazines, an example of which is chlorpromazine, come next, while piperazines, such as procloperazine, are generally not considered to be retinotoxic. Patients under therapy with phenothiazines may develop pigmentation of the skin, cornea, and conjunctiva upon exposure to the sun. One may also see pigmentation of the lens, which can progress to cataract formation. Pigment may also be scattered throughout the fundus. A severe depression of visual acuity may occur as a result of these agents.

The visual fields of persons under prolonged therapy with phenothiazine derivatives are said to show both central scotoma and peripheral constrictions. Obviously, those patients undergoing massive treatment with these drugs are scarcely good candidates for visual field studies. Slow, usually incomplete recovery may occur upon stopping the drug.

High and prolonged dosages of ethambutol and related drugs used in the treatment of tuberculosis may cause a toxic amblyopia. Strangely, ethambutol toxicity is far more prevalent in males than in females and tends to occur when a dose of 35 mg/kg or greater is administered for six months or longer. Some feel that systemic infirmities, such as diabetes mellitus or alcoholism, predispose to

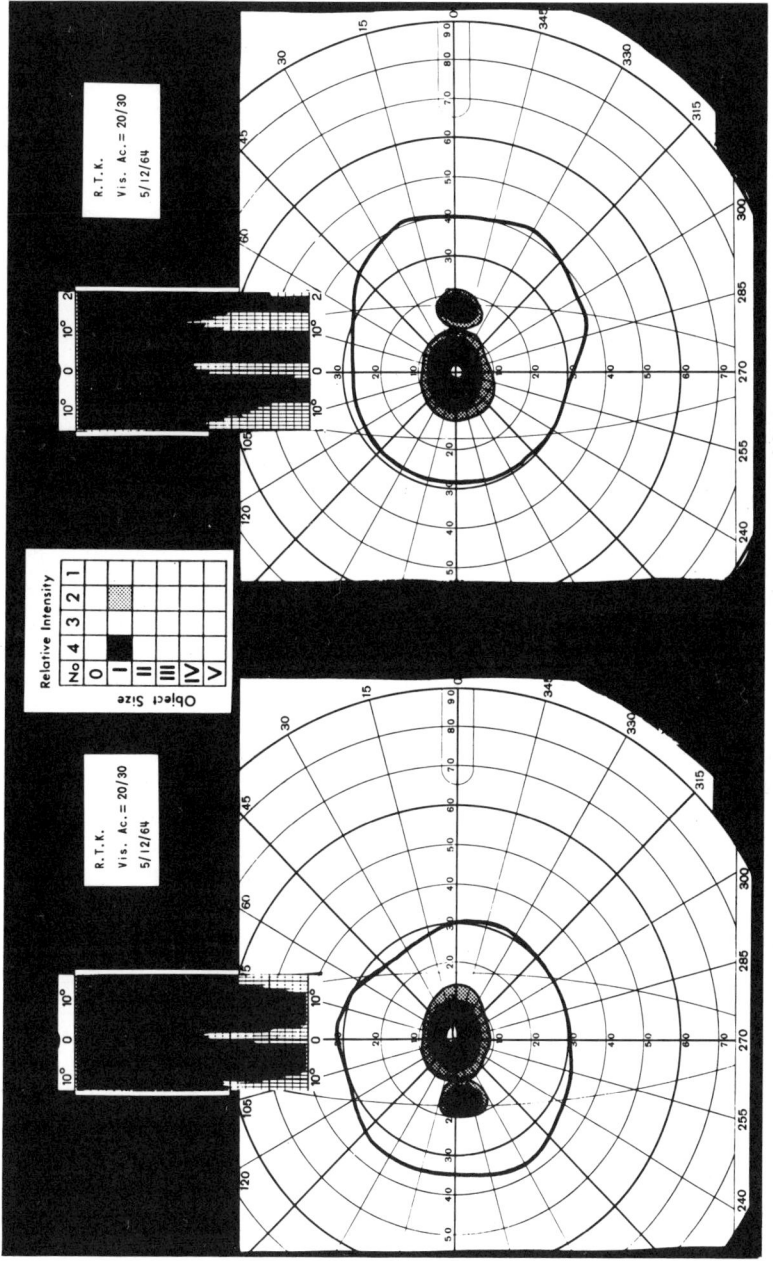

Figure 8-13 Visual fields of the patient with chloroquine retinopathy in Figures 8-11 and 8-12. Note the "bulls-eye" or "donut" character of the scotoma.

the development of symptoms. There are essentially no ophthalmoscopic findings, and all parts of the field may be affected. An early sign of this toxicity is color blindness, particularly to green, which provides the ophthalmologist with a convenient way of screening for toxicity during therapy. Obviously, checks of visual acuity and an occasional visual field should also be done while this drug is being administered. Another potentially retinotoxic antituberculous drug, isoniazid, is thought to work its retinopathic mischief by antagonism of the vitamin B-complex, especially vitamin B_6.

Other toxic drugs that are worth mentioning because of their widespread use include digitalis, sulfonamides, several antibiotics, salicylates, and ergot. Digitalis may cause colored vision, scintillating scotomata, and later a central scotoma that usually recedes when the dosage is reduced. Sulfonamides have also been implicated in causing central scotomas which rapidly improve with withdrawal of the drug.

Chloramphenicol, no longer so widely used as it once was, may cause both central and peripheral changes in the field. Disc edema, a few hemorrhages, and exudates in the retina have been observed. Little improvement occurs upon withdrawal of the drug, although some patients have been reportedly helped by treatment with B-complex vitamins.

Clindamycin, which has been used experimentally in the treatment of ocular toxoplasmosis, has been noted to cause an optic neuritis upon retrobulbar injection, which may progress to a permanent optic atrophy if the dose is high enough. This was not noted with systemic administration, nor with other forms of periocular injection.[33]

Ergot, which is commonly prescribed in the treatment of migraine headaches, may cause a peripheral contraction as well as central scotoma in those patients who become acutely intoxicated. Recovery is usually incomplete. Ergot poisoning can be aggravated by a state of poor nutrition or diabetes.

Salicyates, quinine, and streptomycin are dissimilar drugs that cause similar toxic effects. All are accompanied by deafness, tinnitus, and bilateral peripheral contraction of the visual field. With quinine in particular, retinal artery spasm and disc edema suggest the use of stellate ganglion blocks in the treatment of severe cinchonism. However, if one stops the administration of either quinine or salicylates, the prognosis for recovery is not too bad. In the case of quinine, there may be incomplete recovery, whereas in that of salicylates the recovery is always complete. Numerous other drugs have been implicated in visual field loss, and these are listed in Appendix C.

Vitamin B_{12} in the form of hydroxycobalamine normally is involved in the detoxification of cyanide to thiocynate. Other B-complex vitamins, such as thiamine, may be involved in the process also. A chronic cyanide intoxication may occur if these vitamins are present in decreased amounts, if cyanide is present in increased amounts (such as with smoking), or if another relative defect exists in the detoxification pathway. Additionally, absence of the B-complex vitamins will interfere with other metabolic pathways and thus aggravate visual problems.

Some variation on the above theme is thought to occur in at least four amblyopias.[8,35] These are tobacco-alcohol amblyopia (a dietary deficiency plus cyanide excess);[15] nutritional amblyopia (a profound dietary deficiency of all the B-vitamins plus others); pernicious anemia (an inability to absorb vitamin B_{12} from diet); and Leber's hereditary optic atrophy[36] (an ill-defined and hereditary enzyme deficiency). All of these may be improved by treatment with parenteral hydroxycobalamine or cyanocobalamine coupled with improvement of diet, provided therapy is begun early enough. The cyanide detoxification pathway is implicated in tobacco amblyopia, pernicious anemia, and Leber's disease by the finding of abnormally low serum thiocyanate levels, and again in pernicious anemia by the proven defects in vitamin B_{12} absorption. Nutritional amblyopia is associated with more profound metabolic insults due to the severe lack of all vitamins and may be irreversible later in the course. How important the lack of vitamin B_{12} is in the production of nutritional amblyopia is somewhat speculative.

Tobacco amblyopia, also known as tobacco-alcohol amblyopia, is usually considered to be the most characteristic toxic amblyopia causing bilateral central scotomas. Much has been written concerning the etiology of this disease. Smoking a pipe or cigars is reputed to be more effective in causing the problem than other forms of tobacco use; cigarette smoking, for example, is rarely implicated. Most of the patients tend to be past middle age, on the average about 55 years old. Allegedly, persons from some nationalities, social classes, and occupational groups are more susceptible than others. But those who are most afflicted are heavy drinkers and smokers, many of whom are somewhat arteriosclerotic, have poor dietary habits, or have, in addition, aggravating problems such as diabetes mellitus or pernicious anemia.

The classical treatment for this disease has been vitamin B-complex, but studies done in the late 1950s point specifically to vitamin B_{12} deficiency as a key cause.[15] The disease seems to respond very well to an adequate diet and therapy with hydroxycobalamine,[6] even when patients are allowed to continue smoking and drinking. It is thus difficult to classify this amblyopia as toxic since the better evidence indicates that it is nutritionally controllable.

The visual field defect is typically centrocecal in position (Fig. 8-14), and by the time the field loss is seen clinically, it is usually bilateral. Traquair points out that characteristically within the scotoma there are one or two areas of greater density that may become connected as the scotoma increases in size. In advanced cases, the scotoma may be absolute in parts, although complete blind-

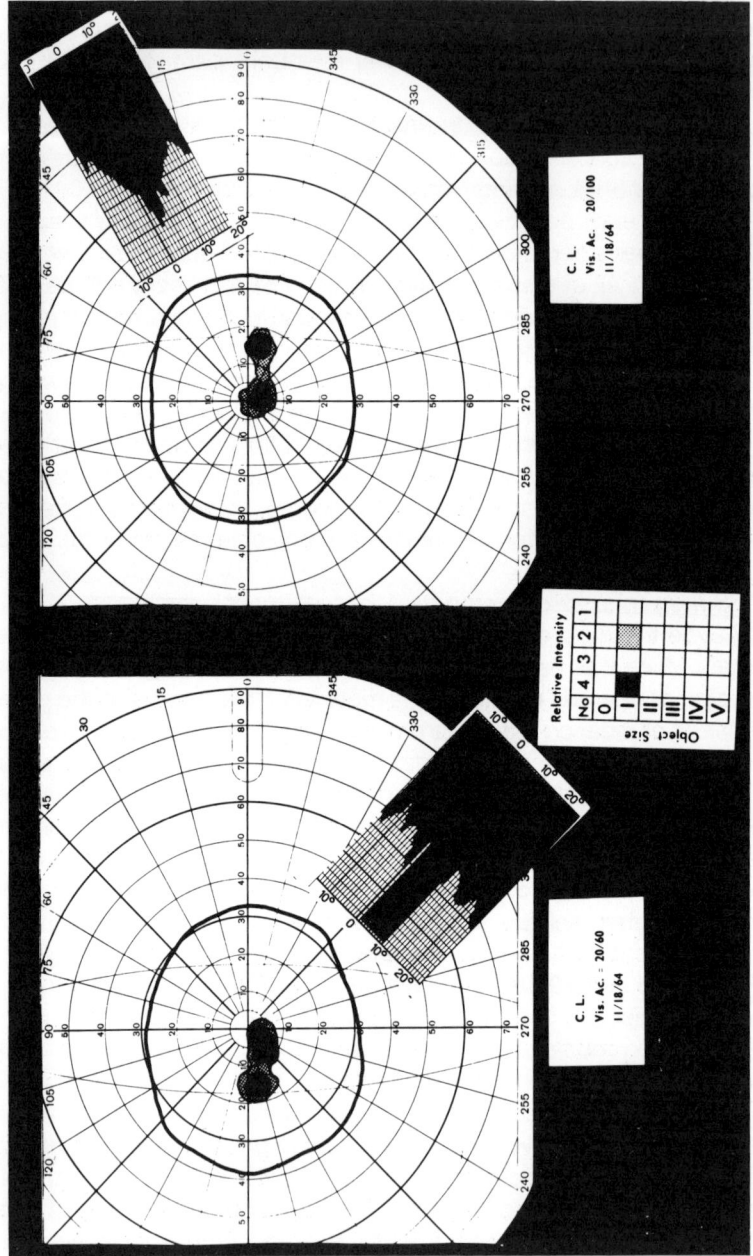

Figure 8-14 Tobacco-alcohol amblyopia. The patient was a white male in his early fifties who had a fondness for cigars and cocktails. Treatment with multivitamins and a correction of his dietary indiscretions caused the scotoma to resolve completely.

ness never seems to occur. If the patient's nutritional deficits are corrected, the damage is completely reversible, with the visual field defects disappearing in the reverse order of their appearance.

Pernicious anemia is very similar in etiology. It is a megaloblastic anemia characterized by gastric achlorhydria, glossitis, and multiple neurological involvements, including subacute combined degeneration of the spinal cord. It is essentially due to a failure to absorb vitamin B_{12} from the gastrointestinal tract and may be prevented or reversed by administration of this vitamin. The disease may occur at any age, but it is more common after 30.

The ocular signs of pernicious anemia usually consist of retinal hemorrhages, including occasionally both retinal and disc edemas. Optic nerve involvement may be severe and proceed to optic atrophy. Field defects are characteristically central or centrocecal scotomas, not unlike those seen in tobacco amblyopia. They respond well if treated early with vitamin B_{12} or hydroxycobalamine, although return of vision is by no means invariable.

Nutritional deficiencies, or the antagonism of drugs to the other B vitamins, may contribute to the neuropathy of vitamin B_{12} deficiency. The absence of many of the B-complex vitamins by themselves are capable of causing central scotomas to appear in the visual field. Thus, deficiencies of vitamin B_1 (thiamin), nicotinic acid (niacin), and vitamin B_6 (pyridoxine) have all been implicated in the production of optic nerve disease with central scotomas.[35] Pyridoxine deficiency (because of antagonism) may explain some of the clinical signs seen in isoniazide toxicity as well as those seen in overuse of hydralazine and penicillamine. Other than pharmacological antagonism, it is exceedingly rare to see a vitamin B_6 deficiency in adults, but the same cannot be said of the other B vitamins. Diseases such as beriberi are well known. Prisoners on a defective diet in the Japanese prison camps of World War II developed many visual symptoms. These unfortunates developed photophobia, retrobulbar pain, and diminution of vision early and gradually developed contraction of the peripheral fields and central or centrocecal scotomas. Optic atrophy developed later. If treatment was instituted early enough with thiamin and diet, the symptoms tended to be reversible; otherwise, the scotomas remained permanently.

The final condition to be considered with the pathologies related to vitamin B deficiency is Leber's disease. Leber's hereditary optic atrophy is characterized by bilateral optic atrophy with a predilection for young adult males—although this is not invariable since cases have been noted in females. Others in the family are usually afflicted. There are other hereditary optic atrophies that may be confused with true Leber's disease.

In typical Leber's disease, the patient is invariably normal at birth. The disease is bilateral, although it may not be equally present in the two eyes, particularly at the outset. Initially there is a blurring or "mistiness" of vision. At this stage, the picture may be one of a low-grade optic neuritis with edema, hemorrhages, and exudates of the disc. Shortly thereafter, however, pallor of the disc appears. The papillomacular bundle is typically the most severely involved. There may be some spontaneous improvement in the disease, and the disease may be improved considerably, according to some authors, by administration of hydroxycobalamine.[36]

The visual field changes are similar to those that have been described previously in this section. Each eye develops a central scotoma that is usually absolute centrally. There is usually intact peripheral vision, although this is not invariable. Field changes, once formed, tend to remain stationary through life.

OTHER HEREDITARY DISEASES

Although Leber's disease is perhaps the prototype of hereditary optic atrophy, at least four types have been described: (1) Leber's disease; (2) a recessive congenital or infantile optic atrophy; (3) a dominant form that may be manifested congenitally (really an agenesis); or (4) an infantile type that may not be noted until age six to eight years or that may not be present until adolescence. Although Leber's optic atrophy has been reported to show some improvement with treatment by hydroxycobalamine, Brodrick[5] has called attention to the fact that other types of optic atrophy may not be helped by this treatment.

Congenital forms of optic atrophy are generally quite severe. However, the later-occuring forms are much more benign, and the vision may actually remain as high as from 20/20 to 20/60 in 40% of the cases.[35] All these conditions are bilateral, and the fields characteristically show paracentral scotomas that may or may not encroach on fixation. These may resemble bitemporal defects.[23] Additionally, hereditary optic atrophy may be associated with other ailments to form syndromes. Such may be seen in conjunction with diabetes mellitus, with some of the hereditary ataxias (Marie's disease), and with other neurological syndromes.

There is a huge variety of other heredofamilial degenerative diseases that may affect the visual field. To discuss them in detail is somewhat beyond the scope of this book, but one may consider a prototype disease, that of retinitis pigmentosa. In its pure form, retinitis pigmentosa is a progressive disease in which characteristically there is peripheral bone spicule pigmentary degeneration, pallor of the disc, and narrowed retinal arterioles. One of the early complaints of retinitis pigmentosa is night blindness. As the disease progresses, a ring scotoma may be demonstrated in the near periphery (Fig. 8-15). Eventually the peripheral field disappears, leaving only a small central island that is gradually extinguished (Fig. 8-16). People with retinitis pigmentosa generally have extreme disability from field loss even though their visual acuity may remain 20/20 for many years. Unfortunately, those afflicted can take scant comfort from

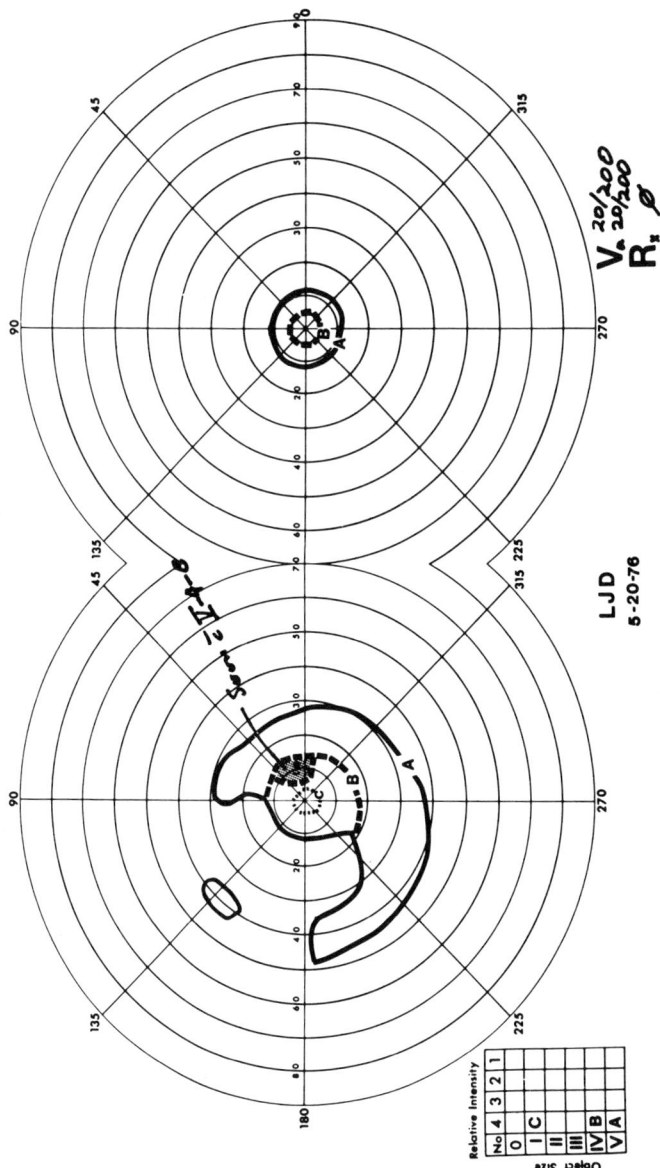

Figure 8-15 Visual field of a patient with retinitis pigmentosa. The right visual field is already advanced. The left eye shows the remnants of a ring scotoma.

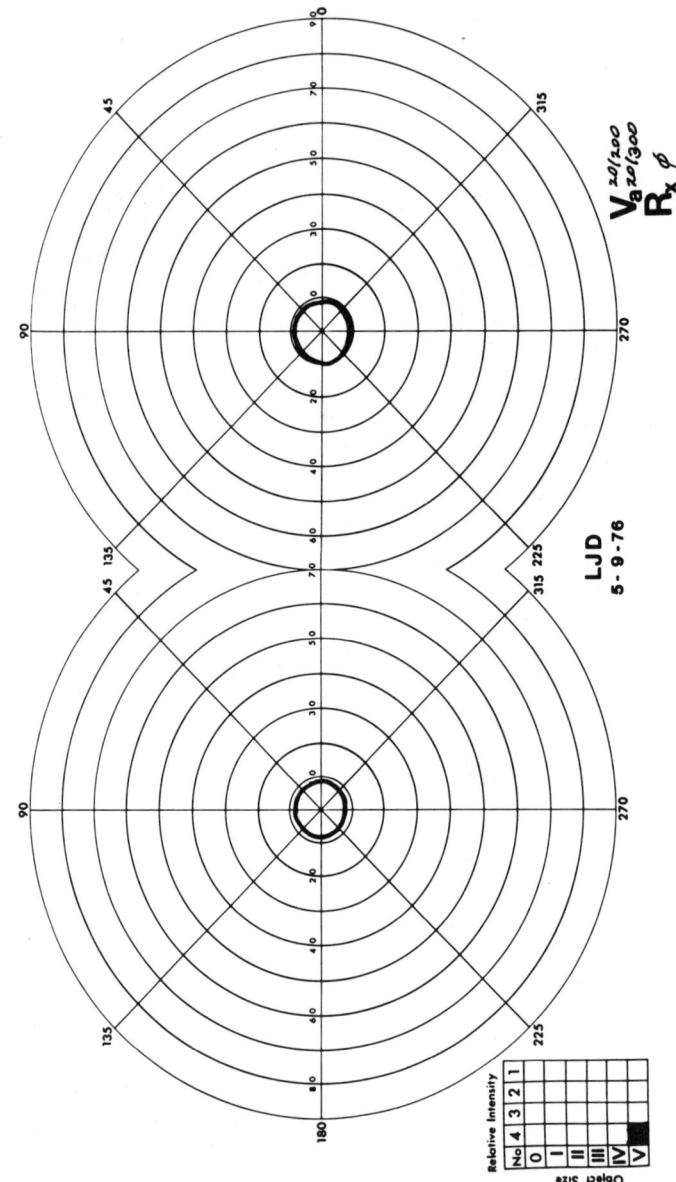

Figure 8-16 Visual field of the patient in Figure 8-15 almost one year later. Both fields are constricted to under 10°.

Condition	Field Defect

1. Night blindness
   a. congenital
   b. Oguchi's disease
	1. Photopic fields normal, progressively constrict with dark adaptation.

2. Albinism	2. Constriction. Occasionally see central scotomas.

3. Hereditary macular dystrophy
   a. juvenile retinoschisis
   b. rod monochromatism
   c. cone dystrophies
   d. Stargardt's disease
   e. fundus flavimaculatus
   f. vitelliform dystrophy
   g. dominant drusen
   h. central areolar choroidal dystrophy
   i. inverse retinitis pigmentosa
	3. Initially central scotoma, but some forms progress to involve periphery.

4. Primary retinal degenerations
   a. retinitis pigmentosa and variants
   b. retinitis punctata albescens
	4. Midperipheral ring scotoma forms, then progresses to severe constriction.

5. Choroidal dystrophies
   a. choroideremia
   b. gyrate atrophy
	5. Similar to retinitis pigmentosa. Severe constriction.

Table 8-1 Hereditary or congenital diseases of the retina and choroid associated with visual field defects.

this promise of good acuity, for the maculopathy and cataracts which not infrequently accompany this disease deprive many of its victims of even this advantage. Retinitis pigmentosa may be associated with a large variety of other syndromes. A listing of many other hereditary disorders that primarily affect the retina is given in Table 8-1.

INFLAMMATORY LESIONS

Optic neuritis is the prototype inflammatory lesion of the visual pathway. Although it may be divided into retrobulbar neuritis and papillitis, this distinction is artificial and differentiates only between the anatomical position of the inflammation rather than the underlying pathology. The condition is most common in young women and is usually unilateral. It is associated with pain or discomfort behind the eye on movement, and usually causes a relative pupillary defect to the Marcus Gunn swinging flashlight sign.

Characteristically, the condition shows a central scotoma that may be either quite small or as large as 40°–50° in diameter (Fig. 8-17). Although the periphery is usually intact, this is not invariably so, and in severe cases the only vision that may remain is light perception. In a few cases, all light perception may be lost temporarily. The central defect is usually absolute and may be surrounded by an area of relative defect. Fiber bundle defects typical of those seen in glaucoma may also be seen, although this is an unusual presentation. In most cases, the visual field recovers slowly over a period of a few weeks to a few months, although complete recovery is not invariable, and some residual visual impairment may remain. Even though the visual acuity has returned to normal, a shallow relative scotoma is frequently found centrally.

Optic neuritis may be associated with a huge variety of diseases.[8, 35] It has already been mentioned that retrobulbar neuritis may be present in vitamin B-complex deficiency. Optic neuritis may be associated with puberty, pregnancy, or lactation, conditions that may also be aggravated by relative B-complex deficiency. Other causes include the menopause, pernicious anemia, diabetes mellitus, syphilis, and as sequelae to a host of acute viral infections. Nevertheless, the most dreaded etiologies are demyelinating diseases such as diffuse sclerosis, opticomyelitis, or, most importantly, multiple sclerosis (MS). Although under half of the patients who have one attack of optic neuritis ever develop the remainder of the signs and symptoms of multiple sclerosis, an attack of optic neuritis is a frequent presenting symptom of the disease. In those cases in which the optic neuritis is bilateral, the visual loss is usually more severe and the likelihood of a demyelinating disease such as multiple sclerosis or Devic's disease is much higher. Nevertheless, in the great majority of the cases of optic neuritis, no amount of investigation reveals a definite etiology for the visual loss.

Predicting the ultimate outcome of a case of optic neuritis is a matter of concern for both physician and patient alike. The classic approach to determining which patients with optic neuritis will eventually develop multiple sclerosis is simply to wait attentively and to observe what transpires. In more recent times, several authors have pointed to the association of certain tissue antigens in patients with multiple sclerosis.[16, 17, 24, 27] HLA-B7 and HLA-A3 are the most commonly mentioned histocompatibility antigens. This pattern is not seen in other forms of optic neuritis and thus appears to be of value in differentiating the disease. Another group[24] reexamined this question by utilizing the LD-7A (now HLA-D7) antigen in mixed lymphocyte culture. They found an increased frequency of this antigen in patients with optic neuritis who did not develop other findings as well as in patients with multiple sclerosis, and they thus felt that

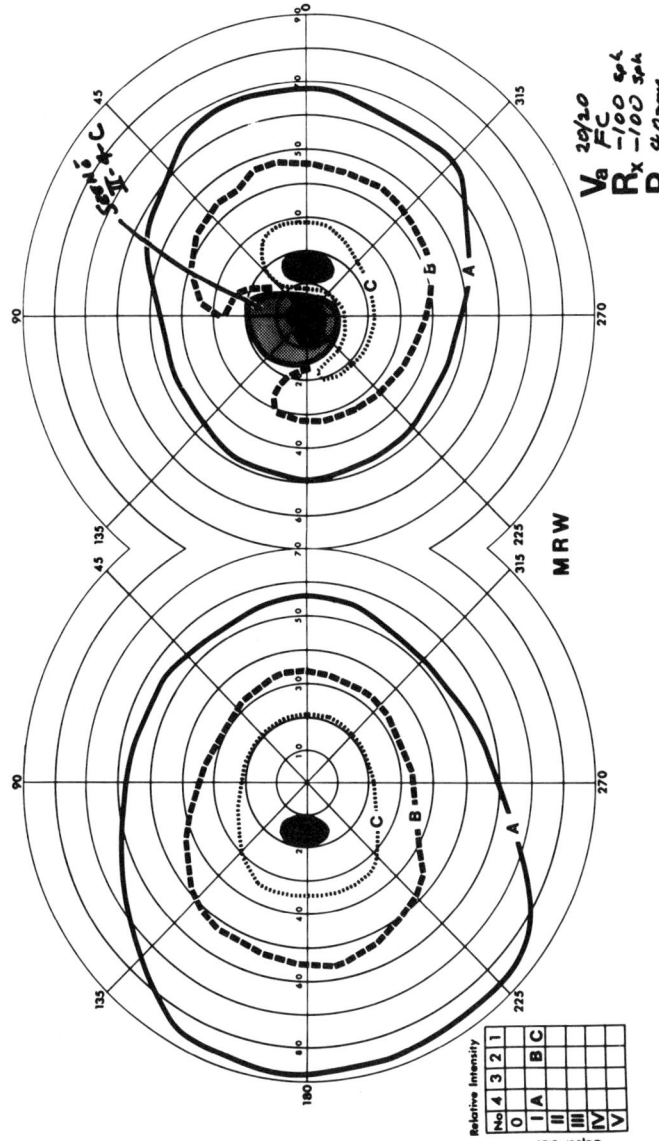

Figure 8-17 Visual field of a young woman with retrobulbar neuritis of the right eye. This field defect completely resolved.

tissue typing offers little information as to the ultimate prognosis. Other antigens that have been mentioned are HLA-Dw2 and one known as B-group 4.[24] Other authors have pointed out that patients with MS show elevated cerebrospinal fluid antibodies to measles virus and an oligoclonal IgG-globulin pattern on agar gel electrophoresis.[20] Finally, in patients with MS, there is a defective cell-mediated immunity to measles.[7,34]

It was initially reported that this defect could be corrected, along with a clinical improvement in the MS patient, with transfer factor* therapy.[18] More recent reports based on double-blind studies have disputed the therapeutic value of transfer factor.[24] Nonetheless, this defect of MS patient leucocytes to measles antigen may provide a test capable of the early diagnosis of MS. Other promising tests involve the migration of macrophages or erythrocytes under the influence of an electric field in the presence of small amounts of linoleic acid. These tests are currently under evalution.[24–26]

No discussion of optic neuritis is complete without a description of those conditions that may mimic it, so-called pseudo-optic neuritis. The most frequent member of this group, ischemic optic neuropathy, has already been discussed. Like optic neuritis, the treatment is palliative, so a confusion between the two entities is of little moment. A more important category is expanding lesions of the anterior or middle cranial fossae, where decisive therapy may be available. The etiologic agents include meningiomas, pituitary adenomas, craniopharyngiomas, nasopharyngeal carcinomas, lymphoma or Hodgkin's disease, metastatic carcinoma and even ectopic pinealomas.[8] Any of these may present with a central scotoma and thus be confused with retrobulbar neuritis. Tumors of the orbit may also cause pseudo-optic neuritis, but here the visual field defect is more likely to involve the periphery in addition to the central defects. Tumors differ from optic neuritis in the following ways:

1. There is no retrobulbar pain.
2. Tumors show a gradual, progressive course.
3. Tumors have x-ray abnormalities.
4. Tumors show an altered neurological status.

Meningioma is perhaps worthy of a few extra comments. This is most common in middle-aged women and gives rise to several syndromes, dependent on the tumor's location. Those confined to the orbit may produce exophthalmos and extraocular muscle paresis, while those within the cranium produce symptoms depending upon their configuration. The diffuse meningioma of the sphenoid ridge may also cause bony hypertrophy which in turn causes ex-

---

*Transfer factor is a small nucleoprotein that provides a way to transfer cellular immunity from one individual to another. It is a controversial subject, and some authorities even deny its existence.

ophthalmos and visual loss, while localized tumors cause blindness by simple compression of the nerve. One well-known syndrome is the Foster-Kennedy syndrome. In this syndrome, one eye shows primary optic atrophy, due to direct compression by the tumor, and the fellow eye shows papilledema, due to the increased intracranial pressure. Another common syndrome is due to meningioma of the olfactory groove, which produces anosmia and headache in addition to visual loss (which may be manifest as the Foster-Kennedy syndrome).

HYSTERIA AND MALINGERING

Malingering and hysteria constitute a problem of increasing proportions for the ophthalmologist. Always the bane of the military ophthalmologist, increasingly generous insurance settlements and successful lawsuits have spurred an increase in the incidence of probable malingering which we see in our consultation practice. The subject in all its ramifications is large, and differentiation of the two is difficult and at times may be impossible. In general, the malingerer has some obvious gain not found in the hysteric, but secondary gain, such as sympathy or the avoidance of an unpleasant duty, may suffice. In cases where patients have actually received some injury—physical or psychological—either is possible, and at times the only persons who "know for sure" what the diagnosis is are the patients themselves. Also, the examiner should be wary of real intracranial pathology, for the literature is replete with case reports of "hysterics" who later developed diffuse scleroses, tumors, or other pathology.

If the condition is unilateral, several tricks in addition to perimetry may be of help. Frequently, the affected eye allegedly has vision far below the level for reading, so the central light sense should be affected. Most commonly, the field test does not show a central scotoma, so the examiner should attempt to verify that the visual acuity is normal. A prism may be placed base up before the affected eye while the subject attempts to read; if the vision in that eye is truly good, the vertical diplopia will cause the subject to falter. The Cuignet bar test is another useful ploy, in which a pencil is held midway on a line between the subject's nose and the paper, the hand held steady, and the patient asked to read. If the patient is able to read an entire line, reading vision is present in both eyes. Should the vision be very poor, have the patient look into a mirror with the "blind" eye while the good eye is covered, then rotate the mirror through a small angle. This maneuver will produce a corresponding movement of the eye if it has enough visual capacity to permit fixation. A related ploy is to have the subject read, then place a base-out prism of moderate strength ($10^{\triangle}$) before the affected eye. An inward movement of the eye with insertion of the prism and an outward movement with its removal signify the ability to fixate.

The classic visual fields of the hysteric are the spiraling field and the tubular field. Despite a reduced visual acuity, hysterics seldom simulate a central scotoma.[35] Ring scotomas, however, may be seen. Malingerers most frequently choose a tubular field, although we have seen central scotomas and hemianopic defects simulated by knowledgeable malingerers.

The spiraling visual field can only be seen if the preferred examination technique of random stimulus presentation is abandoned in favor of regular presentation. Assuming that changing adaptation status can be ruled out, the spiral pattern is characteristic of the neurasthenic or hysterical patient.

Tubular fields are best plotted on the tangent screen. Here, the same size isopter (usually around 5° to 10°) is plotted, regardless of the distance the subject sits from the screen. Moreover, approximately the same isopter will frequently be plotted with all sizes of test objects; that is, the edge of the central visual island will have a very steep slope. This fact permits tubular fields to be suspected with a bowl perimeter by changing stimulus size or brightness. Finally, Cogan[8] notes the constriction may be a function of the size of the screen on which one tests the field. If a larger or smaller tangent screen is used, the size of the defect will change in proportion.

There are several techniques for uncovering simulation at the bowl perimeter. Aulhorn (personal communication) frequently presents statically a spot 10° to 20° outside of the corresponding isopter and asks the patient if he or she can see it. Upon receiving a negative response, the patient is enthusiastically told he is right, he cannot see the spot. Then, while carefully observing the patient's eye through the fixation telescope in the perimeter, the perimetrist asks the patient to look in the direction of the spot until he sees it. Naturally, the patient will be able to look directly at it only if he or she can see it. Occasionally, the patient will oblige the perimetrist long enough to permit a rough determination of the actual isopter limits. This does not work so well if only a restricted area (e.g., a quadrantanopsia) is in question. Obviously, a central scotoma *cannot* be tested by this method.

Pupillomotor perimetry provides another check. For the purpose of detecting simulation or hysteria, the patient's eye should be illuminated from the side to permit observation of the pupil through the fixation telescope. If possible, the blind spot is mapped in the routine fashion and a large, bright test spot presented in its center. If no pupillary response is seen, then the stimulus is increased until the brightest stimulus that does *not* cause a pupillary response when projected into the blind spot is found. This is then projected into an area of the field known to be good and the pupil response noted. Defective areas of the field may then be explored with the spot. Should it not be possible to find the blind spot with certainty, an alternate calibration spot is 60° out in the nasal field.

Pupillomotor perimetry has its pitfalls. The calibration process must be carefully done, else the response may be due to scattered light within the eye, and not to direct light from the stimulus itself. Secondly, the central field is most effective in producing a pupillary response, and more peripherally no response is seen in known normals. The technique is thus most applicable to processes that involve the central field or severely contracted fields.

There are other techniques for the evaluation of malingering available to those with specialized equipment. The visually evoked occipital response, particularly to pattern stimuli, is one such test. Another is to condition the patient by means of mild electric shocks to a certain orientation of a Landolt Ring, then record the galvanic skin response (GSR) as various orientations and sizes of rings are presented. Recognition of the selected orientation in the successfully conditioned subject is accompanied by a change in the GSR, thus permitting a rough determination of acuity. Obviously, such methods are not within the grasp of the average practitioner, but may be available at university or military referral centers where problem cases can be sent for evaluation.

REFERENCES

1. Armaly MF: Selective perimetry for glaucomatous defects in ocular hypertension. Arch Ophthalmol 87:518, 1972
2. Aulhorn E, Harms H: Early visual field defects in glaucoma. Acta XX Congress of Ophthalmology (Munich, Glaucoma Tutzing Symposium, 1966). Basel, Karger, 1967
3. Becker B, Shin DH, Palmberg PF, Waltman SR: HLA antigens and corticosteroid response. Science 194:1427, 1976
4. Becker B, Shin DH: Response to topical epinephrine. Arch Ophthalmol 94:2057, 1976
5. Brodrick JD: Hereditary optic atrophy with onset in early childhood. Br J Ophthalmol 58:817, 1974
6. Chisholm IA, Bronte-Stewart J, Foulds WS: Hydroxycobalamine versus cyanocobalamine in the treatment of tobacco amblyopia. Lancet 2:450, 1967
7. Ciongoli AK, Platz P, Dupont B, Svejgaard A, Fog T, Jersild C: Lack of antigen response to myxoviruses in multiple sclerosis. Lancet 2:1147, 1973
8. Cogan DG: Neurology of the Visual System. Springfield, Illinois, Charles C Thomas, 1970
9. Drance SM: Visual field defects in glaucoma, in: Symposium on Glaucoma. Transactions of the New Orleans Academy of Ophthalmology. St. Louis, CV Mosby Co., 1975
10. Drance SM: Low tension glaucoma and its management, in: Symposium on Glaucoma. Transactions of the New Orleans Academy of Ophthalmology. St. Louis, CV Mosby Co., 1975
11. Drance SM: The glaucomatous visual field. Br J Ophthalmol 56:186, 1972

12. Duke-Elder S, MacFaul PA: Non-mechanical injuries, in Duke-Elder S (ed): System of Ophthalmology, London, Henry Kimpton, 1972
13. Fraunfelder FT: Drug-Induced Ocular Side Effects and Drug Interactions. Philadelphia, Lea & Febiger, 1976
14. Grant WM: Toxicology of the Eye. Springfield, Illinois, Charles C Thomas, 1962
15. Heaton JM, McCormick AJA, Freeman AG: Tobacco amblyopia; a clinical manifestation of vitamin B12 deficiency. Lancet 2:286, 1958
16. Jersild C, Hansen GS, Svejgaard A, Fog T, Thomsen M, Dupont B: Histocompatibility determinants in multiple sclerosis, with special reference to clinical course. Lancet 2:1221, 1973
17. Jersild C, Svejgaard A, Fog T, Ammitzbøll T: HL-A antigens and diseases; I. Multiple sclerosis. Tissue Antigens 3:243, 1973
18. Jersild C, Platz P, Thomsen M, Hansen GS, Svejgaard A, Dupont B, Fog T, Ciongoli AK, Grob P: Transfer-factor therapy in multiple sclerosis. Lancet 2:1381, 1973
19. LeBlanc RP, Becker B: Peripheral nasal field defects. Am J Ophthalmol 72:415, 1971
20. Link H, Norrby E, Olsson J: Immunoglobulins and measles antibodies in optic neuritis. N Engl J Med 289:1103, 1973
21. Lynn JR: Testing the visual field in glaucoma, in: Symposium on Glaucoma, Transactions of the New Orleans Academy of Ophthalmology. St. Louis, CV Mosby Co., 1975
22. Lynn JR: Correlation of pathogenesis, anatomy and patterns of visual field loss in glaucoma, in: Symposium on Glaucoma. Transactions of the New Orleans Academy of Ophthalmology. St. Louis, CV Mosby Co., 1975
23. Manchester PT, Calhoun FP: Dominant hereditary optic atrophy with bitemporal field defects. Arch Ophthalmol 60:479, 1958
24. Maugh TH: Multiple sclerosis; genetic link, viruses suspected. Science 195:667, 1977
25. Maugh TH: Multiple sclerosis; two or more viruses may be involved. Science 195:768, 1977
26. Maugh TH: The EAE Model; a tentative connection to multiple sclerosis. Science 195:969, 1977
27. Naito S, Namerow N, Mickey MR, Terasaki PI: Multiple sclerosis; association with HL-A3. Tissue Antigens 2:1, 1972
28. Read RM, Spaeth GL: The practical clinical appraisal of the optic disc in glaucoma. Trans Am Acad Ophthalmol Otolaryngol 78:255, 1974
29. Ronne H: Über das Gesichtfeld beim Glaukom. Klin Monatsbl Augenheilkd 47:12, 1909
30. Shin DH, Becker B: HLA-A11 and HLA-Bw35 and resistance to glaucoma in white patients with ocular hypertension. Arch Ophthalmol 95:423, 1977
31. Shin DH, Becker B, Waltman SR, et al: The prevalence of HLA-B12 and HLA-B7 antigens in primary open-angle glaucoma. Arch Ophthalmol 95:224, 1977
32. Shin DH, Becker B: The prognostic value of HLA-B12 and HLA-B7 antigens in patients with increased intraocular pressure. Am J Ophthalmol 82:871, 1976
33. Tate GW, Martin RG: Clindamycin in the treatment of human ocular toxoplasmosis. Can J Ophthal 12:188, 1977

34. Utermohlen V, Zabriskie JB: Suppressed cellular immunity to measles antigen in multiple-sclerosis patients. Lancet 2:1147, 1973
35. Walsh FB, Hoyt WF: Clinical Neuro-ophthalmology. Baltimore, Williams & Wilkins, 1969
36. Wilson J: Leber's hereditary optic atrophy; possible defect of cyanide metabolism. Clin Sci 29:505, 1965

9
The Principles and Practice of Automatic Perimetry

Perimetry is done not by the perimeter but by the perimetrist.
                                                            Traquair

I would like to emphasize that perimetry, particularly kinetic perimetry, is an art.
                                                            Goldmann

The quotations that serve as an epigraph to this chapter mark not only a departure in style from the rest of this book, but underline the fact that automatic perimetry represents a departure in thinking and technique from classical manual perimetry. As we emphasized earlier, and as Aulhorn has stated,[1] a good perimetrist remains in contact with the patient to allay inattentiveness or unsteady fixation or incipient anxiety. The perimetrist continually monitors the results and repeats the exam in an area several times if unusual amounts of scatter appear, all the while taking care not to prolong the exam so the patient becomes tired and uncooperative. During the clinical session, the perimetrist must maintain a standard of technical excellence in the performance of the mechanical aspects of the field exam. Obviously, all perimetrists are not equally good at performing this juggling act, and for this reason the results from one perimetrist to the next may not be exactly comparable. It seems obvious at first glance that if one could just replace the perimetrist with a mechanical device to present the stimuli and record the responses, far more predictable results could be obtained.

Unfortunately, this is not so straightforward as it appears at first glance. Merely mechanizing a manual perimeter has never been truly successful, and it has only been lately, since the advent of small, cheap computers, that quality automatic perimetry has become an economically viable possibility. Even though the computer brings a measure of sophistication not found in simple electromechanical devices, a departure from the usual design is frequently necessary in order to achieve comparable results to those of the human perimetrist. For example, it is not practical to have the computer carry on congenial patter with the patient to keep him alert. However, it is possible, through the use of forced choice and feedback techniques, to accomplish this same goal. Also, exam strategies that make a great deal of sense in the manual case make no sense at all for the automatic perimeter. For example, manual static perimetry is usually carried out by choosing a fixed location and presenting a series of subthreshold stimuli, each stimulus one step brighter than the last and at the same spot, until a stimulus is seen. This is done in the manual case because of the difficulty of keeping records, as well as the impracticality of changing the test location between each stimulus presentation. In the automatic perimeter, such a strategy is nonsense. In the first place, it is of no moment whether the spot moves from one time to the next. In the second, because one can stimulate anywhere in the field one time and not return there for several seconds, it is no longer difficult to avoid local adaptation, and the use of suprathreshold stimuli becomes permissible, in fact even desirable. Both Lynn[28] and Aulhorn[1] have noted that the use of frequent suprathreshold stimuli not only spurs patient interest by allowing him to make frequent responses, but it helps to minimize anxiety, and, if the stimuli are presented in a random fashion, serves to encourage improved fixation. On the contrary, if most of the stimuli are presented under threshold, the long intervals during which the patient is not called upon to make a response practically guarantee that the patient will become anxious and glance frequently about the perimetry bowl in the hopes of seeing a stimulus.

Similarly, the use of an appropriate response device can enhance the worth of an automatic test. It has long been known by the psychophysicist that forced-choice methods are most exact techniques for measuring visual thresholds,[6] although Heijl[22] noted that forced choice in his automatic static perimeter seemed to introduce more scatter. Lynn and Tate [29,30] had exactly the opposite experience. The latter investigators utilized a joy stick in which the patient was supposed to move the stick from its central position in a direction corresponding to the direction of the test object relative to fixation. If the response was within acceptable limits of error, the patient was rewarded by hearing a pleasing tone. If, however, his response was inexact and he responded incorrectly, an unpleasant buzz sounded, thereby immediately informing him of his failing. Initially, it was noted that almost every perimetry subject received his fair share of computerized reprimands, but in short order they improved their performance to a very acceptable level. Greve[16] also has utilized a forced choice response device in his automatic perimeter, whereby the patient must report whether he sees two, three, or four stimuli. Greve reports that most patients have no problem in learning to use the device, although a few older persons are not testable with his device, and he said at the 1976 meeting of the International Perimetry Society that many subjects did not like the test. Jernigan[26] utilized a forced choice in which the patient simply looked at the test spot and eye position monitors recorded whether or not he had made a correct move. Although this could be potentially tiring for large saccades, such innovative approaches emphasize that automatic perimetry can and should utilize techniques far different from those employed in the manual perimeter.

The use of a computer also makes possible many innovative schemes of presenting data. Weber and Spahr[39] have discussed a number of these, and they are illustrated in Figure 9-1. In addition, the computer can be used to compare visual fields from one time to the next, and the examiner can choose to plot out only the rate or specific area of change. The theoretical possibility exists to store the results of every visual field a patient has had on magnetic tape, disc, or other suitable storage medium, and each time a new field is performed, to compare it to all previous fields. In this fashion, areas of change that are an established trend, as opposed to fluctuations from one time to the next, can be identified easily. Within a given field, by simply measuring a threshold several times over a small population of points, one can obtain a measure of the accuracy in terms of threshold fluctuation.[4] Finally, automatic perimetry is not limited by the burden of the expenditure of time by technically skilled persons, and therefore, with appropriate programming, mass screening programs can be carried out, which have been shown to be quite productive in discovering pathology, even in a supposedly normal population.[17] Thus, automatic perimetry represents a new technology that has considerably enlarged the horizons beyond which a clinician of a generation ago dared not dream.

STIMULUS PRESENTATION

Multiple techniques of presenting a stimulus are possible. Our initial perimeter, as well as that of Chaplin,[9] utilized spots presented on a television screen for the stimulus. This idea, though appealing, is ill conceived because of the difficulties in making spot size and brightness reproducible. Also, the use of a phosphorus screen, such as found on most cathode ray tubes (CRTs), ties spot size and brightness inextricably together; the brighter the spot, the larger the spot, due to an effect called "blooming" of the phosphor. Thus, the choice of a CRT deprives the examiner of choosing spot size and spot brightness independently. Another approach has been taken by Heijl.[22-25] This group has embedded a grid of light-emitting diodes (LEDs) in a screen. These LEDs are driven by

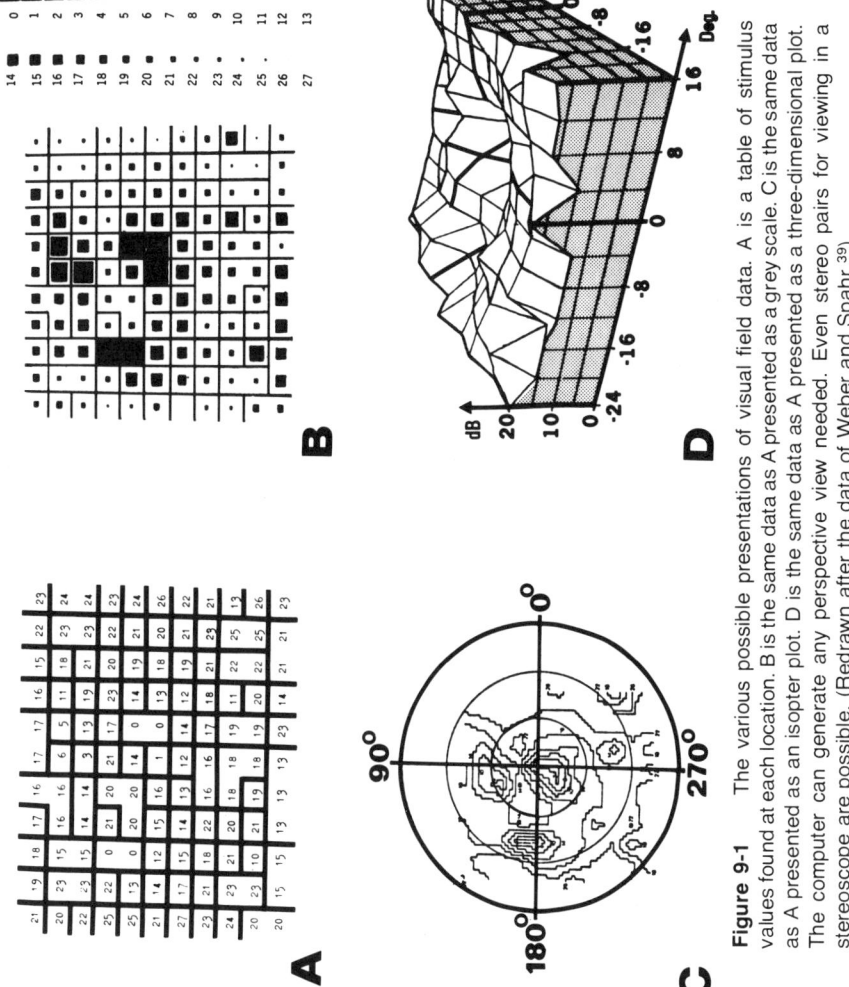

Figure 9-1 The various possible presentations of visual field data. A is a table of stimulus values found at each location. B is the same data as A presented as a grey scale. C is the same data as A presented as an isopter plot. D is the same data as A presented as a three-dimensional plot. The computer can generate any perspective view needed. Even stereo pairs for viewing in a stereoscope are possible. (Redrawn after the data of Weber and Spahr.[39])

a high-frequency pulse current of a variable duty cycle,* thereby permitting variable brightnesses to be achieved at each spot. This scheme has several advantages as well as disadvantages. First of all, there is likely to be some small individual variation from one light-emitting diode to the next. Second, the positions of the light-emitting diodes are fixed on the screen, and it is not possible to alter them, short of moving the diodes manually. Third, the brightness range available in light-emitting diodes is limited, although developments in this field are made daily, and light-emitting diodes of a greater range may soon be on the market.

Despite the innovations possible, the best quality automatic perimeters today still utilize a projection system not at all unlike that found on the best manual bowl perimeters. The Perimetron by Coherent Radiation, the Octopus by Interzeag, the Automated Tübinger by Oculus, and our own second generation automatic perimeter (the rights to which are also owned by Interzeag) all utilize this technique. Projection offers the advantages of an easily calibratible light source, the ability to utilize various colors of stimuli, the ability to control the size and brightness independently of one another, and the ability to position the spot anywhere on the screen, thereby allowing theoretically the possibility of both kinetic and static perimetry. Although new technologies that may someday be suitable to perimetry are now on the horizon, projection is likely to remain the technology of choice for some years to come.

RESPONSE DEVICE

The designer of automatic perimeters has a wide choice of response devices. One option is the simple yes-or-no response, typified by a pushbutton, in which a patient presses a button if he sees a light, and does nothing if he does not. As previously mentioned, it has been well established in the psychophysical literature that some type of forced choice response is more accurate, and indeed, it is our experience that this permits the rejection of a significant number of false responses, as well as having the effect of improving the overall accuracy of response.

When one chooses a forced choice device, three types are theoretically available, although to our knowledge only two have been implemented in automatic perimeters to date. The first type is a joy stick (Figs. 9-2 and 9-3). The joy stick device that we used divides the screen into 28 pie-shaped sectors

---

*Duty cycle is the ratio of the duration of a pulsed current to the total time from the leading edge of one pulse to the leading edge of the next. Thus, a pulsed current that is on for 25 milliseconds out of every 100 milliseconds has a duty cycle of 25%.

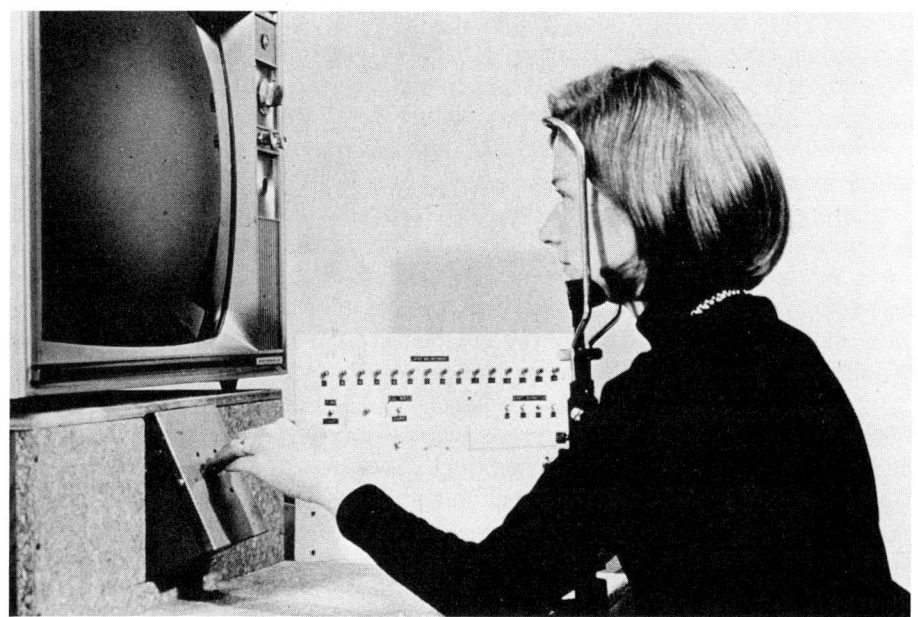

Figure 9-2 Our prototype automatic perimeter that utilized a modified television set as a stimulus and a joy stick as a response device.

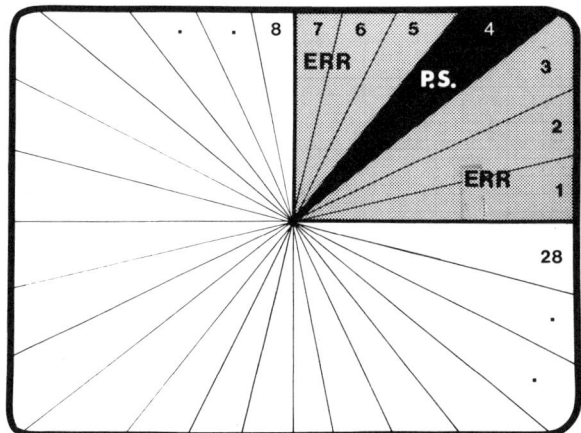

Figure 9-3 Allowable joy-stick error. Schematic diagram to illustrate algorithm for determining if the subject responded accurately with the joy stick. A stimulus is presented up and right of fixation, thus implying the joy stick is subsequently moved into sector 4 (black area marked P.S.). A response inaccuracy of three sectors on either side of the predicted sector is allowed (grey areas marked ERR), so a response by moving the joy stick into any sector from 1–7 is acceptable. All other responses are rejected. The number of allowable error sectors is selectable by the operator.

276   *Principles of Quantitative Perimetry*

centering on fixation. Through simple trigonometry, it is possible to assign any spot which is presented on the screen to one of those 28 sectors. The task given the subject is simply to push the joy stick in a direction that corresponds to the position of the spot relative to fixation. Naturally, the subject is unable to do this perfectly, and it is necessary to allow a number of errors in sectors on either side of the predicted sector. This scheme is outlined in Figure 9-3. Given the anatomy of the hand, however, there is a bias in the probable error that a respondent will make (Fig. 9-4). For example, if the subject is using his right hand and attempts to push the stick directly to the right, anatomical considerations are likely to produce a much larger counterclockwise error than a clockwise one. Thus, by knowing which hand the patient is using and in which sector the light is to appear, it becomes possible to compensate and allow for this bias by specifying different allowable errors on either side of the predicted sector. For example, one may say that for a given sector one will allow a three-sector counterclockwise but only a two-sector clockwise error. The magnitude of the likely error is naturally somewhat related to the age of the patient and his ability to comprehend, as well as to his physical status. Obviously, a person who has severe limitation of motion in the hand cannot perform an adequate forced-choice test, and in this case it is necessary to instruct the computer to accept any response as correct. Likewise, older and senile persons have had large errors, which we have had to take into account. As a general, overall average,

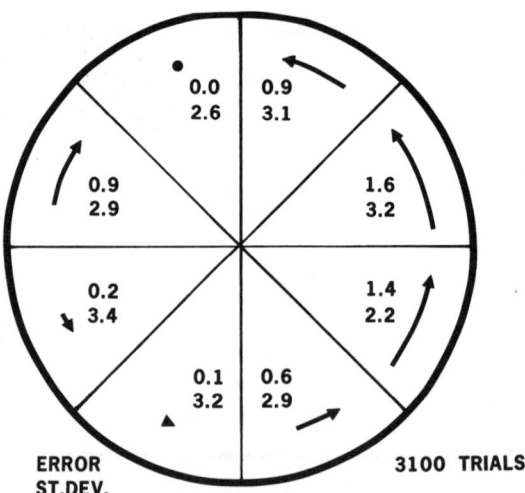

Figure 9-4   Error data for 3100 trials of a joy-stick movement with the right hand. Note that to the right, there is a tendency for a large counterclockwise error, while to the left a smaller error is seen. The left hand tends to mirror these results.

forty degrees on either side of the predicted sector is more than ample for almost anyone.

The second technique implemented applies only to multiple-stimulus perimeters. Multiple-stimulus perimetry has been discussed briefly; it is the sort used in many screeners, such as the Harrington-Flocks, or, more elegantly, in the Freedman Analyzer. Greve[18] has studied the use of multiple-stimulus static perimetry to screen the periphery. He has constructed an automatic perimeter[16] that is essentially an automated Freedman Analyzer. With this device, the subject is asked to indicate by means of a control lever whether he saw two, three, or four stimuli. Greve found that, on the average, only about 4% of the patients were unable to utilize his machine effectively; most of those were over sixty-one years of age and were otherwise infirm. Considering the additional intellectual task of counting the number of stimuli that one sees, this is superior performance indeed.

The final technique, that of temporal forced choice, has not yet been implemented on anyone's machine to our knowledge. Temporal forced choice is the preferred method of many psychophysical investigators, who obtain multiple thresholds at each point. Indeed, if several thresholds are not to be determined, temporal forced choice loses a great deal of its appeal. This would add a measure of accuracy, but it would also prolong the clinical exam, and this problem likely accounts for the fact that no one has utilized it clinically. The temporal forced choice procedure consists of presenting a stimulus in one of three (or more) time intervals and requiring the subject to choose in which of the three time intervals he saw the stimulus, if indeed he saw it at all; and if he did not see it, in which time interval he thinks it most likely appeared. That is to say, he has to choose an interval whether he saw the spot or not. One can visualize a perimeter in which three notes of a musical scale are presented aurally, with the stimulus flashed during one of the notes. The subject must then respond, in a fashion similar to that employed by Greve, as to whether the stimulus appeared in interval one, two, or three (or high, medium, or low pitch). For general clinical use, this technique has the additional drawback of requiring the subject to respond whether the stimulus is seen or not. This is likely to be confusing to many patients, particularly the elderly. If ever implemented in automated devices, this technique is likely to be used for research purposes only.

The form of the response device, however, need not necessarily be a joy stick or a push button. Jernigan[26] has done work with a perimeter that utilizes eye movements as the end point. The subject is instructed to look at each spot as it appears, and an eye-movement monitor senses the direction and speed of motion of the subject's eyes. With these data, the machine can decide whether or not the subject actually saw the spot. If the subject thinks he sees the spot, but actually does not, the machine will sense saccades in several directions, a direct tip-off that the response is an error. We examined this technique manually with a number of subjects, who found it somewhat tiring to refixate after each saccade if the saccades were over 15° to 20° in length. Therefore, we personally have reservations as to whether the technique would be useful for full field perimetry. One tantalizing possibility is to combine a moveable fixation point (see discussion below) with the eye movement response to stimuli, but this is less likely to be successful than one might suppose. The reason for this is that when the subject is tested, say in the far right field, it is obvious that almost anywhere the stimulus appears next, it will involve a left saccade. Therefore, much of the value of the test is lost. As of this writing, Jernigan's device has only been implemented commercially in a screener, although plans are afoot to develop a proper, full-field quantitative perimeter based on his technique.

Finally, it should be remarked that a number of attempts have been made at purely objective responses. Harms[19-21] and Bresky et al[7] have thoroughly investigated a pupillometer perimeter. Aulhorn and Campos (personal communication) are currently building an improved pupil perimeter, in which a computer will monitor the pupil and decide whether or not the spot was in fact "seen." This machine has several innovations designed to minimize the problem of spurious responses due to intraocular light scatter.

The visually evoked response offers promise for use in the future. Cappin[8] has utilized a local visually evoked response to screen for field defects in glaucoma. Actual perimetry, however, has been carried out by Müller et al.[31,32] This group has utilized an array of flickering lights and signal averaging to obtain useable VERs as far temporally as 100°. By utilizing their technique, they have been able to plot out completely objective visual fields that agree excellently with subjectively plotted fields on the Goldmann Perimeter. Although this technique is still in its infancy, it holds much promise for the future. It should be particularly well adapted to children and senile oldsters who are otherwise unable to respond accurately.

FIXATION MONITORING

The standard for monitoring fixation on automatic perimeters ranges from none at all on the automatic Tübinger[1-3] to an elaborate compensation in which the test spot is moved to compensate for vagaries in fixation in the Lynn-Tate Perimeter.[29,30] How far in this regard one should go is a matter of economics, expediency, and philosophy. One end of the pole is championed by Aulhorn et al who feel that good fixation is adequately stimulated by the use of frequent, suprathreshold, randomly appearing test spots. Indeed, in the initial report presented about the machine,[2] the results that she was able to obtain did compare favorably with manual perimetry. Tate has been tested with this machine and did not feel any particular need to glance about the perimetry bowl, although he is a practiced subject and presumably capable of good fixation. The same was true of our initial machine, in which fixation control was not employed. It was nevertheless our experience that a certain percentage of the patients would fix poorly, particularly those who had a poor central light sense to begin with. The middle ground is used by the group in Bern,[34] where fixation is monitored by a computer; when fixation wanders sufficiently, the computer disregards the responses. A similar technique is used in the Perimetron, as well as in several other automatic perimeters that are either under development or on the market in other countries.

What we immodestly feel is one of the more innovative approaches is one that we ourselves have described.[29, 30] In this technique, the fixation is monitored by a device that can determine eye position to within a quarter of a degree or less, and the test spot is moved instantaneously to compensate for any small deviations from fixation in such fashion that the retinal image of the test spot remains stationary, despite eye movements. This technique, of course, has several limitations. For example, it is not practical to build a projection device that allows full saccades, simply because the velocity achieved during a full saccade from full right to full left is quite fast, on the order of 800 arc degrees per second. Fortunately, the saccadic velocity is a function of the length of the saccade, and only modest velocities, on the order of 100 arc degrees per second, are achieved if saccades of under 10 degrees are permitted. Even this velocity is very expensive to track, so initially commercial embodiments of this concept will be even more restrictive. Another limitation is the fact that if fixation is allowed to wander outside the central 10 to 15 degrees or so, torsional effects appear, and it is not too easy to compensate for these. It may be argued that the amount of torsion is known for a given eye position, but one cannot rely on persons with neurological diseases to have intact oculomotor systems. Therefore, it is best to limit the gaze with this device to the central 10 degrees of the field. It is not envisioned that this technique will be very useful for perimetry of the central one or two degrees. Indeed, even a half of a degree error in spot position could cause an artifactitious decrease in the absolute central light sense at fixation in the normal. Such a small error is, however, not important if the test spot is as much as 1° eccentric. In those patients with poor central fixation from any number of causes, the technique will likely be quite valuable. One can easily visualize machines of the future in which fixation compensation such as this, coupled with powerful objective techniques, such as the VER perimeter of Müller, will produce a new generation of automatic perimeters capable of examining anyone who can keep his eyes open and "fixate" within a 10° radius circle.

METHOD OF APPROACHING THRESHOLD

In classical manual static perimetry, the technique for seeking a threshold is known in the psychophysical literature as the *method of ascending limits*. That is, a stimulus starts infrathreshold and is progressively increased in one-step increments until it is just perceived, at which point the perceived stimulus is considered to be threshold, the test terminated at that spot, and the attention of the perimetrist turned to the next spot to be tested. Although classical, this technique has little else to be said for it, since it represents a waste of the perimetrist's and patient's time, but it is necessitated by the manual approach. In other realms of psychophysics, other threshold techniques are available. Cornsweet, for example, has pointed out[10] that the staircase-method (also called the von Békésy technique) provides an efficient technique in some cases, and that an even better result is obtained when the so-called double staircase is employed. In this technique, two series of stimuli start off with one supraliminal, the other infraliminal, and approach threshold through two intertwining series that appear to the subject as one. From the standpoint of anxiety of the patient, the intermixing of suprathreshold with subthreshold in a test is certainly desirable, and indeed mandatory, as we indicated earlier in this chapter. The important question is how to apply this technique most efficiently.

In order to arrive at the optimum stimulus technique in perimetry, one should realize that if a spot, which is thought to be approximately at threshold, is seen, then the likelihood that the actual threshold is far below it is small; whereas if such a spot is unseen, then the likelihood that the real threshold, as altered by disease, etc., could be far above it is comparatively great. Thus, if one starts from a fairly reasonable estimate of threshold to begin with, it makes little sense to vary the stimulus by a constant amount, regardless of whether or not the last test was seen.

This has long been recognized in audiometric circles, where techniques such as von Békésy's staircase and, more recently, the parametric estimation by sequential testing (PEST), have been used for some time.[33,38] PEST is a so-called adaptive procedure, which allows rapid and efficient psychophysical testing. In general, the step size between stimuli is dependent upon the history of what has gone before at that location. One set of rules provided by Taylor[38] suggests that the step size be halved on every reversal of direction, but that if more than two steps are taken in a given direction, then all subsequent steps should double their predecessors in size. Although there are a number of other rules concerning the likely location of threshold and so forth, the point is that variable stimulus step techniques have proven extremely efficient for locating thresholds in the least number of trials, at least in the audiometric studies reported.

Lynn[28] utilized a similar idea. In his algorithm, the predicted threshold level was used as a starting point, the predicted level being the average normal field threshold for a person of the patient's age. If the stimuli was not seen, it was made four steps brighter; if it was seen, it was made two steps dimmer. Once one stimulus level that was not seen and one stimulus level that was seen were found, then threshold was determined by a simple binary search between these two stimulus levels at this location. This proved to be a relatively efficient technique for finding thresholds.

A more elaborate analysis of the perimetric environment has been done by the group at Bern.[4,5,12] They, too, preferred to start from a suprathreshold spot and to utilize variable intervals between stimuli. They have reported very efficient determinations of thresholds in using their technique. In practice, their technique seems to yield, on the average, about the same overall efficiency as that proposed by Lynn. In all of the proposed techniques, it is very important that two tests not be presented in sequence at a given location; several other locations should be tested before coming back to any given location. We found this most convenient to do by use of a random number generator, testing each spot in the field before returning to retest any given spot in the queue.

Although these techniques determine a threshold in the classical sense, any single determination of threshold gives us no measure of variability. Bebie et al[4] has pointed out that the variation in threshold can be divided into short-term and long-term fluctuations; the short-term variation being on the order of 0.18 log units, whereas the total variation (the sum of short- and long-term) is on the order of 0.25 log units of luminance. This, of course, varies widely among individual observers. If one is to obtain a measure of the reliability with a minimum of additional efforts, two threshold determinations must be carried out on a number of points, instead of only single measurements. Bebie recommends that approximately ten such double determinations provide a minimum accurate measurement of the deviation.* Should the variability be large, as might well be expected in inexperienced subjects, it may well be worth while to make several threshold determinations at a given spot, similar to the method of Heijl et al,[24] who essentially used a modification of the up-and-down staircase method and followed it through several reversals. Should it become obvious that more trials are necessary, it is a simple matter once the first estimate of threshold is found to test it by the staircase technique, until several repetitions of the threshold are determined. An average threshold for that point may be com-

---

*This can be calculated by the formula

$$\sigma = \sqrt{K^{-1} \sum_{i=1}^{K} 0.5 \, (S_i - S_i^1)^2}$$

where σ is the variation, K is the number of double determinations, and S_i, S_i^1 are the first and second threshold determinations, respectively, at the retinal point k in the same session.

puted, which will be considerably more reliable than a single trial in the instance of an untrained or otherwise poor subject. However, this increase in accuracy is not without its price. This technique will certainly increase the time of the exam, perhaps necessitating the testing of fewer spots, but it may be necessary with some subjects.

The foregoing has dwelt upon static techniques for finding a threshold, since most of the literature available today deals with this case. Kinetic perimetry also presents a viable alternative, and a reasonable technique for proceeding in an automatic fashion has been given by Lynn and Tate.[30] The basic technique here (Figure 9-5) consists of tracking inward kinetically with the test spot from the periphery and registering the location where it is seen. Initially, the track of the spot runs radially toward fixation. However, once several spots along the periphery are determined (usually a minimum of 4 to 6), a straight line is then calculated which links these spots together, and the perpendicular bisector of this line calculated. This perpendicular bisector serves as the track for the next test spot to follow. The second order test spot, presumably more accurate than the first because it very likely approached the isopter in a more nearly perpendicular direction, is then used in a similar fashion with other spots on the

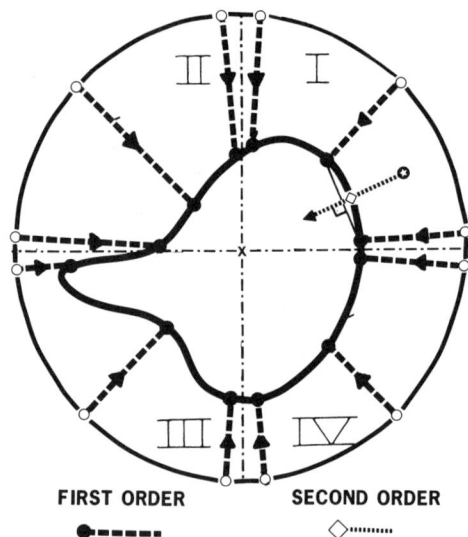

Figure 9-5 Algorithm for plotting an isopter. In this illustration, 12 first-order points are brought in from the periphery (open circles) toward fixation until they contact the isopter (filled circles). In quadrant I, one second-order point is shown. A line is constructed between two first-order points and the test is brought in along the perpendicular bisector from a starting point about 15° outside the predicted isopter (starred circle) until the isopter is reached (open square). The remaining second and higher order points are determined in this fashion.

periphery to help determine the track for third and fourth order test spots. This technique, however, is not at all unlike that used in the best manual kinetic perimetry.

OBJECTIVE ANALYSIS OF THE VISUAL FIELD AND THE DETECTION OF SCOTOMAS

Scotoma detection depends on the thoroughness of the basic field examination, regardless of whether static or kinetic tests are utilized. If static tests are used, the discovery of scotomas increases with increasing the coverage of the field and with increasing the precision by which thresholds are determined at each test location. If kinetic tests are used, then the search for scotomas depends upon the recognition of abnormal isopters. As commented upon elsewhere in the book, abnormally wide spacing between isopters, concavities of isopters, or excessive scatter in an isopter all may tip off the human perimetrist or his computerized counterpart to the location of possible scotomas. This problem has several ramifications. It has long been appreciated by visual scientists that the projection of the retina onto the visual field chart is not at all linear. In fact, the periphery is disproportionately magnified.[11,13] Frisen has pointed out[13-15] that if the visual field is translated so that the blind spot rather than the fixation point serves as the center of the projection, then the visual field, at least for the central isopters, is very well approximated by an ellipse. This is indeed fortunate, because the well-known mathematical and symmetrical properties of an ellipse make a variety of statistical tests possible for determining whether or not the isopters contain abnormalities. Although the details of his technique are beyond the scope of this section, basically they amount to the mathematical equivalent of transforming the isopter so that it is an ellipse, tracing the ellipse on tracing paper, and folding it around various axes of symmetry to make sure that there are no local areas of indentation or other asymmetries in the ellipse. Some of his techniques are actually simple and elegant enough to be done by hand, as just described, while others require the use of a computer. Nevertheless, once abnormal isopters are identified, the spaces between isopters in the area of the abnormality can then be explored with static test spots by whatever technique the investigator desires.

Another approach based on static perimetry is that championed by Fankhauser's group in Bern.[12,27,36,37] They have advocated the calculation of what the value of each point in the field should be from the data gathered during the perimetric exam. A screening mode is then entered in which a point is presented either several steps above the predicted threshold or several steps below it (the exact interval being chosen to correspond to a 90% probability of being seen or unseen). These "high" or "low" test objects are arranged throughout the field in a checkerboard pattern of alternating highs and lows. Thus, if one tests the field with one test at each location in addition to those locations tested to threshold, and if a checkerboard pattern of hits and misses occurs exactly as predicted, there is a fair amount of assurance that the actual threshold corresponds relatively closely to the predicted threshold. Those intervals in which the checkerboard pattern disappears in either direction, either because of an abnormal number of hits or an abnormal number of misses, may be abnormalities or bordering on abnormalities and should be investigated further with additional threshold-seeking stimuli. The exact rationale for this approach is outlined by Koch et al[27] and rests to some extent on a mathematical discipline known as information theory. This technique has proved to be excellent in normal or nearly normal fields but is of small value in fields with extensive damage. In such fields, the majority of the field is identified as abnormal, and the advantage of speed is thus lost. For this reason, we understand, the group in Bern has abandoned this approach.

Once an area of scotoma has been identified, there are several options

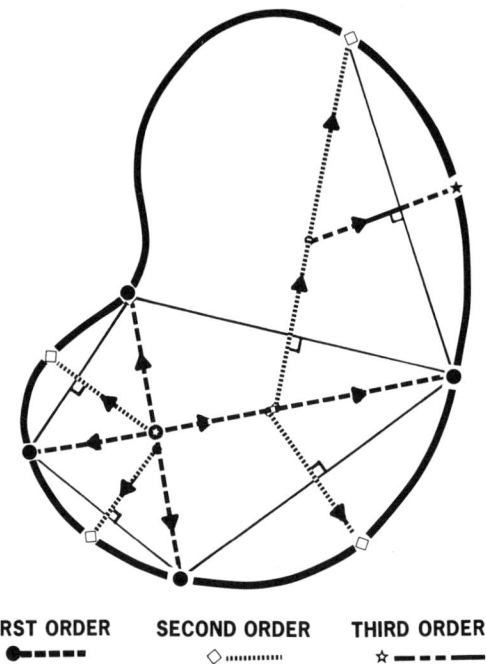

Figure 9-6 Algorithm for exploring a scotoma. Once one point within the scotoma is found (starred circle), four first-order test probes determine the first four boundary points. Again lines are drawn connecting adjacent points and second-order points are sent out along the perpendicular bisector from a point lying on the track made by one of the first-order points. Higher order boundary points are determined in an analogous fashion.

concerning how it can be plotted. Lynn and Tate[30] have outlined several methods. In the approach that is conceptually simplest, the area is simply blanketed by a grid of static tests that are tested to determine threshold, with the brightness of the floor of the scotoma serving as the starting intensity. An alternative approach utilizes kinetic perimetry to explore the scotoma. From an arbitrary starting spot within the scotoma, kinetic probes are extended up, down, right and left. The points at which these mark the edge of the scotoma are then used to construct straight lines from whence perpendicular bisectors are constructed in a manner totally analogous to the method utilized for determining the border of a peripheral isopter. The only difference is that each second-order test spot must start from a line already explored and known not to be seen by one of the first-order test spots. This scheme is illustrated in Figure 9-6. Another permissible variation is to use a circular track of radius equal to the eccentricity at the point shown to lie within a scotoma. This capitalizes on the arcuate nature of many scotomas.

SUMMARY

The field of automatic perimetry has bloomed in the last few years because of the availability of new technology in the form of more sophisticated computers and because of the heightened interest of many centers in perimetric testing. Thus, the simulation of the perimetrist by computer is economically feasible. Although some of the capabilities of the modern automatic perimeters that are now becoming available seem quite miraculous to those of us who have spent many hours slaving over a Goldmann in darkened rooms, the new technology really only scratches the surface of what will become available in the next five to ten years. Nevertheless, the ophthalmologist should be aware that, for the moment at any rate, modern automatic perimeters are capable of testing almost anyone who could be successfully tested with manual perimetry. Of course, not all patients are testable with the same system, especially if it is a rapid and efficient one. It is easy to get in the spirit of thinking that the computer will somehow take an inadequate patient and make him capable. If a person is difficult or impossible to test manually, he or she will still be difficult, if not impossible, to test automatically. Automatic perimetry offers only reproducibility, reliability, and the availability of a skilled perimetrist to those who are otherwise unable to find one. When you think about it, that is already a long and significant step.

REFERENCES

1. Aulhorn E: Über die Automatisierung der Perimetrischen Untersuchung. Die Wahl der Untersuchungsstrategie aus Augenarztlicher sicht. Biomed Tech 20:307, 1975

2. Aulhorn E, Durst W: Comparing investigation with automatic and manual perimetry in different visual field defects. International Perimetry Society Symposium, Tübingen, West Germany, 1976
3. Aulhorn H, Gauger E, Hagmeyer HT: Über die Automatisierung der Perimetrischen Untersuchung. Biomed Tech 20:309, 1975
4. Bebie H, Fankhauser F, Spahr J: Static perimetry; accuracy and fluctuations. Acta Ophthalmol 54:339, 1976
5. Bebie H, Fankhauser F, Spahr J: Static perimetry; strategies. Acta Ophthalmol 54:325, 1976
6. Blackwell HR: Studies of psychophysical methods for measuring visual thresholds. J Opt Soc Am 42:606, 1952
7. Bresky RH, Charles S: Pupil motor perimetry. Am J Ophthalmol 68:108, 1969
8. Cappin JM, Nissim S: Visual evoked responses in the assessment of field defects in glaucoma. Arch Ophthalmol 93:9, 1975
9. Chaplin GBB, Edwards JH, Geyde JL, Marlowe S: Automated system for testing visual fields. Proc IEE 120:1321, 1973
10. Cornsweet TN: The staircase-method in psychophysics. Am J Psychol 75:485, 1962
11. Drasdo N, Fowler CW: Non-linear projection of the retinal image in a wide-angle schematic eye. Br J Ophthalmol 58:709, 1974
12. Fankhauser F, Koch P, Roulier A: On automation of perimetry. Albrecht von Graefes Arch Klin Ophthalmol 184:126, 1972
13. Frisen L: The cartographic deformations of the visual field. Ophthalmologica 161:38, 1970
14. Frisen L: On objective analysis in kinetic perimetry. Acta Ophthalmol 48:1195, 1970
15. Frisen L, Frisen M: Objective recognition of abnormal isopters. Acta Ophthalmol 53:378, 1975
16. Greve EL, Groothuyse MT, Verduin WM: Automation of perimetry. Doc Ophthalmol 40:243, 1976
17. Greve EL, Verduin WM: Mass visual vield investigation in 1834 persons with supposedly normal eyes. Albrecht von Graefes Arch Klin Ophthalmol 183:286, 1972
18. Greve EL: Static perimetry. Ophthalmologica 171:26, 1975
19. Harms H: Grundlagen, Methodik und Bedeutung der Pupillenperimetrie für die Physiologie und Pathologie des Sehorgans. Albrecht von Graefe's Arch Ophthalmol 149:1, 1949
20. Harms H: Hemianopische Pupillenstarre. Klin Monatsbl Augenheilkd 118:113, 1951
21. Harms H: Möglichkeiten und Grenzen der pupillomotorischen Perimetrie. Klin Monatsbl Augenheilkd 129:518, 1956
22. Heijl A, Krakau CET: An automatic perimeter. Acta Ophthalmol 125:23, 1975
23. Heijl A, Krakau CET: An automatic perimeter for glaucoma visual field screening and control. Albrecht von Graefes Arch Klin Ophthalmol 197:13, 1975
24. Heijl A, Krakau CET: An automatic static perimeter, design and pilot study. Acta Ophthalmol 53:293, 1975
25. Heijl A: Automatic perimetry in glaucoma visual field screening. Albrecht von Graefes Arch Klin Ophthalmol 200:21, 1976

26. Jernigan ME: A new technique for objectively plotting visual fields. Ann Ophthalmol 6:335, 1974
27. Koch P, Roulier A, Fankhauser F: Perimetry; the information theoretical basis for its automation. Vision Res 12:1619, 1972
28. Lynn JR: Method for examination of visual fields. US Patent 3,644,732, issued May 23, 1972
29. Lynn JR, Tate GW: Computer controlled apparatus for automatic visual field examination. US Patent 3,883,234, issued May 13, 1975
30. Lynn JR, Tate GW: Automatic visual field examination including fixation monitoring compensation. US Patent 3,883,235, issued May 13, 1975
31. Müller W, Haase E, Henning G, Berndt R: Untersuchungen zur objektiven Perimetrie. Albrecht von Graefes Arch Klin Ophthalmol 190:329, 1974
32. Müller W, Haase E, Henning G: Vergleichende Untersuchungen von subjektiv und objektiv ermittelten Gesichtsfeldern. Albrecht von Graefes Arch Klin Ophthalmol 194:143, 1975
33. Pollack I: Methodological examination of the PEST (parametric estimation by sequential testing) procedure. Percept Psychophys 3:285, 1968
34. Spahr J: Zur Automatisierung der Perimetrie. Albrecht von Graefes Arch Klin Ophthalmol 188:323, 1973
35. Spahr J: Optimisation of the presentation pattern in automated static perimetry. Vision Res 15:1275, 1975
36. Spahr J, Fankhauser F: Automatisierung der Perimetrie. Ophthalmologica 170:106, 1975
37. Spahr J, Fankhauser F, Bebie H: Fortschritte in der Automatisierung der Perimetrie. Klin Monatsbl Augenheilkd 168:84, 1976
38. Taylor MM, Creelman CD: PEST; efficient estimates on probability functions. J Acoust Soc Am 41:782, 1967
39. Weber B, Spahr J: Automatisierung der Perimetrie. Acta Ophthalmol (kbh) 54:349, 1976

10
The Use of Perimetry: The Last Word

In the preceding nine chapters, we have presented to the reader the background in the underlying physics, psychophysics, and art that go into creating good, useful visual fields. At this point, it is probably appropriate to give the reader some insight into how visual fields may be useful in managing a chronic disease. Since both authors have an interest in glaucoma, and since glaucoma is the most common indication for quantitative visual fields, we have chosen to present a brief scheme of how to manage glaucoma in the form of a flow chart (Fig. 10-1). This flow chart is somewhat schematic and has the sin of brevity in that it ignores other possible diagnoses and fails to explore the details of therapy. These sins would be mortal if this were a treatise on the care of glaucoma rather than one on the use of visual fields. Nevertheless, it does illustrate the principle of how visual fields may be useful, and we ask that the flow chart be viewed in that light and its shortcomings, if not overlooked, forgiven.

The patient enters the chart in Block 1 with an initial workup of applanation tensions, visual fields, and stereo photographs of the disc. For the purpose of this discussion, it is assumed that the pressure will be over 20 and the chamber angles open, so that the patient has either ocular hypertension (no visual field defects) or primary open-angle glaucoma in some stage of development. This decision is made in Block 2. If the patient has a visual field defect, the field is then used to determine how much damage has been done (Block 7). If the field defects are massive, the patient is put on enough medical therapy to lower intraocular pressure to below 20, if possible. If it is possible to get the pressure below 20 (Block 8), we feel it is a good idea to check diurnal pressure curves to find out if there are any periods of diurnal pressure elevation or depression. If there are elevations (Block 9), the medication should be adjusted so that the peaks are abolished. If the pressure is found to be low during certain times of day or night, cumulative toxicity of therapy can be diminished by discontinuing or decreasing therapy at those times. If the intraocular pressure can be significantly lowered—but not to below 20—or once the medication regimen is adjusted so that the peaks are as level as possible with the medications that can be tolerated, one then repeats the fields frequently to follow the patient. At this point, it is essential to know if the change in visual fields has stabilized (Block 10). If it has, one simply continues on the current regimen and continues to follow the patient. If it has not, the physician must determine if the patient is on maximum tolerable medications. If the physician feels that there is room for an increase in therapy or a change in therapy is likely to be productive, then this change is made and the patient is again followed through a loop that leads to Block 5. If the patient is determined to be on maximum tolerable medications, then surgery is indicated. Obviously, if the visual field defects in Block 10 are not stable, and if the patient is already on maximum medications, the patient will end up in the same spot.

On the other hand, it there is no visual field defect at the beginning in Block 2, one then checks at Block 3 to learn whether there are any risk factors, as outlined in Chapter 8. If in the physician's opinion the patient is at risk from his intraocular pressure, an attempt should be made to lower the intraocular pressure with the minimum amount of medication possible to achieve a reasonable level. In such a patient, lowering the intraocular pressure about 4 to 6 mm of mercury is probably a significant change in pressure and may or may not arrest progression. Whether risk factors are present or not, one arrives at Block 4. If the disc is easily followable, that is, if it is not overhanging or not too deeply cupped (for us, a cup/disc ratio that is less than about 0.6), then it is probably acceptable to follow disc photos predominantly and do fields less often. If the disc cannot be easily followed, then the fields form the predominant means of following the patient, although the disc must never be ignored. Once again, this logic has been given in Chapter 8.

Regardless of the method one uses to follow the patient, one arrives at Block 5 again, just as in the last path. The same logic of increasing medication or resorting to surgery if field change continues is followed. Obviously, once surgery is performed (Block 11), the patient must still be followed in a similar fashion, because the surgery may not produce a sufficient lowering of pressure to accomplish the goal of arresting field loss.

There is absolutely nothing magical about this scheme. Ignoring that it makes no provision for such entities as low-tension glaucoma, secondary glaucomas, or a disease (other than glaucoma) that mimics glaucoma, it is purely the common-sense approach that most practitioners already follow, to a greater or lesser extent. The point is that, for us, most of the therapeutic decisions are based on the *stability* of the visual field, or the lack thereof. In our clinic, we are blessed with high-quality fields, and therefore feel perfectly secure in trusting

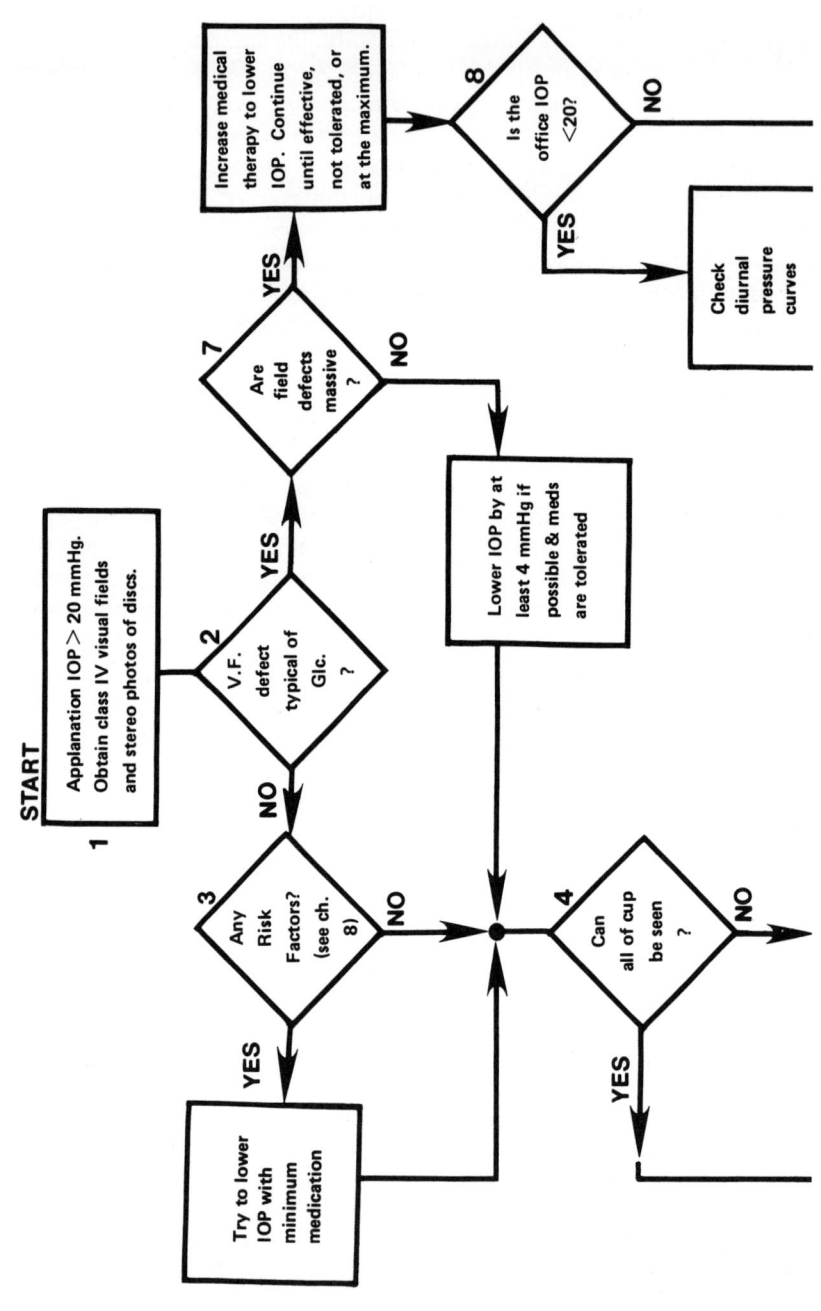

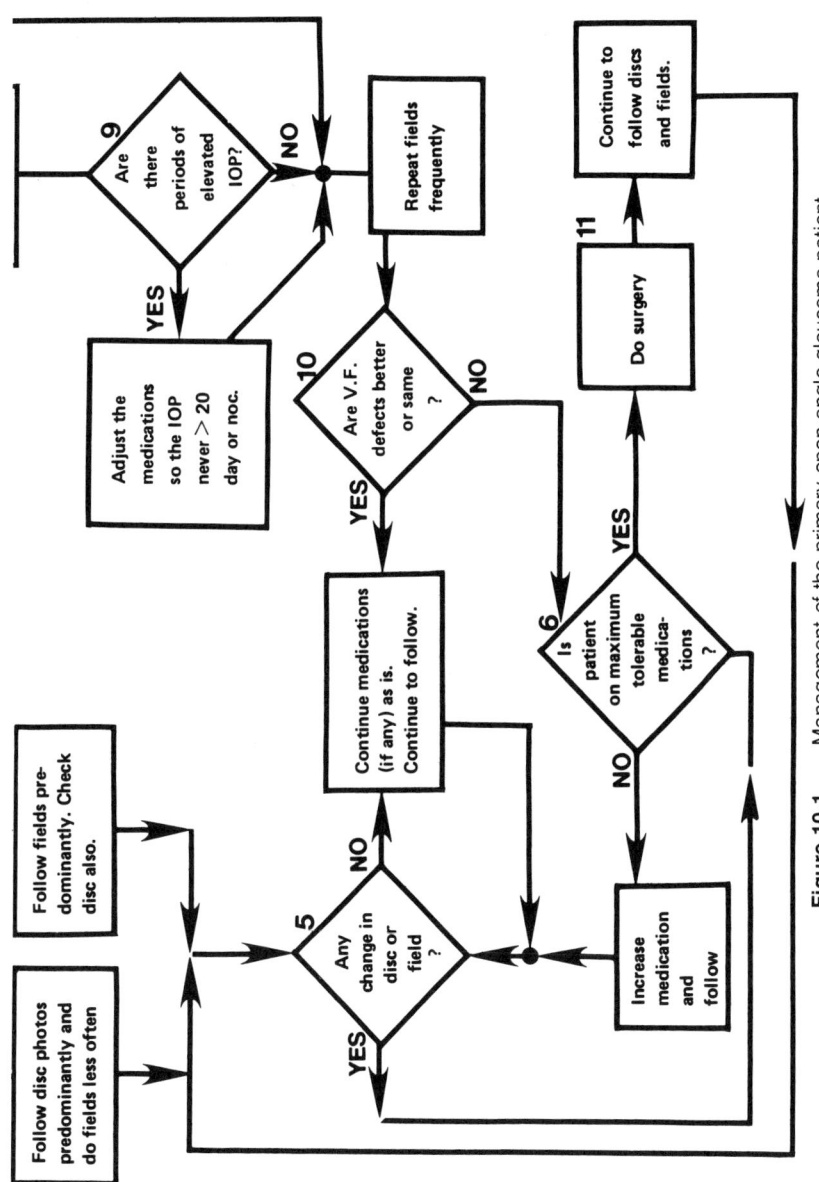

Figure 10-1 Management of the primary open-angle glaucoma patient.

them and in managing the patient accordingly. We are also painfully aware that this is not the case in many other offices for we can remember from our training periods many a patient around whom several residents and staff members would stand and sort through a sheaf of visual fields that looked like they were gathered from ten different patients. As they tried to decide whether or not there was sufficient change to recommend surgery, the patient's vision slipped slowly and irretrievably away. Those visual fields were of absolutely no use to anyone. They cost the patient money, they caused confusion and insecurity for the physician, and they wasted the time of the person who did them. The point of the discussion is simply this: if one wishes to use visual fields to follow the patient with chronic ocular disease, they can certainly be a potent and helpful aid in many cases. But the moment the word "follow" instead of "diagnose" is used, a whole new ball game is begun. Fields that are done sloppily with insufficient isopters and insufficient control of a host of variables that have been enumerated at length earlier in the book, are almost as bad as no fields at all, and if they signal improvement falsely, they are far worse. Granted, the maintenance of the machine and the repeated calibrations are a continuing effort that can seem overwhelming when the physician himself tries to do the test and see thirty or more patients a day as well. To spend an hour or more doing a visual field on a difficult patient while those patients still waiting grow even more irate, is indeed a very poor expenditure of physician time. For this reason, we advocate that either a perimetry technician be hired, trained, and continuously monitored or the physician consider an automatic perimeter as preferred alternatives to neglecting good visual field exams entirely. Granted, visual fields are not spectacular money-makers, and patients do not always enjoy or appreciate them. But they do enable the physician to measure the damage to the patient's vision in a quantitative fashion, and it is this damage that is the bottom line of many diseases, such as glaucoma, rather than any other variable, such as intraocular pressure. The physicians who take the time to become skilled in this art will find not only that the quality of their patient care has improved but also that their sense of security in managing difficult patients has increased. Their patients will have the benefit of neither being needlessly overtreated nor denied stronger medication or surgery when the need is clearly there. Practicing the best medicine possible is always an effort, but it is also what our profession is all about.

Appendices

Appendix A

The Criterion Effect and Signal Detection Theory

Ira H. Bernstein

One of the most basic and important points about a perimetric examination (or, for that matter, any other type of medical examination) is that the results provide only indirect evidence about what a patient actually sees or experiences. And the results that one obtains are influenced potentially by several spurious variables that have nothing to do with the state of health of a patient's visual system. Here we will describe one such spurious influence, the *criterion effect.*

The criterion effect refers to differences in the willingness of patients to report that a target was seen—which is quite independent of how healthy the eye is—and how those differences affect estimates of the patients' thresholds. More specifically, it refers to how differences in the willingness to respond affirmatively (or, conversely, negatively) to an examiner's questions affect the results of a visual field test.

To understand the concept of a criterion effect, consider the incidence of reported symptoms when a patient is being given a physical examination prior to (1) being drafted into the armed services versus (2) being evaluated medically for a job the patient greatly desires. More than likely, far more symptoms will be reported in the former case. This obviously has nothing necessarily to do with the actual differences in the health of a person who is facing conscription rather than the employment he wishes. The difference in incidence of reported symptoms indicates instead that a person has something to gain by reporting symptoms in the former situation (he may be given a physical exemption), whereas in the latter situation he has something to lose (he may be judged to be physically unqualified). The difference is not simply due to "lying" in any denotative meaning of the word. Rather, it is due to the ambiguity created for the patient by the test situation, an ambiguity that cannot be totally ignored by the medical examiner in either case. This situation is especially true in perimetry. Seeing versus not seeing a target is not a direct, physical all-or-none situation.

Some readers may be tempted to conclude that the ambiguity we describe is inevitable in any life situation where verbal or subjective data are used and that such data are unquantifiable in any meaningful way. We will argue, on the contrary, that such a conclusion can be shown to be incorrect. Let us begin by drawing a basic distinction and noting its logical consequences.

In order to consider how well a patient can, in fact, see a target of a specific nature, say a Goldmann test object I-4-e under specified test conditions, we must distinguish between the patient's *sensitivity* (sensory capacity) and his *criterion* (bias or willingness to report the presence of the target). We must also recognize that these two influences *jointly* determine what data one will obtain. The theory of signal detection offers a detailed and useful treatment of this topic, to which John Swets, Wilson Tanner, Jr., and Theodore Birdsall have provided a sound and basic introduction.

One of the articles by Swets, Tanner, and Birdsall[4] is entitled "Decision Processes in Perception." The key word in the title is "decision." As an ophthalmologist, one must realize that data concerning visual functioning are influenced by a patient's decision making as well as the state of his or her visual system. The terms "decisional" and "criterion effect" can be used with nearly equal interchangeability in the present context.

As an introduction to the topic, we will present the example of a decision-making game that these authors used to illustrate some important concepts in statistical decision making. The game involves the rolling of three dice. Two are ordinary in the sense that the sides contain the numbers 1 through 6. The third is different. It contains the number 0 on three sides and the number 3 on the remaining three sides. You are given the sum of the three numbers and are asked to say whether the third or *special* die was a 0 or a 3.

A moment's reflection will tell you that the outcomes can vary from a sum of 2 (the two ordinary die each are 1 and the special die is 0) through 15 (the two ordinary dice each are 6 and the special die is 3). Some outcomes leave no doubt as to the state of the third die. If the sum is 2, 3, or 4, the special die must be a 0, since the minimum outcome of the ordinary die is 2 and the sum of all three when the special one is a 3 must therefore be at least 5. Likewise, if the sum is 13, 14, or 15, the special die must therefore be 3, since the two ordinary dice cannot sum to more than 12.

Any outcome between 5 and 12, however, leaves you in doubt. Suppose the sum were 5. This could be produced because the special die is a 0 and the other two are a 2 and a 3, a 3 and a 2, a 4 and a 1, or a 1 and a 4. (If you have difficulty seeing why there are four rather than two combinations, imagine one of the ordinary dice is red and the other is green; thus we may have the result that red equals 3 and green equals 2 *or* the result that red equals 2 and green equals 3, etc.) But a 5 can be obtained because the special die is 3 and the other two dice are each 1. Although a 5 can be produced when the special die is either 3 or 0,

The Criterion Effect and Signal Detection Theory

there are four times as many ways it can come about when the third die is 0; we can therefore say that the odds favoring the outcome that the special die is a 0 are 4:1 (or, alternatively, the odds favoring the outcome that the special die is a 3 are 1:4).

Your task in the dice throwing situation is to convert the *sum* which you are given to a *yes-no* (binary) decision. ("Yes" will be assumed to correspond to the judgment that a 3 was thrown and "no" to the judgment that a 0 was thrown on the special die, although the reverse could be assumed with no loss of generality.) In signal detection terms, this corresponds to converting your perception of the sum into a decision as to whether a *signal* was present above and beyond the random effects of the ordinary dice, called *noise*. To do so requires a *decision rule*.

In order to consider what decision rule might be used to take one of a set of outcomes (the numbers 2 through 15) and convert it into a "yes" or "no" answer, we need to consider the probabilities of the various outcomes. These have been presented in Table A-1. We will let x denote the observed sum. The second column in the table, symbolized "P(x/0)," is the probability of obtaining that sum given that the third die is in fact a 0. Note that the two other dice can be combined in 36 different ways since each of the two dice can fall in 6 different ways. We therefore divide the number of different ways the two normal dice can

x	P(x/0)	P(x/3)	$L(3) = \dfrac{P(x/3)}{P(x/0)}$	FAR	HR
2	1/36	0	0/1 (0)	36/36	36/36
3	2/36	0	0/2 (0)	35/36	36/36
4	3/36	0	0/3 (0)	33/36	36/36
5	4/36	1/36	1/4	30/36	36/36
6	5/36	2/36	2/5	26/36	35/36
7	6/36	3/36	3/6	21/36	33/36
8	5/36	4/36	4/5	15/36	30/36
9	4/36	5/36	5/4	10/36	26/36
10	3/36	6/36	6/3	6/36	21/36
11	2/36	5/36	5/2	3/36	15/36
12	1/36	4/36	4/1	1/36	10/36
13	0	3/36	3/0 (∞)	0/36	6/36
14	0	2/36	2/0 (∞)	0/36	3/36
15	0	1/36	1/0 (∞)	0/36	1/36

Table A-1 Dice game example. Probabilities of the various outcomes, x (the sum of the spots on the three dice), given that the special die was a 0, P(x/0), and that the special die was a 3, P(x/3); the likelihood of a 3, $L(3) = P(x/3)/P(x/0)$; the hit rates (HR), and the alse alarm rates (FAR).

fall by 36 to obtain the probability that they will fall that way. The third column, symbolized "P(x/3)," is the corresponding probability of obtaining that sum given that the special die is in fact a 3.

The fourth column, symbolized "L(3x)" is the likelihood of a 3 given the sum, x. It is obtained by dividing the value of P(x/3) by P(x/0). In this example, where it is just as probable that a 0 will be thrown as a 3, this quantity is the "odds" in favor of a 3.

A key point is that as x increases from 2 to 15, the values of L(3x) increase from 0 to infinity. In other words, the larger the value of x, the more the odds favor the occurrence of a 3 for the third die. Under these conditions, it can be shown that the best thing a person can do is to choose a value of x and answer "yes" if the observed sum is equal to that number or higher and answer "no" if the observed sum is less than that number. This value of x is called the *criterion value*. (Note that we could also state the decision rule so that a person says "yes" only when the x that is observed is larger than the criterion value and respond "no" when it is equal to or less than the criterion value and wind up with the same results.)

Since any given value of x between 5 and 12 inclusive can arise when the special die is a 3 (signal plus noise) or a 0 (noise alone), the person in this game must make errors. One way to describe his performance is to obtain the probability he will say "yes," given that the third die is a 3, which is called the *hit rate*, as well as the probability he will say "yes," given that the third die is a 0, which is called the *false alarm rate*. Note that we do not need to compute the probability that the person will respond "no" to a 0, the *miss rate*, separately, since it is 1.0 minus the hit rate; nor the probability that the person will respond "no" to a 3, the *correct rejection rate*, since it is 1.0 minus the false alarm rate. The fifth and sixth columns of Table A-1 contain the hit and false alarm rates. Note that the hit rate is obtained by adding the values of P(x/3) from the criterion value of x in question through 15 in this example, and the false alarm rates are obtained by adding the corresponding values of P(x/0).

Any value of x can serve as a criterion value. However, if the economic consequences of the four outcomes and the probability of signal are defined, one value will serve to maximize a person's winnings. This value of x is called the *maximum expected value criterion*.

In order to understand this concept, let us actually convert this game into a betting situation. Suppose I agree to pay you $1.00 for every hit and correct rejection, and charge you $1.00 for every miss and false alarm (this is called a *symmetric* payoff). Under these conditions, it can be shown that a criterion value of 9 will maximize your winnings. You will say "yes" on 72% of the trials on which a 3 is thrown and on 28% of the trials on which a 0 is thrown (your hit and false alarm rates, respectively, which may be found in Table A-1). You will therefore have miss and correct rejection rates of 28% and 72%. Your expected outcome on any one trial is the sum of these probabilities times their respective reward or penalty. This equals (.72 × +$1.00) for hits + (.28 × −$1.00) for false alarms + (.28 × −$1.00) for misses + (.72 × +$1.00) for correct rejections. This equals an outcome of +$.88 a trial. You may wish to verify that this is the maximum expected value by using the hit and false alarm rates from Table A-1 for another criterion value. For example, a criterion value of 6 will limit your expected gain to +$.50 a trial. Note that the difference in expected winnings for a criterion value of 6 and one of 9 is *not* one of quality of the information that you have to go by in making a decision; it is identical in both cases. Rather, it represents a difference in how that information is used.

Suppose we change the bet by charging you $5.00 for a false alarm while leaving the other payoffs as they were. What should you do to maximize your winnings? The answer is to say "yes" less often by adopting a higher criterion value (12 to be exact, since its expected value of $.39 a trial is a maximum). Conversely, if the reward for a hit were $5.00 and the other payoffs were $1.00, you should say "yes" more often by adopting a lower criterion example (6 for a payoff of $4.39 a trial). Likewise, if a signal were more probable, e.g., four faces of the special die had the 3s, the rational thing to do is to say "yes" more often and vice versa if a signal were less probable, e.g., only two sides had a 3. In short, a rational individual is sensitive to the economics and the prior odds (outcome probabilities in the absence of information like x). There is no reason to believe that a patient would act any differently when confronted with ambiguous information, a point to which we will return after completing our discussion of this dice game.

In Figure A-1 we have plotted the distribution of P(x/0) and P(x/3). (This is adapted from a similar figure that appears in Swets, Tanner, and Birdsall.) This illustrates the concepts of the noise and signal plus noise. That is, the various probabilities of respective distributions given the special die of 0 and 3. Note that the signal plus noise distribution is, in this case, simply a shifting over of noise distribution by 3 units. In figure A-2 we have presented what is called a receiver operating characteristic curve (ROC curve) by plotting hit rate along the y-axis and false alarm rate along the x-axis. Though this does not make the relation between P(x/3) and x and between P(x/0) and x as explicit as Figure A-1 does, it does have a very important property. Each point on the ROC curve describes the outcome (in hit and false alarm rates) obtained with an unchanging ability to discriminate between the two states of nature (3 and 0 in the dice-throwing example) but different criteria for reporting "yes." As Table A-1 illustrates, a hit rate of 10/36 and a false alarm rate of 1/36 (which obtains when a person says "yes" to a value of x that is 12 or more) is neither better nor worse than a hit rate of 33/36 and a false alarm rate of 31/36, which is obtained with a criterion of 7.

You may note that the ability to discriminate between the two alternatives is

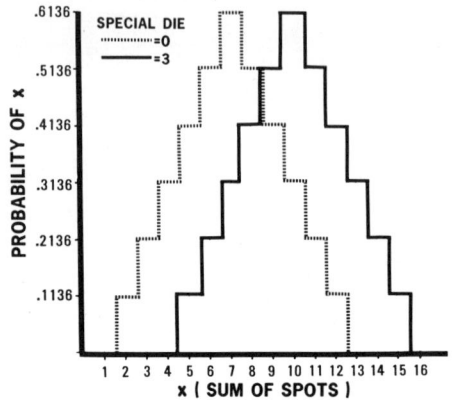

Figure A-1 The probability distribution of x (the sum of the spots on the three dice) when the special die is a 0 (dotted lines) and when the special die is a 3 (solid lines).

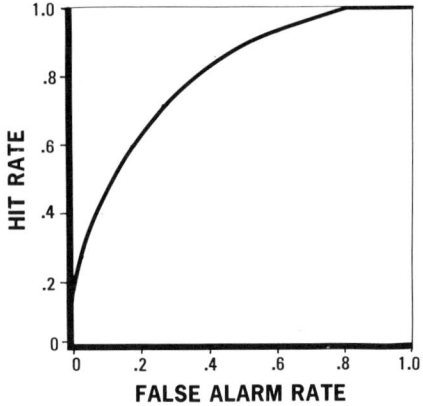

Figure A-2 The receiver operating characteristic (ROC) curve (hit rate as a function of false alarm rate) obtained from the data of Table A-1.

inversely related to the overlap of the two distributions. Consider a change in our dice-throwing example in which the signal is equal to 1 rather than 3. This has been plotted in Figure A-3, where it can be seen that the signal plus noise distribution is shifted over 1 rather than 3 units from the noise distribution. Note, however, that if a person adopts a criterion of 8, for example, in this latter case he will have a hit rate of 21/36. This is the same hit rate obtained with a criterion of 10 in the first-named problem. It illustrates the *criterion effect* as an apparent increase in performance (hit rate) caused solely by a shift in criterion. The difference is that a person could obtain a hit rate of 21/36 and a false alarm rate

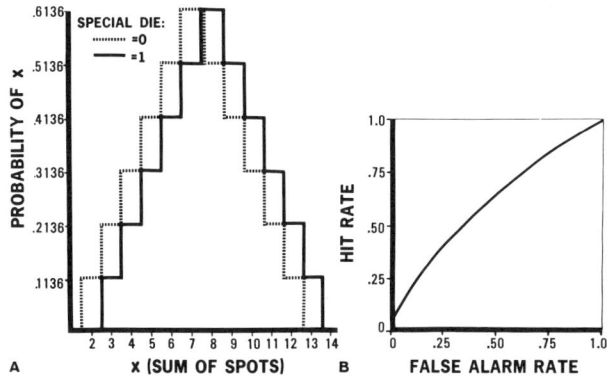

Figure A-3 **A** The probability distribution of x (the sum of the spots on the three dice) when the special die is a 0 (dashed lines) or a 1 (solid lines). **B** The receiver operating characteristic (ROC) curve corresponding to these data.

of only 6/36 when the special die was 3, whereas he would obtain a false alarm rate of 15/36 when the special die is a 1 in the new problem. What this tells us is that a hit rate by itself is insufficient; it needs to be associated with a false alarm rate to determine whether any difference between testings is due to a change in sensitivity (change in overlap of the distributions) versus a change in criterion (change in location of the criterion value). In any situation, a subject can obtain a hit rate of any desired amount by a suitable choice of criterion. A patient's perceptual capabilities are thus insufficiently indexed by a single quantity like the hit rate; the hit rate needs to be specified relative to the false alarm rate in order to control for the effects of differences that are to be attributed to the criterion.

How this may be done is a topic of some discussion. One fairly simple pair of measures to obtain as indices of sensitivity and bias are the eta (η) and beta (β) measures, respectively.[3] The quantity eta equals the square root of the product of the false alarm and miss rates (the product of probabilities of the two types of error) divided by the product of the hit and correct rejection rates (the product of the two types of correct decisions). Thus:

$$\eta = \sqrt{\frac{\text{false alarm} \times \text{miss rate}}{\text{hit rate} \times \text{correction rejection rate}}} = \sqrt{\frac{\text{false alarm rate} \times (1 - \text{hit rate})}{(1 - \text{false alarm rate}) \times \text{hit rate}}}$$

The quantity beta is the square root of the ratio of the product of the miss and correct rejection rates (the product of the two probabilities of saying "no") to the product of the hit and false alarm rates (the product of the two probabilities of saying "yes"):

$$\beta = \sqrt{\frac{\text{miss rate} \times \text{correction rejection rate}}{\text{hit rate} \times \text{false alarm rate}}} = \sqrt{\frac{(1 - \text{hit rate}) \times (1 - \text{false alarm rate})}{\text{hit rate} \times \text{false alarm rate}}}$$

There are other alternatives, but a discussion of these is beyond the scope of this appendix. A point to remember when using the eta index is that it is a measure of overlap or similarity of noise and signal plus noise distributions. The larger its value, the *poorer* performance is. A person who is just guessing will have an eta equal to 1.0. Likewise, beta is a measure of the tendency to say "no." It will equal 1.0 when a person is as likely to say "yes" as "no." This is called a *symmetric criterion* (which would be obtained in the case of Fig. A-1 and A-3 if the criterion were at the point of intersection of the two distributions).

Having considered this dice-throwing game as an introduction to decision making, we will now turn to a situation similar to ones that are commonly employed in psychophysical laboratories. An individual is told that a dim flash of light will be presented to the fovea on a randomly selected half of the trials and will not be presented on the remaining half. He is told to say "yes" or "no" accordingly. Although the individual attempts to be as accurate as possible, the low level of stimulus input prevents him from being perfectly accurate. What will happen (and you might wish to perform this experiment on yourself to get a better feel for what we are describing) is that the sensations produced will vary widely on trials in which the flash is presented (your instincts may be to assume incorrectly that the equipment is malfunctioning), and they will also vary quite widely on those trials in which the flash is not presented. Indeed, you will feel more certain that a flash was present on some no-flash trials than on some trials on which a flash was actually present. In short, the flash, though it is of constant magnitude, is superimposed upon a random process. Just as in our dice-throwing game, the *average* sensation evoked by the signal will be greater than the *average* sensation evoked by noise alone. However, trial-to-trial variation makes the concept of overlapping distributions that is central to signal detection theory applicable to any situation in which there is a difficult-to-detect stimulus present.

The concept of a threshold was introduced centuries ago to describe the minimal amount of stimulation needed to see (hear, feel, etc.) a target under specified conditions. Because statistical fluctuations in the magnitude of threshold estimates have also been known for a long time, it became customary in psychophysics to define the threshold as that target energy that can be seen half the time. (More generally, the threshold can be applied to the judgment of stimulus difference, but we are concerned here only with a threshold obtained by judging a stimulus relative to the absence of stimulation.)

The concept of a threshold needs to be sharply differentiated from that of a criterion. A threshold is generally conceived of as a biological limit. A criterion is a cognitive concept and can be varied at will in most situations. Moreover, any threshold measure is of limited utility in the absence of false alarm rate specification. The proper form of specification is to ask the question, "How intense must a stimulus be in order to evoke a hit rate of, say, 0.5 while evoking a false alarm rate of, say, 0.1?" Even so, any definition of threshold will be arbitrary since we could just as well define it as a hit rate of 0.6 and a false alarm rate of 0.01. To repeat, any attempt to define how well the visual system functions without at least an implicit notion of the criterion used to obtain the result is meaningless!

One of the major problems that we hope is apparent to the reader is that data obtained in a clinical situation do not provide any estimates of false alarm rate and hence the patient's criterion is unassessed. As a matter of fact, since a given target is rarely presented at the same meridian more than once, the probabilistic nature of the situation is typically not apparent. The point that differences obtained during two testing sessions may reflect differences in response criteria as well as changes in patient's condition needs to be understood even though it is quite difficult to decide between them. (The two are not exclusive; a patient may get worse and adopt a different criterion.)

In our dice-throwing example, we used a very unrealistic example of how noise is statistically distributed. The outcome of rolling dice is conceptually simple and the quantities may be verified easily. However, it is somewhat more realistic to assume that the shapes of the distributions are normal (Gaussian or bell-shaped) and that the signal plus noise distribution has greater variance (more spread) than the noise distribution. The mathematics of this model, as well as numerous others that are evaluated by signal detection theorists for application to various situations, may be found in various sources.[1-3]

A situation illustrative of this unequal variance-Gaussian model, which also illustrates how signal detection theory may be applied to biological measures, is as follows. Assume that you were trying to diagnose whether or not each of a number of people had an infection, using only their temperature as diagnostic information. A sample of normal people would yield a spread of temperatures about an average of 98.6°F (37°C). These people comprise the noise distribution. The temperature of people with the infection in question would in general be elevated. However, a person whose normal temperature runs low and who had only a mild infection might also have a normal temperature. Because the effects of the infection are not constant from person to person, the signal plus noise distribution would be more variable than the noise distribution. This situation is illustrated in Figure A-4. The left-hand side contains the distributions; the right-hand side the ROC curves that can be derived. The point is that your ability to decide whether a person is normal or infected is imperfect because people from both classes are represented at any given temperature. As you get more and more data (white cell count, etc.), a combined measure allows better dis-

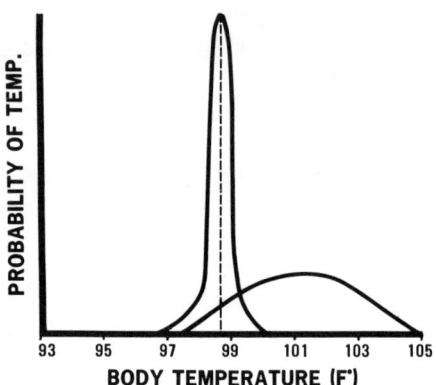

Figure A-4 Hypothetical distributions of body temperatures for normals and people with infections.

crimination (less overlap), but no matter what the outcome, so long as the distributions overlap, errors of diagnosis will occur. The adequacy of the diagnostic procedure here, as in the previous example, cannot be stated in terms of the hit rate alone (percentage of sick people so identified) but also requires false alarm data (percentage of normals identified as sick).

Thus far, we have shown that a given hit rate can be obtained in any situation albeit at the cost of different false alarm rates, depending upon the difficulty of the discrimination. We have also shown how different criteria lead to different hit and false alarm rates even though the underlying data are the same. In addition, we have shown how an explicit payoff and prior odds lead to an optimal criterion value in the sense of one that makes the most money for the individual given the information at hand. What we have not considered, and what is important for any medical situation, is what happens when there is no explicit payoff. The result is that the patient creates a payoff *implicitly* based upon his perception of the situation to establish his criterion. The criterion of course can vary from situation to situation and is what underlies the probable difference in incidence of reported symptoms discussed early in this appendix. The social interaction between patient and physician will determine the former's perception of the payoffs. For example, most patients evaluate false alarms more negatively than they do misses since the former are associated with "hallucinations," the latter merely with understandable lapses of attention.

We may summarize the role of signal detection theory as follows. The ophthalmologist should be aware that any form of diagnostic data is fallible and criterion effects are an important source of fallibility. In particular, the ophthalmologist should be sensitive to the possibility that changes in a patient's fields (or any other test) between successive testing may or may not reflect any real change in those conditions that are of medical interest. A patient's behavior and that of the ophthalmologist are governed by decisional rules and the perceived consequences of those rules.

REFERENCES

1. Egan JP: Signal Detection Theory and ROC Analysis. New York, Academic Press, 1975
2. Green DM, Swets JA: Signal Detection Theory and Psychophysics. New York, Wiley, 1966; reprinted, New York, Krieger, 1974
3. Luce RD: Detection and recognition, in Luce RD, Bush RR, Galanter E (eds): Handbook of Mathematical Psychology, vol 1. New York, Wiley, 1963
4. Swets JA, Tanner WP, Birdsall TG: Decision processes in perception. Psychol Rev 68:301, 1961
5. Tanner WP, Swets JA: A decision-making theory of visual detection. Psychol Rev 61:401, 1954

Appendix B

The Differential Diagnosis of Visual Field Defects

The following is a list of various types of visual field defects that may be found, along with the major causes of each of them.

I. Prechiasmal Patterns

Defect	Differential Diagnosis	Comment and Associated Defects

A. Nerve fiber bundle defects include:
Bjerrum (arcuate) scotoma*
Paracentral scotoma
Baring of blind spot
Nasal step of Rönne
Vertical step of Lynn
Ring (double Bjerrum)
Central and temporal visual islands
	A. The lesion may be as far posterior as the chiasm.
	  1. Lesions of retina and papilla
	    a. Glaucoma
	    b. Juxtapapillary choroiditis
	    c. Myopia with peripapillary atrophy
	    d. Coloboma of disc
	    e. Optic pits
	    f. Papilledema, and optic atrophy secondary to increased intracranial pressure
	    g. Drusen of optic disc
	    h. Papillitis
	    i. Retinal arterial plaques on disc
	    j. Occlusion of branches of central retinal artery
	  2. Anterior optic nerve
	    a. Ischemic infarct and segmental atrophy secondary to vascular disease
	    b. Carotid or ophthalmic artery occlusion
	    c. Cranial arteritis
	    d. Retrobulbar neuritis
	    e. Electric shock
	    f. Exophthalmos
		A. Glaucoma is more frequent than all other causes combined.
		– See Harrington[2] for additional information on DDx.
		– Lesions in optic nerve usually include a central scotoma, but not invariably.
		– Lesions involving dorsum sellae or pituitary most typically have other presentations.
		– Always suspect vertical step as a pathway (not retinal) lesion.
		– In glaucoma, look for small hemorrhages on disc, which herald the appearance of sector field defects. See Drance and Begg.[1]

*Other synonyms for arcuate scotoma include Seidel, cuneate, scimitar, and comet scotomas. Most of these terms are obsolete.

I. Prechiasmal Patterns

Defect	Differential Diagnosis	Comment and Associated Defects

	3. Posterior optic nerve and chiasm
	   a. Meningioma of optic foramen or dorsum sellae
	   b. Pituitary adenoma
	   c. Opticochiasmatic arachnoiditis	

B. Constricted visual field	B. 1. Glaucoma
	2. Refractive problems (central only)
	   a. Incorrect basic refraction
	   b. Incorrect addition for age and refraction
	   c. Cataract
	   d. Decrease in corneal transparency
	3. Small pupil, especially with cataract
	4. Age
	5. "Functional" patient problems
	   a. Lack of orientation or experience with test
	   b. Slow reaction time
	   c. Malingering or hysteria
	6. Retinitis pigmentosa (see F-2)
	7. Central retinal vein occlusion
	8. Endocrine exophthalmos
		B. – Refractive problems affect central field more than periphery in general.
		– The small pupil is particularly troublesome with glaucoma or ocular hypertensive patients who have just been started on miotic therapy. Thus, should obtain baseline fields both before and within one month after starting this therapy.
		– In patients with very slow reaction times, etc., also moving the target from seeing to nonseeing may verify problem by intrasopter disparity at $10°$ or more. When this occurs, etiology is "functional."
		– Syphilis may simulate a wide variety of problems, including glaucoma, chiasmatic or postchiasmatic lesions.
		– Toxic amblyopia may cause

9. Syphilitic optic atrophy 10. Postneuritic optic atrophy 11. Congenitally small optic nerve 12. Drusen of disc 13. Toxic amblyopia 14. Orbital tumors compressing optic nerve 15. Total retinal detachment 16. Opticochiasmatic arachnoiditis 17. Posthemorrhagic optic atrophy 18. Midline occipital tumors with only macular function remaining	peripheral constriction, central scotoma or both. — Total retinal detachments partially inhibit function before evident destruction. The smaller and dimmer the test object that is visible preop, the better the prognosis for visual function after surgery.

C. Irregular or solitary field defects

C. 1. Diabetic retinopathy 2. Hematologic and vascular diseases (many) 3. Chorioretinitis, various etiologies 4. Sickle cell retinopathy 5. Trauma 6. Tumor 7. Nevi 8. Eales disease 9. Myopic degeneration 10. Opticochiasmatic arachnoiditis	C. — Size, shape, and slope of lesion correspond to the size, shape, and activity of fundus lesion. — Nevi may show no defects unless carefully searched for by static techniques. Malignant tumors (e.g., melanoma) usually show a larger scotoma than the area occupied by the tumor because of surrounding zone of subretinal fluid.

D. Peripheral defects

D. 1. Retinal detachment 2. Tumor with or without retinal detachment 3. Retinoschisis	D. — Retinoschisis shows an absolute cut with smooth, sharp, steep margins, most commonly nasal in the field, temporal in the fundus.

I. Prechiasmal Patterns

Defect	Differential Diagnosis	Comment and Associated Defects
	4. Trauma 5. Cranial arteritis 6. Myopic degeneration 7. Hysteria 8. Pterygium 9. Cataract 10. Miscellaneous (see Sect. I-C)	– Untreated retinal detachment shows a relative defect from the periphery with a shallow slope, (unless due to a giant tear with "foldover") or interlacing of red and blue color isopters. Retinal detachments due to tumor have steeper slope than rhegmatogenous detachments and often do not extend completely to periphery. – Cranial arteritis may cause central scotoma, peripheral sector defects or arcuate scotoma.

E. Central scotoma including centrocecal scotoma	E. 1. Maculopathies, various etiologies
	2. Optic neuritis
	   a. retrobulbar neuritis
	   b. optic papillitis
	3. Toxic amblyopia
	4. Vascular
	   a. Venous occlusions
	   b. Cranial arteritis
	   c. Occlusion of cilioretinal artery
	5. Myopic degeneration
	6. Papilledema (esp. chronic)
		E – Central scotoma is often combined with sector defects in venous occlusions, due to macular edema, and is most common in superior temporal branch vein occlusions. The incidence of pre-existing glaucoma in branch vein occlusions is about 20%. Many eyes with venous occlusion also develop neovascular glaucoma.
		– The ambylopia of pernicious anemia, tobacco amblyopia, Leber's atrophy, and nutritional amblyopia are

7. Trauma
8. Nutritional amblyopia
9. Pernicious anemia amblyopia
10. Hereditary optic atrophy (Leber)
11. Pituitary tumor
12. Compression of optic nerve by tumor
13. Opticochiasmatic arachnoiditis
14. Total retinal detachment after repair
15. Optic pits

thought to be due to a failure to detoxify cyanide. Treatment with B-group vitamins, including hydroxycobalamine, may be helpful.
— With optic neuritis, may have Marcus Gunn pupil, pain on movement of eye, and disc edema (papillitis). It may be associated with demyelinating disease, diabetes mellitus, syphilis, arachnoiditis, acute viral infections, sinusitis, puberty, pregnancy, lactation, and menopause, among others. It is idiopathic in the majority of cases.
— Pituitary tumors may cause small, bitemporal central scotomas as their presenting sign which may be confused with the above defects.

F. Arcuate, ring, or sector defects not following nerve fiber bundle pattern

F. 1. Chloroquine toxicity
2. Retinitis pigmentosa (early)
3. Artifact due to lens holder
4. Trauma
5. Compression of nerve (e.g.: tumor, etc.)
6. Vascular occlusion

F. True or pseudoretinitis pigmentosa has been reported in Ushers syndrome, Bassen-Kornzweig syndrome, Kern-Sayers syndrome, Lawrence-Moon-Biedl syndrome, status dysraphicus, Friedreich's ataxia, Refsum's syndrome, Leber's amaurosis, myotonic dystrophy, Hurlers syndrome, postviral (esp. rubeola, rubella, and cytomegalic inclusion disease), and postsyphilitic neuroretinitis and drug toxicities.

I. Prechiasmal Patterns

Defect	Differential Diagnosis	Comment and Associated Defects
G. Enlargement of blind spot	G. 1. Glaucoma 2. Medullated nerve fibers 3. Coloboma of Disc 4. Myopia 5. Papilledema 6. Drusen of disc 7. Pseudopapilledema 8. Juxtapapillary choroiditis 9. Posterior ectasial or staphyloma of retina above or below disc 10. Toxic agents	G. Most of these defects are easily differentiated on ophthalmoscopy and may be combined with other field defects.

H. Junctional scotoma	H. 1. Optic neuritis
	2. Pituitary tumor
	3. Craniopharyngioma
	4. Vascular
	   a. Ischemia
	   b. Aneuryism of circle of Willis
	5. Meningioma of sphenoid ridge
	6. Arachnoiditis
	7. Gliomata of frontal lobe
		H. Junctional defects are those that occur in the posterior optic nerve and involve the fibers of the genu of the chiasm from the fellow eye. This causes a contralateral superior-temporal field defect, and an ipsilateral prechiasmatic pattern or blind eye.

II. "Qualified" Hemianopsias

A. Altitudinal hemianopsia	A. 1. Ischemic optic atrophy
	2. Vascular occlusion
	   a. Branch retinal vessels
	   b. Vessels supplying optic nerve
	3. Retinal detachment
	4. Trauma (anywhere along pathway)
	5. Syphilitic optic atrophy
	6. Posthemorrhagic optic atrophy
	7. Compression of optic nerve by orbital tumor
	8. Hypotension with infarction of occipital cortex
	9. Glaucoma
		A. Trauma to occipital lobe is more likely to produce an inferior altitudinal defect than a superior defect, since in the latter case, death is likely to occur due to damage to supratentorial venous sinuses.

B. Binasal hemianopsia	B. 1. Glaucoma 2. Retinoschisis 3. Postneuritic optic atrophy 4. Chronic papilledema 5. Internal hydrocephalus 6. Bilateral internal carotid aneurysms 7. Cataracts 8. Pterygium 9. Bilateral drusen of disc	B. True binasal defects are extremely rare. The reason for their occurrence in cases of internal hydrocephalus is poorly understood.

III. True Hemianopsias

A. Bitemporal hemianopsia

A. 1. Pituitary tumor
    a. Chromophobic adenoma
    b. Eosinophilic adenoma
    c. Basophilic adenoma
2. Craniopharyngioma
3. Other tumors
    a. Meningioma
    b. Nasopharyngeal carcinoma
    c. Glioma of chiasm or frontal lobe
    d. Ganglioneuroma
    e. Ependymoma
    f. Infundibuloma
    g. Chordomas
    h. Osteochondroma
    i. Ectopic pinealoma
    j. Metastatic
4. Aneurysm
5. Internal hydrocephalus
6. Demyelinating disease
7. Opticochiasmatic arachnoiditis
8. Inflammation
    a. Influenza
    b. Scarlet fever
    c. Rheumatic fever
    d. Poliomyelitis
    e. Tuberculosis
    f. Syphilis
    g. Sarcoidosis
    h. Sphenoidal sinusitis

A. – Pituitary lesions tend to cause slowly enlarging peripheral defects.
– Chromophobic adenomas cause symptoms of hypopituitarism (loss of libido, amenorrhea, hypothyroidism, etc.) and may cause field loss early in their course.
– Eosinophilic adenomas cause gigantism or acromegaly and are smaller, thus causing field defects late in their course.
– Basophilic adenomas are associated with Cushing's syndrome, are very small, and rarely cause field changes.
– Craniopharyngioma, as well as glioma of chiasm and optic nerve are seen most commonly in childhood.
– Aneurysm is associated with ophthalmoplegia and deep pain.
– Internal hydrocephalus may cause distention of third ventrical and thereby cause chiasmatic compression.
– Symmetrical bitemporal field defects are the exception, rather than the rule.
– Completely normal nasal half-field is common in at least one eye.
– Myopes may show a superior temporal contraction which fills with stronger minus lenses. This is due to partial chorodial ectasia.
– Bilateral (midline) anterior occipital cortical lesions may cause defects in both uniocular

9. Trauma
10. Myopia
11. Bilateral occipital cortical lesion
12. Bilateral tilting of disc
13. Bilateral ischemia of optic nerve
14. Bilateral drusen of disc
15. Functional enlargement of pituitary
16. Hereditary optic atrophy

  fields. This is uncommon.
  — Manchester and Calhoun[3] have reported bitemporal field defects in a family with dominant hereditary optic atrophy.

B. Inferior homonymous quadrantanopsia

  1. Ischemia of optic radiation usually 2° to carotid disease.
  2. Other causes (see Sect. III-D).

  B. This pattern most often seen on a vascular basis, since the upper fibers receive their blood supply from middle cerebral artery, but the lower fibers also are supplied by branches of posterior cerebral artery. This may be a scotoma or a defect that includes central and peripheral field ("breaks through to periphery").

C. Superior homonymous quadrantanopsia

  1. Damage to Meyer's loop in temporal lobe.
  2. Lesion elsewhere, most likely in geniculocalcarine path (see Sect. III-D).

  C. Temporal lobe lesions produce in the visual field superior homonymous wedges that eventually grow to become a quadrantanopsia. This is the "pie-in-the-sky" field defect. Posttraumatic quadrantic defects involving occipital lobe seldom involve horizontal meridian, most likely because the cortex subserving this area is protected in calcarine fissure.

III. True Hemianopsias

D. Homonymous hemianopsia

D. Lesions of:
1. Optic tract
2. Lateral geniculate body
3. Optic radiation
4. Visual cortex

D. See Tables 7-4 and 7-5 for associated systemic signs and symptoms of hemianopic lesions. Macular sparing is more common with vascular lesions of occipital lobe or optic radiation.
— Patients with hemianopsias often complain of bumping into objects on side of defect, difficulty in reading (particularly right-sided defects) or finding start of line of print (left-sided defects). Many think that the defect is confined to one eye on the side of the defect and are unaware that both eyes may be involved.

IV. Shifts, Rotations, and Magnifications

A. Blind spot closer to field center than normal

A. 1. Aphakia
2. Extreme hyperopia
3. Central scotoma with eccentric fixation

A. In aphakia, all central isopters are concentrically contracted due to magnification effects. In central scotomas, the other isopters are shifted laterally along with the blind spot.

B. Blind spot further from field center than normal

B. 1. High myopia
2. Central scotoma with eccentric fixation

C. Blind spot displaced superiorly or inferiorly

C. 1. Cyclovertical muscle/nerve palsy
2. Central scotoma with eccentric fixation

C. Most common cause is superior oblique dysfunction. Eccentric fixation above or below a scotoma is comparatively rare.

REFERENCES

1. Drance SM, Begg IS: Sector haemorrhage. Probable acute ischaemic disc change in chronic simple glaucoma. Can J Ophthalmol 5:137, 1970
2. Harrington DO: The Bjerrum scotoma. Trans Am Ophthalmol Soc 62:324, 1964
3. Manchester PT, Calhoun FP: Dominant hereditary optic atrophy with bitemporal field defects. Arch Ophthalmol 60:479, 1958

Appendix C

Toxic Agents that Affect the Visual Field

In this appendix are listed numerous toxic agents that have been reported to affect the visual field. The list is probably not all-inclusive, although certainly the major offenders are listed here. Some prominent agents are listed by themselves, whereas their less-well-known brethren are lumped together as a group. Thus, aspirin and salicylates appear as separate headings. With some of the agents, it is not easy to find detailed case reports, and such information as is available is listed. Thus, there are several agents that are noted to cause retinal vascular disorders, but none of the other categories. Although it is not unreasonable to assume that these agents would cause other problems (certainly scotomas), we have chosen—in the absence of specific information—to let the reader speculate along with us on the exact pattern the visual field defect may take.

Drug	Central scotoma	Scotomas	Maculopathy	Macular edema	Constriction of visual fields	Blindness	Cortical blindness	Enlarged blind spot	Hemianopsia	Hearing difficulties or tinnitus	Optic atrophy	Retrobulbar or optic neuritis	Peripheral neuropathy	Retinal degeneration	Retinal vascular disorders
Acetaminophen						•									•
Acetanilid						•									•
Acetazolamide	•	•		•											
Acetohexamide												•			
Acetophenazine		•			•	•						•			
Acetyldigitoxin		•										•			
Alcohols		•			•	•									
Allopurinol	•	•	•												
Alseroxylon											•				
Aluminum nicotinate	•	•		•											
Aminosalicylic acid											•	•			
Amitriptyline						•						•			•
Amodiaquine	•	•	•		•	•						•		•	•
Amphetamine															•
Amyl nitrite															•
Analine dyes	•				•										
Antimony compounds						•					•				
Antipyrine						•					•				
Arsenic					•										
Aspidium (Filix mas)					•	•			•		•				
Aspirin		•			•	•			•		•				
Aurothioglucose						•									
Aurothioglycanide						•									
Barbiturates	•	•			•	•	•				•	•			•
Bendroflumethiazide						•	•								
Benoxinate						•									
Benzine and coal tar derivatives	•				•										
Benzphetamine															•
Benzthiazide						•	•								
Bishydroxycoumarin						•									
Bromide		•									•				
Bromisovalum		•			•							•			
Bupivacaine						•					•	•			
Butacaine						•									
Butallylonal		•			•	•					•	•			•
Butaperazine		•			•	•					•				

	Central scotoma	Scotomas	Maculopathy	Macular edema	Constriction of visual fields	Blindness	Cortical blindness	Enlarged blind spot	Hemianopsia	Hearing difficulties or tinnitus	Optic atrophy	Retrobulbar or optic neuritis	Peripheral neuropathy	Retinal degeneration	Retinal vascular disorders
Butethal		●			●	●					●	●			●
Capreomycin					●										
Caramiphen		●										●			
Carbinoxamine					●										
Carbon bisulphide	●				●										
Carbon dioxide					●	●			●						●
Carbon monoxide				●		●	●			●					
Carbon tetrachloride										●		●	●		
Carbromal		●			●							●			
Carisoprodol					●	●									
Carphenazine		●			●	●									
Chloral hydrate						●						●			
Chloramphenicol	●	●			●	●					●	●			
Chlorisondamine						●									
Chloroform						●	●								
Chloroprocaine						●					●	●			
Chloroquine	●	●	●		●	●								●	●
Chlorothiazide						●	●				●				
Chlorphentermine															●
Chlorpromazine		●			●	●					●				
Chlorpropamide		●										●			
Chlortetracycline								●							
Chlorthalidone						●	●								
Clindamycin	●										●	●			
Clomiphene		●			●						●				●
Cobalt		●			●						●				
Cocaine						●									
Corticosteroids and analogs	●	●	●		●	●			●		●		●		
Cycloserine											●	●			
Cyclothiazide						●	●								
Demeclocycline								●							
Deserpidine											●				
Desipramine						●						●			●
Deslanoside		●										●			
Dextroamphetamine															●
Dibucaine						●									
Diethazine		●			●	●					●				

	Central scotoma	Scotomas	Maculopathy	Macular edema	Constriction of visual fields	Blindness	Cortical blindness	Enlarged blind spot	Hemianopsia	Hearing difficulties or tinnitus	Optic atrophy	Retrobulbar or optic neuritis	Peripheral neuropathy	Retinal degeneration	Retinal vascular disorders
Diethylcarbamazine						•									
Diethylpropion															•
Digitalis	•	•			•	•					•	•			
Digitoxin		•										•			
Digoxin		•										•			
Diiodohydroxyquin	•	•	•	•		•					•	•			
Diphenhydramine						•									
Diphenylhydantoin						•									
Diphenylpyraline						•									
Disulfiram	•	•				•						•			
Doxycycline								•							
Dyclonine						•									
Emetine		•			•	•									
Epinephrine	•	•	•							•					
Ergot and alkaloids	•	•			•	•		•	•		•				•
Ethambutol	•	•	•	•					•		•	•			•
Ethanol	•												•		
Ethchlorvynol	•	•			•	•						•			
Ether						•	•								
Ethionamide												•			
Ethopropazine		•			•	•					•				
Ethoxzolamide	•	•	•												
Fluphenazine		•			•	•					•				
Gentamicin						•									
Gitalin		•										•			
Gold and gold compounds						•									
Griseofulvin	•	•	•	•		•									
Guanethidine															•
Hexamethonium	•	•		•	•	•			•		•				•
Hexethal		•		•		•					•	•			•
Hydrochlorothiazide						•	•								
Hydroflumethiazide						•	•								
Hydroxychloroquine	•	•	•		•	•					•			•	•
Ibuprofen		•				•			•			•			
Iodoform	•	•													
Imipramine						•						•			•

	Central scotoma	Scotomas	Maculopathy	Macular edema	Constriction of visual fields	Blindness	Cortical blindness	Enlarged blind spot	Hemianopsia	Hearing difficulties or tinnitus	Optic atrophy	Retrobulbar or optic neuritis	Peripheral neuropathy	Retinal degeneration	Retinal vascular disorders
Indomethacin	•	•	•	•		•		•						•	
Iodine and compounds	•	•		•		•			•		•	•		•	•
Iodochlorhydroxyquin	•	•	•	•		•					•	•			
Iron compounds											•	•		•	
Isocarboxazid						•									
Isoniazid		•			•	•			•		•	•			
Kanamycin													•	•	
Ketamine						•									
Lanatoside C		•										•			
Lead	•	•											•		
Lidocaine						•					•	•			•
Lithium carbonate		•				•									
Manganese					•										
Mepivacaine						•						•			
Meprobamate					•	•									
Mesoridazine		•			•	•					•				
Methacycline															
Methamphetamine															•
Methanol	•					•									
Methazolamide	•	•		•											
Methdilazine		•			•	•						•			
Methotrimeprazine		•				•						•			
Methyclothiazide								•							
Methyl acetate						•						•			
Methyl bromide	•														
Methyl chloride	•														
Methylene blue						•						•			
Methylergonovine															•
Methysergide		•													•
Minocycline								•							
Morphine		•			•	•				•					
Nalidixic acid						•									
Niacinamide	•	•	•												
Nialamide						•						•			
Nicotinic acid	•	•	•												
Nicotinyl alcohol	•	•	•												
Nitroglycerin						•					•				•

	Central scotoma	Scotomas	Maculopathy	Macular edema	Constriction of visual fields	Blindness	Cortical blindness	Enlarged blind spot	Hemianopsia	Hearing difficulties or tinnitus	Optic atrophy	Retrobulbar or optic neuritis	Peripheral neuropathy	Retinal degeneration	Retinal vascular disorders
Nitrous oxide						●	●								
Nortriptyline						●						●			●
Nystatin												●			
Opium and derivatives	●	●			●	●			●						
Optochine	●				●										
Oral contraceptives	●	●	●			●			●		●	●			●
Ouabain		●										●			
Oxygen		●			●	●									●
Oxyphenbutazone						●					●	●			
Oxytetracycline								●							
Paraldehyde										●					
Paramethadione		●													
Penicillamine	●											●			
Penicillins						●									
Perazine		●			●	●					●				
Pericyazine		●			●	●					●				
Perphenazine		●			●	●					●				
Phenacaine						●									●
Phenacetin						●									●
Phendimetrazine															●
Phenelzine						●									
Phenmetrazine															●
Phentermine															●
Phenylbutazone						●					●	●			
Phenylephrine	●			●											
Piperacetazine		●			●	●					●				
Piperocaine						●									
Polythiazide								●							
Prilocaine						●					●	●			
Primidone		●			●	●					●	●		●	
Procaine						●					●	●		●	
Prochlorperazine		●			●	●					●				
Promazine		●			●	●					●				
Promethazine		●			●	●					●				
Proparacaine						●									
Propiomazine		●			●	●					●				
Propoxycaine						●					●	●			

Drug	Central scotoma	Scotomas	Maculopathy	Macular edema	Constriction of visual fields	Blindness	Cortical blindness	Enlarged blind spot	Hemianopsia	Hearing difficulties or tinnitus	Optic atrophy	Retrobulbar or optic neuritis	Peripheral neuropathy	Retinal degeneration	Retinal vascular disorders
Protriptyline						•						•			•
Quinacrine		•						•				•			
Quinidine		•			•	•									
Quinine	•	•	•	•	•	•				•	•				•
Quinoline	•				•										
Rescinnamine											•				
Reserpine											•				
Salicylates		•			•	•				•	•				
Sparsomycin	•														
Stibocaptate						•					•				
Stibophen						•					•				
Streptomycin	•	•				•				•	•	•			•
Sulfonamides	•	•			•	•	•					•			•
Syrosingopine											•				
Tetracaine						•									
Tetracycline								•							
Thallium	•												•		
Thiethylperazine		•			•	•					•				
Thiopropazate		•			•	•					•				
Thioproperazine		•			•	•					•				
Thioridazine	•	•			•	•					•				
Thyroid	•	•									•	•			
Tobacco/alcohol	•	•													
Tolazamide												•			
Tolbutamide												•			
Tranylcypromine						•									
Trichlormethiazide							•								
Trichloroethylene		•			•	•		•			•	•			•
Tricresyl phosphate						•					•		•		
Trifluoperazine		•			•	•					•				
Triflupromazine		•			•	•					•				
Trimeprazine		•			•	•					•				
Trimethadione	•														
Tripelennamine						•									
Tryparsamide					•	•						•	•		
Vitamin A								•							
Vitamin D										•		•	•		

REFERENCES

Cogan DG: Neurology of the Visual System., Springfield, Illinois, Charles C Thomas, 1970

Duke-Elder A, MacFaul PA: Nonmechanical injuries, in Duke-Elder S (ed): System of Ophthalmology. London, Henry Kimpton, 1972

Fraunfelder FT: Drug-induced Ocular Side Effects and Drug Interactions. Philadelphia, Lea & Fabiger, 1976

Grant WM: Toxicology of the Eye. Springfield, Illinois, Charles C Thomas, 1962

Walsh WB, Hoyt WF: Clinical Neuro-opthalmology. Baltimore, Williams & Wilkins, 1969

Index

Acuity, visual, 8
Adaptation process, retinal, 97–100
   local, 32, 119–121
   neural, 99
   photochemical, 99
   signal pooling in, 99–100
Adler F, 117
Alcohol, visual changes from, 248, 250, 255, 319
Age, and baring of blind spot, 238
Agnosia
   topographic, 224
   visual, 224
AIMARK Projection Perimeter, 141–142
Albedo, 68
Alexandridis E, 107
Amacrine cells, retinal, 75, 78–80
   receptive fields in, 91–94
Amblyopia
   nutritional, 310–311
   toxic, 248–258
      agents causing, 318–324
      visual fields in, 308
Amsler Grid, 121–122, 144
Anatomy
   of chiasm, 206
   of lateral geniculate body, 216
   of optic radiations, 219
   of optic tracts, 213
   of retina, 4–7, 75–76
      in nerve fiber layer, 199–201
Anemia, pernicious, 257, 310

Angular size of test objects, 3
Anton's syndrome, 227
Aphakia, visual field in, 316
Aphasias, 224
Apostilbs, 64
Arc perimeters, 141
Armaly MF, 237
Arsenic, toxic effects of, 248, 319
Arteritis, cranial, 246
   visual field in, 310
Astereognosis, 222
Aulhorn E, 107, 108, 113, 119, 120, 122, 123, 230, 233, 236, 241, 242, 266, 270, 271, 278
Aulhorn's curves, 7, 100
Automatic perimetry, 144, 149–150, 270–285
   eye-movement monitoring in, 277–278
   fixation monitoring in, 278–279
   forced choice responses in, 271–272
   joy stick used in, 271, 274–276
   method of approaching threshold in, 280–283
   multiple-stimulus use in, 277
   objective responses in, 278
   response devices in, 274–278
   and scotoma detection, 283–285
   stimulus presentation in, 272–274
   temporal forced choice in, 277
   and visually evoked responses, 278
Autoplot, 139–140

Background luminance and Talbot brightness, 118
Baumgartner E, 124
Bebie H, 281
Becker B, 237
Begg IS, 307
Berens Test Targets, 136
Beriberi, 257
Bernstein I, 295–305
Best W, 119
Bipolar cells, retinal, 78, 80
  receptive fields in, 87–91
Birdsall T, 296, 299
Bjerrum scotoma, 240
Black body, 59
Bleaching of retinal photopigments, 98–99
Blind spot
  baring of, 237–238
    lesions with, 307
  campimetry of, 31
  demonstration of, 11
  enlargement of, 312
  examination of, 192
  and scotomas, 37–38
  shifts of, 316
Blindness, cortical, 227
Bloch's law, 107
Blood supply
  of optic nerve, 204
    ischemic lesions of, 244–246
  of retina
    defects in, 201–203
    occlusions of, 246–248
Blur, affecting perimetric thresholds, 113–115
Border contrast, effects of, 112–113
Bowl perimeters, 130–134
Boycott BB, 75
Bresky RH, 278
Brightness, of retinal image, 69
Brodrick JD, 258

Calhoun FP, 315
Calibration, of Goldmann Perimeter, 159, 160
Camera, compared to eye, 1–4
Camera film, compared to retina, 4
Campimetry
  compared to perimetry, 23–26
  kinetic, 31
Campos EC, 278
Candela, 63
Cappin JM, 278
Cataract, visual changes in, 199
Center-surround organization, retinal, 81–83
  testing in humans, 84
Central islands, lesions with, 231, 307
Central scotoma device, 169, 181–184, 195
Cerebral arteries, compression of, 222
Chamlin M, 188
Chaplin GBB, 272
Chiasm
  anatomy of, 206
  compression of, patterns in, 209, 210, 211
  field defects with lesions of, 206–210
Chloramphenicol, toxicity of, 254, 320
Chloroquine, toxicity of, 248, 250–251, 320
Choroidal circulation, defects in, 203
Cibis P, 120, 121
Cinchonism, 254
Clindamycin, toxicity of, 254, 320
Cogan DG, 266
Color blindness, from ethambutol, 254
Color perimetry, 71–75, 187–189
  clinical use of, 74–75
  monochromatic light in, 72–74
  stimulus problems in, 71–72
Completion phenomenon, 121–122
Computer use, with automatic perimetry, 144, 149–150, 271, 272
Cones and rods, 5–7. See also Receptor cells
Confrontation fields, 189–190
Congruity, 44–52, 210–213
  operational model for, 50
Constricted visual fields, lesions with, 308–309

Contractions, 37–38
  concentric, disorders with, 236–237
  in glaucoma, 236–240
  from toxins, 249
    chloroquine, 251
    phenothiazine, 252
Copenhagen DR, 83, 97
Cornsweet TN, 189, 280
Cortex, visual, 224
  lesions in, 224–228
  organization of receptive fields in, 101–103
Crescent, temporal, 44
Criterion effect, 123–124
  and signal detection theory, 295–305
Critical flicker frequency, 117–119
Critical fusion frequency, 117, 119
Cuignet bar test, 265
Cut or contraction, 37–38

Dark adaptation, 73–74, 98, 100
  curve of normal subject, 100
Decision-making, factors in, 296–302
DeLange Dzn, 117
Devic's disease, optic neuritis in, 262
Diabetes, visual field changes in, 199, 201, 309
Differential diagnosis of field defects, 306–316
Diffraction, 68
Digitalis, visual changes from, 250, 254, 321
Dimethylazines, toxicity of, 252
Disharmony
  photochromic, 188
  photometric, 111–112
Disproportion, in color perimetry, 188
Donaldson Perimeter, 133
Double simultaneous stimulation, effects of, 122
Dowling JE, 75, 78, 98
Drance SM, 230, 236, 240, 242, 245, 307
Drifts, slow, 112
Drusen of disc, binasal hemianopsia in, 208

Dubois-Poulsen A, 111, 112
Duty cycle, 118, 274
Dyad, synaptic, 78

Edema, in retinal venous occlusions, 248
Ehinger B, 75
Electron microscopy, of retina, 75–80
Electrophysiology of retina, 80–97
  comparative studies in, 84
Electroretinogram, increment threshold for, 98
Emery JM, 205
Energy transfer, rate of, 59–60
Enoch JM, 113
Erg, 59
Ergot, toxicity of, 254, 321
Errors in perimetry, 192
  and bias of technician, 178
  and failure to patch one eye, 192
  in interpretation of glaucomatous fields, 243
  in joy-stick use in automatic perimetry, 276
Ethambutol, toxicity of, 252–254, 321
Ethanol, visual changes from, 248, 250, 255, 321
Evoked responses, visual, 278
Extinction phenomenon, 122

Fain GL, 99
Fankhauser F, 104, 106, 108, 113, 122, 283
Ferry-Porter law, 117
Field defects, 37–54
  congruity in, 44–52
  cuts or contractions, 37–38
  hemianopsia, 39–44
  scotomas, 37–38
  slope in, 52–54
Finger-count field, 190
Fixation
  monitoring on automatic perimeters, 278–279
  and testing of sensitivity zones, 16
Fixation nystagmus, 112

Fixation point
  in campimetry, 24
  in perimetry, 21
Flicker fusion perimetry, 90–91, 189
  background luminance in, 118
  duty cycle in, 118
  eye response to, 115–119
  and object size, 119
Flow chart
  for patient management, 290–291
  for performing perimetry, 164–165
  for preparing to test with Goldmann Perimeter, 154–155
Flux curve
  luminous or photometric, 62
  radiant or radiometric, 62
Form sense, demonstration of, 10
Foster-Kennedy syndrome, 265
Fovea, 6
Freedman Analyzer, 143–144, 145, 277
French LA, 50–51
Frisen L, 283
Full field devices, 130–134

Galvanic skin response, in evaluation of malingering, 267
Gambs Perimeter, 134
Ganglion cells, retinal, 6–7, 75
  on-off, 82, 83, 94
  receptive fields in, 83, 94–96
  responses to light, 81–83
Gap junction synapses, 80
Geiger H, 122
Geniculate body, lateral, 101, 216–217
  lesions of, 217
Geniculocalcarine pathway, 219
Gennari, White line of, 224
Gerstmann's syndrome, 224
Glaucoma, 230–244
  arcuate scotoma in, 240–241
  atypical field defects in, 242
  contractions in, 236–240
  and errors in interpretation of fields, 243
  hemianopic offsets in, 242
  low-tension, 244–245
  management of, 288–292
  progression of field defects in, 242–243
  risk factors in, 231–232
  visual field changes in, 199–201, 233–236, 307, 308
Goldmann H, 106, 108, 121
Goldmann Perimeter, 17–18, 104, 130–132
  calibration of, 159, 160
  and central scotoma device, 169, 181–184, 195
  guide to use of, 152–178
  and instructions to patient, 161–162, 163
  normal field with, 197
  and one-dot-four-dot test, 179–181, 195
  preparations for testing with, 152–162
  psychological factors affecting results with, 176–177
  for scotoma testing, 167
  size and brightness steps on, 108, 109
  for static perimetry, 185–187
  testing with, 162–169
  troubleshooting with, 169–178
  view from operator's side, 157
  view from patient's side, 156
Graefe A, 30
Greve EL, 108, 112, 122, 148, 271, 272, 277

Hallucinations, peduncular, 222
Harms H, 107, 113, 119, 120, 123, 213, 230, 233, 236, 237, 241, 242, 278
Harrington DO, 307
Harrington-Flocks Screener, 143, 277
Hartline HK, 83
Hayreh SS, 203, 204
Heijl A, 271, 272, 281
Helicopters, campimetric and perimetric analogy, 25–26
Hemianopic offsets in glaucoma, 242
Hemianopic pupil, 213

Index 331

Hemianopsia, 39–44
　altitudinal, 44, 48, 205
　　inferior, in cortical lesions, 227
　　lesions with, 313
　binasal, 44, 47
　　in drusen of disc, 208
　　lesions with, 313
　bitemporal, 40–41, 42, 46
　　in chiasmal compression, 209
　　lesions with, 314–315
　homonymous, 41
　　lesions with, 212, 214–215, 316
　　in postchiasmal lesions, 210
　　right, 43
　left temporal, 45
　unilateral, 44
Hemorrhage, and visual field loss, 245
Hertz, 59
HLA type
　and field loss in glaucoma, 231
　and multiple sclerosis, 262
Homonymous field defects, 41
　congruous, 44–52
Horizontal cells, retinal, 75, 78
　receptive fields in, 86
Horizontal raphe, 200
Hubel DH, 10, 102
Hue, 72
Hydroxycobalamine, in ocular disorders, 257, 258, 311
Hypertensive vascular disease, visual field changes in, 199
Hysterical or malingering patients, 121, 138, 265–267

Illuminance, 63
Illuminated screeners, 144
Image brightness, 69
Indications for perimetry, 145–151
　for Stage I examination, 145, 146
　for Stage II examination, 146
　for Stage III examination, 146–149
　for Stage IV examination, 149
Inflammatory lesions, visual field defects in, 261–265

Integration. See Summation
Intensity
　luminous, 63
　radiant, 60, 63
Internal capsule, optic radiations in, 219
Interpretation of visual field, 191–228
　bilateral defects, 205–228
　in chiasmal lesions, 206–210
　and clues to validity of field, 191–192
　and comparisons with previous fields, 195
　normal field, 197–198
　orientation with ophthalmoscopic findings, 197
　in postchiasmal lesions, 210–228
　in prechiasmal lesions, 198–205
　and sufficiency of data, 192–195
　uniocular defects, 198–205
Intraocular pressure, 244
Irradiance, 60, 63
Irregular field defects, lesions with, 309
Ischemia
　and optic nerve lesions, 244–246, 264
　and retinal circulation occlusions, 246–248
Islands, central, lesions with, 231, 307
Isopters, 13
　in campimetry, 26
　on Goldmann Perimeter, 18
　intermediate, 18–19
　plotting of, 12–15
　scatter zones in, 16
　and three-dimensional model of visual fields, 21

Jenkel-Davidson Lumiwand, 135, 136
Jernigan ME, 272, 277, 278
Joule, 59
Juler Scotometer, 140–141

Kelly DH, 117
Kinetic campimetry, 31
Kinetic perimetry, 26–27
　automatic technique in, 282
　balancing effects in, 29–30

Kinetic perimetry, *continued*
  inherent inaccuracy of, 30–32
  and scotoma detection, 285
  vs static testing, 55, 104–106
Koch P, 284

Lambert's law, 64, 67
Lamina cribrosa, 203–204
Lead, toxic effects of, 248, 322
Leber's disease, 257–258, 310
LeBlanc RP, 237
Lens of eye, compared to camera lens, 3
Light
  adaptation to, 98–99
  luminous efficiency of, 62
  monochromatic, 72
  physics of, 58–59
  velocity of, 59
  wavelengths of. *See* Wavelengths
Light sense, 7
  demonstration of, 10
Luddeke H, 108, 117, 119, 189
Lumen, 63
Luminance, 63, 64
Luminosity curves, relative, 60–61
Luminous efficiency of light, 62
Luminous flux, 62, 63
Luminous intensity, 63
Lumiwands, 135, 137
Lynn JR, 122, 131, 188, 200, 231, 242, 271, 280, 282, 285
Lynn-Tate Perimeter, 274, 278

Mach bands, 113
Macula lutea, 6
  senile degeneration of, visual changes in, 199
Macular sparing, 227–228
Magnesium ion, retinal effects of, 81
Malingering and hysterical patients, 121, 138, 265–267
Manchester PT, 315
McColgin FH, 104
Meningioma, ocular signs in, 264, 265

Meridian, in static perimetry, 35
Mesopic vision, 8
Metameric matching, 72
Meyer's loop, 219
Microsaccades, rapid, 112
Millilambert, 64
Monochromatic perimetry, 72–74
Movement, perception of, 104–106
Müller W, 278, 279
Multiple-stimulus perimetry, 122, 143, 277
Mydriasis, in cerebral artery compression, 222

Nanometer, 59
Nasal step, 237
  lesions with, 307
Nerve fibers, retinal, 199–201
  bundle defects, 307–308
Neuritis, optic, 261–264
  ischemic, 246
  pseudo-optic, 264
Niacin deficiency, 257
Night blindness, in retinitis pigmentosa, 258
Nit, 64
Normal visual field, 197–198
Normann RA, 99
Nutritional amblyopias, 250, 255–257
Nystagmus
  fixation, 112
  optokinetic, abnormal, 222

Occlusions of retinal circulation, 246–248
Offsets, hemianopic, in glaucoma, 242
One-dot-four-dot test, 179–181, 195
Ophthalmic artery pressure, 244
Optic chiasm. *See* Chiasm
Optic disc, stereo photographs of, 231
Optic nerve, 203–205
  atrophy of, hereditary, 257–258
  blood supply of, 204
  ischemic lesions of, 244–246

neuritis of, 261–264
pseudo-optic neuritis, 264
visual field in lesions of, 307–308
Optic radiations, 219
Optic tracts, anatomy of, 213
Optical axis of eye, 15
Optics, physiological, 58–75
Østerberg G, 5
Østerberg's curve of cone distribution, 7, 9

Papillomacular bundle, 200
Parietal lobe
  lesions in, 222, 224
  optic radiations in, 220
Perimetric angle
  nasal, 1
  temporal, 1
Perimetron, 274, 279
Perimetry
  vs campimetry, 23–26
  compared to helicopter mapping of topography, 21
  definition of, 1
  devices in, 130–144
Peripheral defects, lesions with, 309–310
Phenothiazines, toxic effects of, 251–252
Photographic film, compared to retina, 4–10
Photography, stereo, of optic disc, 231
Photometric disharmony, 111–112
Photometry, 3, 58, 63–66
Photon, 58, 70
Photon flux, incident, 71
Photophysics, 58–75
Photopic vision, 8, 61
Photopigments, retinal, bleaching of, 98–99
Photopsias, 227
Photoreceptors, retinal, 5–7. *See also* Receptor cells
Physics, and visual field, 58–75
"Pie-in-the-sky" defect, 219, 221, 315

Pieron's law, 108
Piper's law, 108
Piperazines, toxicity of, 252
Piperidines, toxicity of, 252
Pituitary tumors, visual field in, 314
Planck's constant, 58, 59
Polyak SL, 5
Pressure
  intraocular, 244
  ophthalmic artery, 244
Prochlorperazine, toxicity of, 252, 323
Psychological factors affecting testing, 121–124
  completion phenomenon, 121–122
  criterion effect, 123–124, 295–305
  and effects of training, 123
  extinction phenomenon, 122
  and signal detection theory, 124, 295–305
  in testing with Goldmann Perimeter, 176–177
Psychologists, experimental, 28
Pupil
  diminished pupil phenomenon, 5
  in glaucoma, 243
  hemianopic, of Wernicke, 213
  size changes, effects of, 68–69
Pupillometric perimetry, 278
  in hysteria or malingering, 266
Purkinje JE, 61
Purkinje shift, 74
Pyridoxine deficiency, 257

Quadrantanopsia, 44
  bilateral inferior, 49
  bitemporal, in chiasmal compression, 209
  inferior homonymous, 222
  lesions with, 315
  inferior temporal, in chiasmal compression, 210
  superior homonymous, 219
  lesions with, 315
Quantum physics, 58
Quinine, toxicity of, 254, 324

Radian, 60
Radiance, 60, 63, 71
Radiant flux curve, 62
Radiant intensity, 60, 63
Radiant power, 59
Radiations, optic, 219
Radiometry, 58–62
Raphe, horizontal, 200
Reaction time, slow, and summation, 29–30
Receptive fields
  in amacrine cells, 91–94
  in bipolar cells, 87–91
  in cortical cells, 101–103
  in ganglion cells, 83, 94–96
  in horizontal cells, 86
  in lateral geniculate body, 101
  in receptor cells, 84–85
Receptor cells, retinal, 5–7
  linear response curve of cones, 103
  nonlinear response curve of rods, 103
  pedicles of cones, 80
  receptive fields in, 84–85
  rod-cone break in dark-adaptation curve, 101
  signal pooling by rods, 99–100
  and summation mechanisms, 107
Reflectance, 67–68
Refraction, 68
Refractive scotoma, 115
Retina, 4–10
  anatomy of, 4–7, 75–76
    in nerve fiber layer, 199–201
  blood supply defects in, 201–203
  center-surround organization of, 81–83
    testing in humans, 84
  compared to camera film, 4
  control of sensitivity in, 97–100
  detachment of, visual field changes in, 199, 201, 309, 310
  electron microscopy of, 75–80
  electrophysiology of, 80–97
    comparative studies in, 84
  function of, 7–10
  image brightness in, 69

  intracellular recordings of, 80–81
  and limit of nasal visual field, 1
  local adaptation of, 32, 119–121
  occlusions of circulation in, 246–248
    arterial, 246–248
    venous, 248
  plexiform layers of, 75
  receptive fields in, 83, 84–96. *See also* Receptive fields
  synapses in, 76–80
Retinitis pigmentosa, 258–261, 311
Retinoschisis, visual field in, 309
Rhodopsin, bleaching of, 98–99
Ricco's law, 108
Riddoch G, 104
Riddoch phenomena, 105
Ring scotoma. *See* Scotoma, ring
Rodenstock Perimeter, 134
Rods and cones, 5–7. *See also* Receptor cells
Rönne H, 237
Rotary movement, perception of, 104
Rushton WAH, 99–100

Salicylates, toxicity of, 254, 324
Saturation perimetry, 188–189
Scatter, in perimetry, 16, 109–111, 192
  in automatic perimetry, 271
  in testing with Goldmann Perimeter, 169–178
Scattering of light, in diffraction, 68
Schmidt D, 1
Schmidt TH, 104, 108, 115
Schweigger hand perimeter, 142
Sclerosis, multiple, optic neuritis in, 262–264
Scotomas, 37–38
  arcuate, 201–205
    in glaucoma, 240–241
    lesions with, 308, 311
  central, 205
    in chloroquine toxicity, 251
    lesions with, 307, 310–311
    in optic neuritis, 262
    in phenothiazine toxicity, 252

in retinal venous occlusions, 248
    from toxins, 249
  central scotoma device, 169, 181–184, 195
  detection with automatic perimetry, 283–285
  junctional, 207
    lesions with, 312
  refractive, 115
  ring, 205
    in glaucoma, 243
    lesions with, 307
    in retinitis pigmentosa, 258
    testing with Goldmann Perimeter, 167
Scotometer, Juler, 140–141
Scotopic vision, 8, 61
Screening examinations, 143–144
  indications for, 145, 146
  multiple-stimulus devices in, 122
  results of, 148
Senile macular degeneration, visual field changes in, 199
Sensitivity of eye
  control of, 97–100
  zones of, 15
Shickman G, 117
Sieve effect, 177, 205
Signal detection theory, 124, 295–305
Signal pooling, and adaptation, 99–100
Simultaneous stimulation, effects of, 122
Sloan LL, 108, 113
Slope
  in field defects, 52–54
  and spatial summation, 110
Slow drifts, 112
Solitary field defects, lesions with, 309
Spahr J, 272
Sparing, macular, 227–228
Sperling G, 117
Spiraling visual field, in hysterical patients, 266
Staircase technique, in perimetry, 280, 281

Static perimetry, 26–27, 32–37
  determination of threshold in, 280–282
  Goldmann Perimeter in, 185–187
  vs kinetic testing, 55, 204–206
  limitation of, 32–34
  location of points in, 35
  and scotoma detection, 283–284
  technique of, 35–37
Steradian, 60
Stiles-Crawford effect, 70
Streptomycin, toxicity of, 254, 324
Striate cortex. See Cortex, visual
Stroboscope, use of, 118
Sulfonamides, visual changes from, 250, 254, 324
Summation, 29
  and photometric disharmony, 111–112
  spatial, 29, 100, 106–112
    slope affecting, 110
  temporal, 29, 106–112
Swets J, 296, 299
Synapses, retinal, 76–80
  conventional, 78–80
  gap junction, 80
  ribbon, 77–78
  serial, 80
Syphilis, visual field in, 308

Talbot brightness, 117
  and background luminance, 118
Talbot's law, 117
Tangent screen, 135–139
Tanner W, 296, 299
Tate GW, 84, 231, 271, 279, 282, 285
Taylor MM, 280
Technicians, perimetry, 150–151, 292
  biased, 178
Temporal crescent, 44
Temporal lobe
  lesions in, 222, 224
  optic radiations in, 219
Test objects
  angular size of, 3

Test objects, *continued*
  intensity of, 17–18
  size in flicker studies, 119
Thiamine deficiency, 254, 257
Thioridazine, toxicity of, 252, 324
Threshold of vision, 27–29
  vs criterion, 302–303
  determination in perimetry, 12–15
    adaptive techniques, 280–282
    blur affecting, 113–115
    training affecting, 123
Tobacco amblyopia, 250, 255, 310, 324
Toxic agents affecting visual field, 248–258, 318–324
Tremor, in fixation nystagmus, 112
Training, affecting perimetric threshold, 123
Transfer factor therapy, in multiple sclerosis, 264
Traquair
  island of vision, 21
  junction scotoma, 207
Troland unit, 3, 70–71
Troxler effect, 120
Tübinger Perimeter, 132–133
  automatic, 274, 278
Tubular fields, in malingerers, 266
Tumors
  pituitary, visual field in, 314
  and pseudo-optic neuritis, 264
  visual field in, 309

Uncinate fit, 222
Uniocular defects, 198–205
Uveitis, visual field changes in, 199

Vertical step, lesions with, 242, 307
Visual acuity, 8
Visual field
  classes of defects in, 37–54. *See also* Field defects
  definitions and limits of, 1
Visual pathway
  and anatomy of nerve fibers, 199–201
  retrochiasmal, lesions of, 41, 213
Visually evoked response, use of, 278
Vitamin B complex deficiency, 254–255, 257, 262
Von Békésy staircase technique, in perimetry, 280

Watt, 59
Wavelenghts of light, 58–59
  and color, 71
  and critical fusion frequency, 117
  variable sensitivity to, 60–62
Weber B, 272
Weber's law, 103
Werblin FS, 83, 97, 99
Wernicke's hemianopic pupil, 213
White line of Gennari, 224
Wolf E, 117, 118, 119

Yarbus AL, 121

Zappia RJ, 104
Zinn-Haller circle, 204